Genomic Medicine

Laura J. Tafe • Maria E. Arcila
Editors

Genomic Medicine

A Practical Guide

Springer

Editors
Laura J. Tafe
Dartmouth–Hitchcock Medical Center
Lebanon, NH
USA

Maria E. Arcila
Memorial Sloan Kettering Cancer Center
New York, NY
USA

ISBN 978-3-030-22921-4 ISBN 978-3-030-22922-1 (eBook)
https://doi.org/10.1007/978-3-030-22922-1

This Springer imprint is published by the registered company Springer Nature Switzerland AG
The registered company address is: Gewerbestrasse 11, 6330 Cham, Switzerland

Preface

Molecular pathology is a rapidly evolving scientific discipline that encompasses the development of molecular and genetic approaches to the diagnosis, classification, monitoring, and risk assessment of human diseases. At the core of this discipline is the application of classical, novel, and cutting-edge technologies, developed in biochemistry, cell biology, molecular biology, proteomics, genetics, and bioinformatics, to the evaluation of pathologic processes. With the advent of high-throughput technology in recent years, the evolution of the field has gained such momentum, where it is difficult for the general pathologist, the clinician in practice, or young physicians in training to keep up with even the most basic concepts. While the information is readily available through various sources, it is extensive and is often difficult to find a central location with the "nuts and bolts" for quick reference.

As molecular fellows, we both looked for the ideal high-yield reference book that would compile critical information related to molecular biomarkers for various solid tumor and hematologic malignancy subspecialties. We hoped for a book to be succinct yet comprehensive enough to be suitable for fellows in training and medical professionals with an interest in molecular pathology and biomarkers. Several years passed and many comprehensive books have been published, yet there was still a gap for a quick reference resource. In this first edition of *Genomic Medicine: A Practical Guide*, we aimed to fill this gap and have brought together experts from various areas of molecular diagnostics with the same vision. The book covers many aspects of molecular diagnostics, from techniques to applications and comprehensive summaries of the molecular biomarkers of critical importance in solid and liquid tumors. Attention was also specifically devoted to bioinformatics and next-generation sequencing, as well as preanalytical issues related to molecular diagnostics which are commonly not extensively addressed in the literature.

In the first edition of this book, we concentrated on some of the key solid tumor and hematologic malignancies for which we felt consolidation of information would be most critical. A number of important organ systems such as central nervous system tumors and cutaneous and some head and neck malignancies were not captured in this edition but will be included, along with others in a future planned edition. We also welcome our readers' feedback for other important topics to be covered.

We'd like to thank our authors for generously contributing their efforts and expertise to our vision of this book and our families, friends, and colleagues in supporting us along this journey.

Lebanon, NH, USA Laura J. Tafe
New York, NY, USA Maria E. Arcila

Contents

Contributors

Jose Jasper L. Andal, MD St. Luke's Medical Center, Quezon City and Global City, Philippines

Philippine Orthopedic Center, Quezon City, Philippines

Daphne C. Ang, MD Department of Pathology, St. Luke's Medical Center, Quezon City and Global City, Philippines

Maria E. Arcila, MD Department of Pathology, Memorial Sloan Kettering Cancer Center, New York, NY, USA

Jason C. Chang, MD Department of Pathology, Memorial Sloan Kettering Cancer Center, New York, NY, USA

Alanna J. Church, MSc, MD Laboratory for Molecular Pediatric Pathology (LaMPP), Boston Children's Hospital and Harvard Medical School, Boston, MA, USA

Alejandro Luiña Contreras, MD Joint Pathology Center, Molecular Diagnostics Laboratory, Silver Spring, MD, USA

Brennan Decker, MD, PhD Department of Pathology, Brigham and Women's Hospital, Boston, MA, USA

Jessica L. Dillon, MS, MD Department of Pathology and Laboratory Medicine, Dartmouth-Hitchcock Medical Center, Lebanon, NH, USA

Geisel School of Medicine at Dartmouth, Hanover, NH, USA

Snjezana Dogan, MD Department of Pathology, Memorial Sloan Kettering Cancer Center, New York, NY, USA

Marie-Lisa Eich, MD Department of Pathology, The University of Alabama at Birmingham, Birmingham, AL, USA

Caleb Ho, MD Department of Pathology, Memorial Sloan Kettering Cancer Center, New York, NY, USA

Annette S. Kim, MD, PhD Department of Pathology, Brigham and Women's Hospital/Harvard Medical School, Boston, MA, USA

Konstantinos Linos, MD, FCAP, FASDP Dartmouth-Hitchcock Medical Center, Department of Pathology and Laboratory Medicine, Lebanon, NH, USA

Geisel School of Medicine at Dartmouth, Hanover, NH, USA

Raymundo M. Lo, MD St. Luke's Medical Center, Quezon City, Philippines

Philippine Children's Medical Center, Quezon City, Philippines

Eric Y. Loo, MD Department of Pathology and Laboratory Medicine, Dartmouth-Hitchcock Medical Center, Lebanon, NH, USA

Geisel School of Medicine at Dartmouth, Hanover, NH, USA

Sumit Middha, PhD Department of Pathology, Memorial Sloan Kettering Cancer Center, New York, NY, USA

George J. Netto, MD Department of Pathology, The University of Alabama at Birmingham, Birmingham, AL, USA

Dara S. Ross, MD Department of Pathology, Memorial Sloan Kettering Cancer Center, New York, NY, USA

Vignesh Shanmugam, MD Department of Pathology, Brigham and Women's Hospital/Harvard Medical School, Boston, MA, USA

Lynette M. Sholl, MD Department of Pathology, Brigham and Women's Hospital, Boston, MA, USA

Laura J. Tafe, MD Department of Pathology and Laboratory Medicine, Dartmouth-Hitchcock Medical Center, Lebanon, NH, USA

Geisel School of Medicine at Dartmouth, Hanover, NH, USA

Efsevia Vakiani, MD, PhD Department of Pathology, Memorial Sloan-Kettering Cancer Center, New York, NY, USA

Chad Vanderbilt, MD Department of Pathology, Memorial Sloan Kettering Cancer Center, New York, NY, USA

Part I
General Concepts

Chapter 1
Pre-analytics, Current Testing Technologies, and Limitations of Testing

Alejandro Luiña Contreras, Jose Jasper L. Andal, Raymundo M. Lo, and Daphne C. Ang

Technical Terms and Abbreviations

aCGH	Array comparative genomic hybridization
CNV	Copy number variant
FISH	Fluorescence in situ hybridization
indel	Insertions and deletions
MLPA	Multiplex ligation-dependent probe amplification
NGS	Next-generation sequencing
RT-PCR	Reverse transcription polymerase chain reaction
SNV	Single-nucleotide variant
SV	Structural variants

A. L. Contreras (✉)
Joint Pathology Center, Molecular Diagnostics Laboratory, Silver Spring, MD, USA
e-mail: Alejandro.luinacontreras.civ@mail.mil

J. J. L. Andal
St. Luke's Medical Center, Quezon City and Global City, Philippines

Philippine Orthopedic Center, Quezon City, Philippines

R. M. Lo
St. Luke's Medical Center, Quezon City, Philippines

Philippine Children's Medical Center, Quezon City, Philippines

D. C. Ang
Department of Pathology, St. Luke's Medical Center,
Quezon City and Global City, Philippines

L. J. Tafe, M. E. Arcila (eds.), *Genomic Medicine*,
https://doi.org/10.1007/978-3-030-22922-1_1

Key Points

- Molecular techniques are evolving rapidly.
- Pre-analytical variables can affect the results of an assay.
- Molecular methods can be divided in three broad categories: (1) methods used to detect chromosomal abnormalities, (2) methods used to detect changes in the DNA/RNA sequence, and (3) gene expression profiling.
- Clinicians should familiarize themselves in the different techniques in order to choose the best test to detect the genetic abnormality in question.

Key Online Resources

- My Cancer Genome [1]: https://www.mycancergenome.org/
- AMP Education Resources [2]: https://www.amp.org/education/education-resources/

Introduction

Molecular diagnostic tests have become routine in daily practice, and the landscape of analytical platforms is continuously evolving in the era of personalized medicine. An important aspect of molecular diagnostic tests is that the quality of biomarker information provided by these tests is dependent not solely on the analytical platform utilized but also on the quality of specimens used and the strict adherence to validated protocols. As such, all healthcare professionals need to familiarize themselves with pre-analytic variables that affect tissue for downstream testing, basic details of the platforms used to evaluate for these abnormalities, and limitations for each platform in order to effectively use and understand the provided results.

In this chapter, we will summarize the most common pre-analytic variables affecting samples and some of the most commonly used molecular testing technologies with their limitations.

Pre-analytic Variables in Surgical Pathology

Consideration of pre-analytic variables, including specimen handling, is a crucial requirement for ensuring accurate results of molecular diagnostic testing. The following pre-analytic variables impact subsequent molecular testing of tissue specimens: collection of the specimen, time to fixation (cold ischemia time), fixative type, duration of fixation, postfixation treatments, water quality, digestion, tissue processing time, macrodissection, section thickness, and the need for additional ancillary tests (e.g., immunohistochemistry). In general, nucleic acids from blood or bone marrow aspirate samples are of good quality; however, the appropriate anticoagulants must be used.

Prefixation

Time to fixation (cold ischemia time) is generally defined as the time from tissue removal to initiation of fixation. It should be recognized, however, that hypoxia, ischemia, metabolic stress, and tissue degradation start as soon as the first major vessel is ligated in surgery and not when the sample is removed. Embolization procedures prior to surgery, which often happened up to 2–3 days before surgery, can have major effects on tissue quality as well. High temperatures in the operating room can also speed up the autolysis process. Many of these factors are not within the control of the laboratory since the operating room staff are tasked with the immediate care of the sample. Proper communication and the establishment of interdisciplinary protocols for tissue handling are important, which take into consideration the type of testing that is to be performed downstream. While established guidelines do not exist for most uses at this time, tissue-handling requirements must be standardized at an institutional level and tracked on every specimen. It is generally recommended for the cold ischemia time to be less than an hour. Ideally, the surgical pathology request form should contain the information by allocating a "Time Specimen Out" and "Time Specimen Fixed" line on the forms for quality control purposes. For samples that are going to be delayed in the operating room, incubating in ice is recommended to preserve RNA.

Based on published literature, the effect of delay to tissue preservation will depend on the type of test to be performed and the target. For instance, DNA extracted from FFPE tissue that was subjected to a cold ischemia time of 1 hour displayed reduced fluorescence in situ hybridization (FISH) signals [3], while a cold ischemia time of 24 hours did not alter PCR amplification success rate [4].

It is believed that a prolonged time prior to fixation results in a time-dependent, autolysis-induced RNA degradation that starts early upon surgical removal of tissue [5]. RNA integrity numbers (RIN) were comparable between FFPE specimens subjected to a cold ischemia time of 0 and 2 hours, and a cold ischemia time of 0 hours versus 12 hours also did not lead to a difference in the relative expression of six transcripts [6, 7]. For immunohistochemical analysis, cold ischemia time of less than 12 hours is recommended to avoid negative effects [3].

The size of the biospecimen before fixation also plays a role in the PCR success rate. DNA extracted from tissue ranging from 3 to 10 mm in diameter has the highest success rate, as opposed to smaller specimens or larger specimens (encountered a higher background) [8].

In summary, the generally accepted cold ischemia time is less than 60 minutes. Unfixed specimens are best sent to the laboratory as soon as possible. The time points of collection and fixation should be established by the individual institution depending on the projected downstream use of the sample and should be available for all personnel and clearly stated in laboratory records [9].

Fixation

Most diagnostic laboratories utilize 10% neutral buffered formalin for routine fixation and have validated tests from FFPE samples. The traditional formalin fixation process causes cross-linking of proteins, leading to shorter DNA fragments, and also random cytosine deamination. These limitations are mitigated by designing assays with shorter amplicon sizes and more robust assay protocols.

Different types of fixation used, temperature of fixation, and fixative delivery method affect downstream DNA analysis. DNA from neutral buffered formalin (NBF), as compared to unbuffered formalin, has greater DNA yields and better success rate in PCR, in situ hybridization (ISH), and genotype determination [10–15]. IHC staining is also optimal when fixed in a buffered 10–15% [16, 17] formalin solution with a neutral pH [18, 19]. Currently, 10% neutral buffered formalin (NBF) is the best and most broadly used and studied fixative. If an alternative fixative is considered, it must be validated against results for the same specimens fixed in 10% NBF. The laboratory director is responsible for the test performance using an alternative fixative. Other fixatives previously used before the molecular diagnostics era, including Zenker's, Bouin's, and B-5, have been shown to be harmful for downstream PCR testing [4].

Duration of fixation and its effects on ISH performance have been extensively studied, and the consensus is that excisional specimens should be fixed in 10% NBF for 6–72 hours, and this information should be documented in the pathology report. Fixation time of less than 72 hours in formalin is preferable for DNA integrity and yield, PCR, ISH, and single-nucleotide polymorphism detection assay performance [4, 10, 12, 20]. Amplification success after prolonged fixation was reportedly influenced by the target sequence, amplicon length, and tissue type [15]. Fixation at elevated temperatures (37 °C) has shown reductions in DNA yield and integrity and PCR success [21, 22], while fixation at 4 °C increased yield of high-molecular-weight DNA and PCR success [23].

Microwave-accelerated or ultrasound-accelerated fixation improves the yield of high-molecular-weight (HMW) DNA and PCR success from FFPE tissue [24–28]. Ultrasound-accelerated fixation also results in a more intense and uniform ISH staining and yielded longer amplicons and higher levels of amplifiable RNA as compared to conventional immersion fixation [27, 28].

For postfixation pretreatments in in situ hybridization (ISH) analysis, tissue processing time and digestion also impact the quality and interpretation. Different digestion enzymes may result in variable signal strengths as well. The ISH product might benefit from longer tissue processing times. The type of slides used (silanized versus positively charged) also affect adherence of tissues. Even water quality impacts the outcome. The use of highly purified water is recommended.

The generally accepted guidelines for fixation recommend 6–72 hours of fixation at 10% neutral buffered formalin. The laboratory records should document the date and time of fixation ideally within the pathology reports [9].

Decalcification

Decalcification methods may have marked adverse effects on nucleic acid analysis. Commonly used methods use acid-based decalcifiers, such as formic acid, hydrochloric acid, or nitric acid. Effects vary based on the concentration used and the length of tissue contact with the decalcifier. When different concentrations of formic acid are compared, decalcification with 5% formic acid for 12–18 hours produced FISH signals, while decalcification in a 10% formic acid solution for 7–10 days abolished the signal [29]. Decalcification with formic acid generally renders nucleic acid unsuitable for downstream testing by PCR methods in the majority of cases.

Recently, studies have shown that decalcification using ethylene diamine tetra acetic acid (EDTA) as opposed to acid methods is a better alternative. It allows amplification of longer PCR products [30], reduces background staining, provides stronger FISH signals [31–33], and provides superior determination of loss and gain of sequences for comparative genomic hybridization [31].

Processing and Storage

There are no studies showing the potential effects of dehydration, clearing, paraffin reagents, and embedding parameters in DNA and RNA yield.

Long-term storage of paraffin blocks has effects on DNA analysis, mostly in the length of amplifiable DNA. One study showed storage of FFPE sections for more than 10 years before DNA extraction and analysis was detrimental to PCR success rates; however, shorter durations have not been investigated [14].

Storage of 2–20 years leads to reduced RNA integrity as determined by RNA integrity number (RIN), as compared to those stored for 1 year or less [4, 20, 34, 35]. Humidity and temperature of the storage facility also plays a role in preserving (or degrading) the nucleic acid integrity.

Tissue Stewardship

A constant pre-analytic variable across all molecular testing technologies for solid tumor malignancies is tumor cellularity or the amount of viable tumor nuclei in the sample relative to the non-tumoral nucleated cells. A corresponding H&E slide should be evaluated by a pathologist to identify the area(s) on the slides for testing and to quantify the amount of tumor in the selected areas. The choice of testing platform may be considered depending on the available sample and in cases wherein a repeat biopsy is not feasible. This limitation can be overcome by tumor enrichment or microdissection. For example, a cell block sample that contains less than 10% is not ideal for a Sanger sequencing assay that requires at least 30–50% tumor. Manual macrodissection or laser capture microdissection may enrich for tumor in these cases. More sensitive test methods may be utilized, such as droplet digital PCR or real-time PCR. These assays have greater analytic sensitivity (0.1% for ddPCR, 1% for rt-PCR), but are usually targeted mutational assays, frequently designed to cover only the most common mutations. It should be recognized, however, that the process of formalin fixation induces DNA damage that leads to low-level mutation detection. Highly sensitive assays may therefore lead to false positive results in such cases. The level of this DNA damage and risk for false positive results should be established at the time of validation of each high-sensitivity assay.

The amount of DNA yield from surgical pathology FFPE tissues to meet test requirements has been demonstrated to require at least nine square millimeters to produce 1ug of DNA in 99% of cases. This amount of DNA is deemed sufficient to meet most multigene assays [36]. It is up to each laboratory to validate the FFPE tissue requirements and DNA yields for each assay as part of the validation as these can be highly variable from assay to assay, laboratory to laboratory, and specimen type. Most laboratories will accept unstained slides for testing. The number of sections/slides and the tumor cellularity requirements will vary depending on the assay.

RNA Pre-analytic Considerations

RNA from formalin-fixed paraffin-embedded (FFPE) tissues is now commonly used in clinical practice. And, similar to DNA, pre-analytic variables that can influence RNA quality include the time to fixation, fixation time, tissue storage time, tumor cell content, and tumor percentage [37–39]. RNA analysis is commonly utilized for gene fusion detection and also gene expression profiling via reverse-transcriptase PCR (RT-PCR).

Pre-analytics of Circulating Tumor DNA or Cell-Free DNA

Liquid biopsy, especially plasma, obtained through a simple blood draw, has recently emerged as an alternative to surgical biopsy using blood samples of cancer patients for the detection of genetic alterations in plasma (cell-free) circulating tumor DNA (ctDNA) [40]. In cancer patients, plasma cfDNA is a combination of cell-free DNA from normal cells and ctDNA. The levels of ctDNA can be highly variable and correlates with tumor size, degree of tumor invasion, disease stage, survival, and disease progression [41]. The cfDNA is usually fragmented to an average length of 140–170 bp and is present in limited quantities in the peripheral blood [42, 43].

Variability in blood collection affects the recovery of cfDNA. Peripheral blood collection tubes with cell stabilization agents that prevent cell lysis for several days are now commercially available, and several studies show the stability of cfDNA when the tubes remain at room temperature. Mehrotra et al., for example, shows that the yields of cfDNA in plasma from PB collected in Streck and K3-EDTA tubes were comparable when separated between 2 and 16 hours [40]. Plasma cfDNA integrity showed higher levels of larger fragments in the cfDNA from K3-EDTA tubes than in the cfDNA from Streck tubes [40]. In another study, blood sampled in Streck tubes, PAXgene® tubes (Qiagen), and cfDNA collection tubes from Roche GmbH (formerly from Ariosa) remained without noticeable contamination by high-molecular-weight DNA after 1 week at 22 °C [44]. Qualitative analysis of cfDNA from different blood collection tubes showed an average cfDNA fragment size of 100–120 bp at 2, 4, and 16 hours, with no HMW DNA [40].

Pre-analytical K2EDTA blood storage before cfDNA extraction in different conditions (room temperature for 4 hours, room temperature for 24 hours, and 4 °C for 24 hours) did not show significant difference in cfDNA concentrations [45]. However, a noticeable contamination by high-molecular-weight DNA, most likely originating from leukocyte lysis, is apparent by 24 hours [44]. Exposure to high temperatures, 39 °C for 5 hours and then 22 °C for another 19 hours, leads to high–molecular-weight DNA contamination in EDTA tubes, but not in the Streck tubes, PAXgene® tubes, and Roche tubes [45]. The mean concentration of cfDNA also increased proportionally in 3 ml compared to 1 ml plasma samples and in 5 ml compared to 3 ml samples by 2.9-fold and 3.44-fold [45].

Landscape of Current Testing Technologies

As a general rule, molecular methods can be divided in three broad categories: (1) methods used to detect large chromosomal or structural abnormalities; (2) methods used to detect small changes in the DNA sequence, including single-nucleotide changes, indels; and (3) gene expression profiling. Currently, several approaches and methodologies exist to detect each of the different types of alterations described above (Table 1.1). The choice of which approach to use is dependent on multiple factors including which type of alteration is being sought, medical necessity (diagnostic, prognostic, predictive), and tissue available for testing. The complexity of these tests can range from simple (interrogating a single variant) to very complex (multiplexed assays and NGS) depending on the need. In addition, each of these methods comes with strengths and limitations which are important to consider when choosing a test.

Table 1.1 Abnormalities detected by method

Method	SNV	Small duplications, insertions, or deletions	Large deletions	Copy number changes	Structural variants	Limits of detection	Turnaround time[a]
Karyotyping	–	–	+	+	+	Low, depends on cell growth	Weeks
FISH	–	–	+	+	+	Up to 0.5% depending on preparation	2–3 days
RT-PCR	+	+/–	–	–	–/+[b]	Below 1%	1–2 days
Fragment analysis and RFLP	+/–	+	–	–	–	~5%	1–2 days
dPCR	+	+/–	–	+/–	–/+[b]	Below 1%	1–2 days
MLPA	+	–	+	+	–/+[b]	~25%	2–3 days
aCGH	–	–	+	+	–	~25%	2–3 days
Allele-specific PCR	+	+/–	–	–	–/+[b]	1–5%	1–2 days
Sanger sequencing with capillary electrophoresis	+	+	–	–	+	~25%	3–5 days
Pyrosequencing	+	+	–	–	–	~5%	2–3 days
Melting curve analysis	+	+	–	–	–	10–20%	2–3 days
NGS-amplicon capture	+	+	+	–	+	5–10%	5–10 days
NGS-hybridization capture	+	+	+	+	+	2–5%	5–10 days
NGS-exon sequencing	+	+	+	+	–/+[c]	10%	5–10 days
NGS-whole genome sequencing	+	+	+	+	+	Depends on assay design	Weeks

RFLP restriction fragment length polymorphism
[a]In some laboratories, short turnaround times are not feasible due to specimen batching or fixed day runs
[b]Will detect specific rearrangements
[c]With difficulty, depending on the assay design

Tests to Detect Chromosomal Abnormalities

Chromosomal abnormalities include structural variants (SV) and changes in the number of chromosomes or copy number variations (CNV). SV are large structural changes and include rearrangements within or between different chromosomes and inversions. The most common tests used to detect structural and numerical abnormalities include karyotyping (G-banding being the most common), fluorescence in situ hybridization (FISH), reverse transcription polymerase chain reaction (RT-PCR), array comparative genomic hybridization (aCGH), multiplex ligation-dependent probe amplification (MLPA), and next-generation sequencing (NGS). An overview of testing modalities used to detect chromosomal abnormalities is provided in Table 1.2. Even though all these tests are designed to detect SV or CNV,

Table 1.2 Tests to evaluate chromosomal abnormalities

Assay	Applications	Will not detect	Limitations	Sensitivity
Conventional karyotype (G-banding) [46]	Detect numerical and structural abnormalities	Small (cryptic) rearrangements; small insertions, deletions, or indels; SNV	Requires fresh tissue; long, turnaround time, low resolution; tumor cells might not grow in culture; necessitates high skills and experience in interpretation; difficult to detect complex rearrangements; might not detect cryptic translocations	Low, dependent on which cells grow
FISH [46, 47]	Detect rearrangements, large deletions and copy number variations of large chromosome segments	Small (cryptic) rearrangements; small insertions, deletions, or indels; SNV	Can only detect rearrangements, deletions, or copy number variations in the specific area of interest; insertions, small deletions, or inversions might not be detected	High, in touch imprints, and cytology specimens can be as high as 0.5%
Reverse transcriptase PCR [46]	Detect specific rearrangements; works well in formalin-fixed paraffin-embedded tissue	May not detect variants of the rearrangement	Can only detect rearrangements in a specific area. Not well suited for rearrangements with multiple fusion partners (e.g., the primer set might not cover the fusion present)	High, 1% to 5% when quantitative PCR is used
aCGH [48]	Can detect copy number at higher resolution	Copy neutral changes like balanced translocations or inversions	Requires normal DNA for comparison	Low, around 25%
MLPA [48, 49]	Can detect copy number, methylation, and point mutations	Copy neutral changes like balanced translocations or inversions	Single base pair changes can affect probe hybridization and be interpreted as a deletion; requires normal DNA for comparison	Low, around 25%

their design is significantly different, and they may not be used interchangeably and/or have different requirements for specimen submission.

Karyotyping (G-Banding)

Karyotyping can be done by several methods, the most common being Giemsa banding (G-banding). It is a cytogenetic technique used to visualize the complete karyotype by staining condensed chromosomes with the Giemsa stain. It is available in commercial laboratories and some hospitals. This technique allows visualization of all chromosomes [50] and is capable to detect copy number variants and large structural abnormalities [51, 52]. It is considered a low-resolution technique and requires prolonged turnaround time (weeks).

This technique suffers from several pre-analytical, technical, and interpretative limitations [53]. It requires rapid delivery of the sample to the laboratory because fresh tissue is needed to culture living cells. Timely delivery is important, but submission of the tissue in suitable culture media helps preserve the cells during delivery when shipping is delayed. During culture, insufficient cells may reach metaphase, yielding inconclusive results, or the culture may be overgrown by normal fibroblasts, which can lead to false negative results. Also, the cells may fail to grow or grow slowly.

The test is dependent on the availability of experienced interpreters and requires high skills. Also, a neoplasm may have numerous complex anomalies making interpretation difficult or mask recurrent rearrangements. Finally, a neoplasm can have cryptic rearrangements that cannot be detected by the test.

Fluorescence In Situ Hybridization

FISH is a molecular cytogenetic technique that uses fluorescence probes to detect specific areas in a chromosome. This technique can be performed in interphase (non-dividing) or metaphase (dividing) cells, in tissues procured fresh, frozen, or formalin-fixed, paraffin-embedded (FFPE). It can also be used in materials from blood smears, touch imprints, and cytology specimens like fine needle aspirations and cytospins, or other samples with minimal cellularity. It is considered a targeted approach, medium-resolution technique and, depending on the laboratory, can have a turnaround time of 1–3 days. It allows direct visualization of the abnormality in individual cells and when interphase cells are prepared from fresh tissue by touch prep or smear can have high sensitivity (up to 0.5% depending on how many cells can be visualized).

FISH is commonly used to detect copy numbers for specific chromosomes, amplifications, and rearrangements. Two methods to detect rearrangements exist. The first method uses break-apart probes, which are probes flanking the gene or region of interest. They detect the rearrangement when the fused signal separates into a split signal. This approach is frequently used for genes that have recurring breakpoints and also rearrange with multiple different partner genes (e.g., *EWSR1*, *ALK*). The second uses fusion probes. Fusion probes flank two genes or regions of interest and detect the rearrangement when the separate signals fuse as a consequence of a rearrangement. With this approach, both partner genes are known.

The major limitation of FISH is its targeted approach, since it needs high suspicion for the specific abnormality being tested, and it is not well suited as a screening tool. In FFPE tissues, analysis may be limited by loss of nuclear material during sectioning (truncation artifact) that may lead to false positive or false negative results. For example, the nuclear material might be lost during sectioning, and it might falsely detect a deletion. This is mitigated by through validation and establishing cutoff values during the validation. These cutoff values may vary by laboratory.

Crushing, poor, or prolonged fixation time (usually more than 72 hours) and decalcification procedures may also affect interpretation and signal intensity. Because the probes are large, up to 500 kilobases (kb), it is not well suited to detect single-base mutations. Also, nomenclature and reporting may be inconsistent among laboratories although the vast majority adhere to standard nomenclature guidelines. The last major limitation is signal fading over time that does not allow for rereview of the slides after prolonged periods. Therefore, photo documentation is recommended.

Reverse Transcription Polymerase Chain Reaction

Reverse transcription PCR (RT-PCR) is well suited to detect chimeric transcripts as a consequence of chromosomal rearrangements [54, 55]. RT-PCR involves the conversion of RNA to complementary DNA (cDNA) sequences for subsequent testing. To detect rearrangements, both genes or one gene partner is needed to detect the fusion transcript [56]. This technique can be performed using formalin-fixed paraffin-embedded tissue, fresh or previously frozen tissues. It is considered a very specific technique, and the turnaround time is usually 1–3 days, similar to FISH.

RT-PCR is a highly sensitive technique that will allow detection of low-level disease down to 1% [57]. When performed in conjunction with real-time PCR, it can be used for quantitation of minimal residual disease to as low as 0.0001% depending on the amount of template used [58].

Because of its specificity, it is not a very good screening tool and requires high level of suspicion for a given rearrangement, like FISH. Another caveat for this test is that it will only detect one variant fusion, unless it is multiplexed [56]. For genes with multiple rearrangement partners or multiple fusion variants, like the *ALK* or *EWSR1* genes, it is difficult to design primer sets that will cover all possibilities. In these instances, it is easier to detect a rearrangement using a break-apart FISH probe or NGS technology, such as RNAseq or sequencing in conjunction with anchored PCR.

Multiplex Ligation-Dependent Probe Amplification

MLPA [59] is a molecular technique that utilizes ligation of specific probes to a target DNA sequence. If successful hybridization occurs, the probes are ligated and then amplified. The assay can be used to detect single-nucleotide polymorphism or point mutations, copy number alterations, deletions, and small rearrangements. The main limitations of this methodology are that it cannot detect copy neutral loss heterozygosity (like uniparental disomy) or balanced rearrangements. It may also have problems detecting mosaicism, tumor heterogeneity, or alterations when there is excessive contamination with normal cells [60]. In addition, because this technique targets specific areas within an exon, point mutations or polymorphisms that hinder hybridization of the probe might be falsely interpreted as a deletion. Lastly, this technique requires a "normal" DNA for a control. The turnaround time is usually 2–3 days and the limit of detection is around 10%.

Array Comparative Genomic Hybridization (aCGH) and Single-Nucleotide Polymorphism (SNP) Arrays

Array comparative genomic hybridization (aCGH) is a molecular cytogenetic technique developed to detect whole genome copy number variations (CNV). It compares the target DNA to a reference sample using fluorescence probes. In order to achieve this, the target DNA and the reference DNA are hybridized in a solid support with immobilized capture probes (the array) [61, 62]. Its main advantages are that it does not need fresh tissue; it is a high-resolution technique; it can interrogate the whole genome and detect aneuploidies, deletions, duplications, and amplifications; and it has the added benefit of detecting submicroscopic chromosomal abnormalities. Its main disadvantage is the inability to detect chromosomal aberrations that do not result in copy number changes (like balanced translocations, inversions, or balanced insertions). It can be performed in fresh, frozen, or FFPE tissues. Lastly, aCGH has low detection limit (around 20%) and long turnaround time (weeks). Some newer arrays are based on single-nucleotide polymorphisms (SNPs) which have several added advantages including the ability to detect copy neutral loss of heterozygosity which is important in some cancers.

Methods Used to Detect Changes in the DNA Sequence

Changes in the DNA sequence that commonly cause disease include single-nucleotide variants (SNV), small duplications, insertions or deletions, and simultaneous insertions and deletions (indels). Numerous methods to detect mutations have been developed, and the most common ones used in routine clinical practice include polymerase chain reaction (PCR) and variants as the basic form of amplification followed by a detection method with or without subsequent sequencing (Table 1.3). Following PCR, detection may involve the measuring of the PCR products by size (fragment analysis, or restriction fragment length polymorphism analysis) or by specific melting curve characteristics (melting curve analysis). Alternatively, the PCR product may be sequenced by various methods including Sanger sequencing,

Table 1.3 Tests to evaluate changes in DNA sequence

Assay	Application	Will not detect	Limitations	Sensitivity
Allele-specific PCR	SNV	Deletions, duplications, insertions, deletions	Specific assay for the specific gene in question may not detect other mutations than the one the assay was designed for	1–5%
Sanger sequencing with capillary electrophoresis [63]	Considered the gold standard for sequencing, can be designed to detect changes in sequence in up to 1000 bp. Will detect insertions, deletions, and indels and rearrangements	Large chromosomal abnormalities, deletions	Low detection limit; labor intensive, costly	Approximately 25%
Pyrosequencing [63, 64]	Easy to implement; very good at detecting point mutations; high sensitivity (around 5%)	Very difficult to detect small insertions and deletions or rearrangements	Difficult to detect sequences with the same base (homopolymers when longer than 6–8 bp in length), requires a short template (around 40 bp, but can be designed up to 400 bp)	Around 5%
Melting curve analysis [63]	Fast and easy to implement; used to detect commonly known mutations		The specific mutation is not known; might require confirmation for unusual mutations	10–20%

pyrosequencing, mass spectrometry genotyping, or next-generation sequencing (NGS). NGS techniques, depending on the capture method, can be used to detect copy number variations, and they are also used to detect mutations, duplications, small insertions, deletions, and indels.

Next-generation sequencing methods are considered highly specific or of high resolution. One limitation that affects all sequencing methods is the size of sequence that can be evaluated at a given time. Depending on the assay, the sequences vary from around 40 bp (pyrosequencing) to up to 1000 bp (Sanger sequencing). However, most of the assays are optimized for DNA fragments ranging in size from 100 to 300 bp to allow use with FFPE tissue, since formalin fixation fragments the DNA.

The following is a description of some of these assays with their limitations.

Allele-Specific PCR

This is a targeted analysis for the detection of specific SNV. It is very specific for the mutation that the assay was designed for. It is also sensitive, and it can detect mutations when present at 1–5% concentrations. Its main limitation is its specificity. It cannot detect other mutations than the one the assay is designed for.

Sanger Sequencing with Capillary Electrophoresis

Sanger sequencing is a PCR technique and it is considered the gold standard for DNA sequencing. RNA can also be sequenced if converted to cDNA. Capillary electrophoresis is the method to separate the DNA strands by size and allow separation of up to 1 bp resolution. Sanger sequencing is well suited to detect SNVs, small deletions, insertions, and indels. It can also detect fusion transcripts, if appropriately designed. If good-quality DNA is used, it can sequence segments up to 1000 bp. The main benefits are that it will detect any mutation or variant in the DNA segment covered by the primer set. The biggest limitations are its costs and it is also labor intensive. It has low sensitivity, at around 20%, but sensitivity can be improved by using locked nucleic acids (LNA-PCR) [65]. Also, this method will not detect CNV. The turnaround time is around 3–5 days.

Pyrosequencing

Pyrosequencing is a sequencing-by-synthesis method that uses a series of reactions to measure the release of inorganic pyrophosphate as each nucleotide is incorporated into the DNA chain [66]. This technique is easy to implement and has fast turnaround time (can be performed in 1 or 2 days), and it is good at detecting SNV and has high sensitivity. It will detect a mutation in approximately 5% concentration. Also, it is well suited to detect mutations in less than optimal DNA, like decalcified bone specimens [67] because it requires short DNA templates (around 40 bp). When using this method, it is difficult to detect sequences with the same base (homopolymers when longer than 6–8 bp in length) and insertions and deletions. Also, it cannot sequence long templates well (more than 400 bp).

Melting Curve Analysis

Melting curve analysis is a technique developed to detect mutations by measuring the changes in fluorescence generated by the different dissociation curves between mutated and wild-type samples [68]. This technique is suitable to detect single base pair substitutions and small deletions and insertions. It can also be used to detect methylation status of a specific region [69]. Its main benefits are that it is a fast, closed-end system that is not labor intensive. The main limitations are that even though it can detect a mutation in the area of interest, it cannot define which mutation is present. Also, in some instances, it might require confirmation by another method [63]. This assay can detect a mutation at approximately 10% concentration.

Next-Generation Sequencing

Next-generation sequencing (NGS) is a group of high-throughput methodologies that allow for low-cost sequencing of the genome or exome, transcriptome profiling (RNA-seq), protein-DNA interactions (ChIP-Seq), and epigenetic modifications. Depending on the manufacturer or platform, the assay may differ in the way the bases are incorporated and detected. The assays will also differ in the way the library is prepared and how the targets are enriched, when a targeted approach is used. The two most common methodologies for base incorporation and detection are sequence-by-synthesis using fluorescence (Illumina® dye sequencing) and hydrogen ions (Ion Torrent®) [70]. The most common target enrichment methods include hybridization or capture based and amplicon based (Table 1.4) [72]. All of these factors affect the performance characteristics of the assays [70–72].

Both methods of base incorporation can detect copy number variations and mutations, small insertions, and deletions. Between these base incorporation methods, dye sequencing appears to have a lower error rate (<0.4%) versus (~1.8%) [70]. The

Table 1.4 Next-generation sequencing approaches [70–72]

Method	Uses	Will not detect	Limitations
NGS-amplicon capture	SNV, small deletions, insertions, small duplications, structural rearrangements depending on design	Copy number alterations Limited capabilities for structural rearrangements Large structural change	Slow turnaround time, complex setup, need for bioinformatics support
NGS-hybridization capture	SNV, small deletions, insertions, small duplications, rearrangements (depending on design)	Large structural changes	Slow turnaround time, cumbersome to setup time, heavy bioinformatics support
NGS-whole exome sequencing	SNV, small deletions, insertions duplications	Structural rearrangements involving introns	Slow turnaround time, cumbersome to setup time, heavy bioinformatics support
NGS-whole genome sequencing	SNV, small deletions, insertions, duplications, structural changes		Expensive, slow, cumbersome to setup time, not practical for everyday use, few automated solutions Heavy bioinformatics support

base content of the template also influences the error rate as dye sequencing has difficulty reading areas rich in GC and ion semiconductor has difficulty detecting homopolymers (sequences with more than 6–8 base pairs) and is not well suited for AT-rich areas in the genome.

Additional limitations affecting next-generation sequencing are related to the general architecture of the DNA templates. The most important of these limitations is the presence of difficult-to-sequence areas in the genome. Areas of high-homology (e.g., pseudogenes), repetitive, and GC-rich regions [73–75] affect assay performance and sensitivity. The reason for poor performance in areas of high homology or repetitive regions of the genome is related to inaccuracies in the mapping to the reference sequence. In CG-rich regions, it has been proposed that the reason for the high error rate might be due to secondary structure formation, lower quality of reads, or high background noise [76, 77].

Additional limitations in next-generation sequencing are related to the analysis of the data which are discussed at length in both the bioinformatics section and dedicated NGS sections of this book. Genomic analysis and bioinformatics pipelines rely on the use of numerous public and private sources for analysis tools for which no specific guidelines and standardization have been applied [78]. This leads to significant variability among laboratories.

The next-generation sequencing limitations noted above are mainly due to the early stages of clinical implementation of these assays and will, in most likelihood, be resolved in the upcoming years. The bioinformatics pipeline limitations should be resolved as the "Standards for Clinical Grade Genomics Databases" is implemented [78].

Gene Expression Profiling

Gene expression profiles are most commonly used in the research setting, but have found clinical use in the prognostication of some malignancies [79]. In essence, these tests quantify the expression of multiple genes (signature panel) in an attempt to predict the likelihood of recurrence and/or selecting individual therapies. Depending on the assay, these may be performed in fresh, frozen, or FFPE tissues. Also, these tests require well-preserved tissue that has not seen prolonged cold ischemia time or is highly necrotic, since they utilize mRNA. The labile nature of RNA from FFPE has been overcome by specific extraction kits that can minimize RNA degradation and remove genomic DNA that can affect downstream applications. At least 30% of invasive tumor is needed to increase accuracy. Turnaround time is test dependent and could be 1–2 weeks. The limits of detection also vary by assay, but the norm is to submit tissue with at least 25% tumor.

Tissue stewardship and selecting and optimizing the use of tissues for ancillary testing are the responsibility of the pathologists in collaboration with other providers. It is essential to understand the pre-analytic variables at play as part of the tissue accrual, optimization, and management process. In addition, there is a spectrum of molecular methods available in clinical laboratories, each designed for different applications and with different strengths and limitations. Keeping all of these factors in mind, an educated decision to select the test that will best serve the patient's clinical need can be made.

References

1. Genetically Informed Cancer Medicine – My Cancer Genome [Internet]. Mycancergenome.org. 2019 [cited 31 March 2019]. Available from: https://www.mycancergenome.org/
2. Education Resources [Internet]. Association for Molecular Pathology. 2019 [cited 31 March 2019]. Available from: https://www.amp.org/education/education-resources/.
3. Khoury T, Sait S, Hwang H, Chandrasekhar R, Wilding G, Tan D, et al. Delay to formalin fixation effect on breast biomarkers. Mod Pathol. 2009;22(11):1457–67.
4. Greer CE, Lund JK, Manos MM. PCR amplification from paraffin-embedded tissues: recommendations on fixatives for long-term storage and prospective studies. PCR Methods Appl. 1991;1(1):46–50.
5. Srinivasan M, Sedmak D, Jewell S. Effect of fixatives and tissue processing on the content and integrity of nucleic acids. Am J Pathol. 2002;161:1961–197.
6. Godfrey T, Kim S, Chavira M, Ruff D, Warren R, Gray J, et al. Quantitative mRNA expression analysis from formalin-fixed, paraffin-embedded tissues using 5′ nuclease quantitative reverse transcription-polymerase chain reaction. J Mol Diagn. 2000;2(2):84–91.
7. Coudry R, Meireles S, Stoyanova R, Cooper H, Carpino A, Wang X, et al. Successful application of microarray technology to microdissected formalin-fixed, paraffin-embedded tissue. J Mol Diagn. 2007;9(1):70–9.
8. Neubauer A, Neubauer B, He M, Effert P, Iglehart D, Frye R, et al. Analysis of gene amplification in archival tissue by differential polymerase chain reaction. Oncogene. 2019;7(5):1019–25.
9. Lott R, Tunnicliffe J, Sheppard E, Santiago J, Hladik C, Nasim M et al. Practical guide to specimen handling in surgical pathology [Internet]. 7th ed. CAP/NSH Histotechnology Committee; 2017 [cited 31 March 2019]. Available from: https://documents.cap.org/documents/practical-guide-specimen-handling.pdf
10. Kösel S, Grasbon-Frodl EM, Arima K, Chimelli L, Hahn M, Hashizume Y, et al. Interlaboratory comparison of DNA preservation in archival paraffin-embedded human brain tissue from participating centres on four continents. Neurogenetics. 2001;3(3):163–70.
11. Nuovo GJ, Richart RM. Buffered formalin is the superior fixative for the detection of HPV DNA by in situ hybridization analysis. Am J Pathol. 1989;132(4):837–42.
12. Ferrer I, Armstrong J, Capellari S, Parchi P, Arzberger T, Bell J, et al. Effects of formalin fixation, paraffin embedding, and time of storage on DNA preservation in brain tissue: a BrainNet Europe Study. Brain Pathol. 2007;17(3):297–303.
13. Barcelos D, Franco M, Leão S. Effects of tissue handling and processing steps on PCR for detection of Mycobacterium tuberculosis in formalin-fixed paraffin-embedded samples. Rev Inst Med Trop Sao Paulo. 2008;50(6):321–6.
14. Coura R. An alternative protocol for DNA extraction from formalin fixed and paraffin wax embedded tissue. J Clin Pathol. 2005;58(8):894–5.
15. Miething F, Hering S, Hanschke B, Dressler J. Effect of fixation to the degradation of nuclear and mitochondrial DNA in different tissues. J Histochem Cytochem. 2006;54(3):371–4.
16. Apple S, Pucci R, Lowe A, Shintaku I, Shapourifar-Tehrani S, Moatamed N. The effect of delay in fixation, different fixatives, and duration of fixation in estrogen and progesterone receptor results in breast carcinoma. Am J Clin Pathol. 2011;135(4):592–8.
17. Hashizume K, Hatanaka Y, Kamihara Y, Kato T, Hata S, Akashi S, et al. Interlaboratory comparison in HercepTest assessment of HER2 protein status in invasive breast carcinoma fixed with various formalin-based fixatives. Appl Immunohistochem Mol Morphol. 2003;11(4):339–44.

18. Williams JH, Mepham BL, Wright DH. Tissue preparation for immunocytochemistry. J Clin Pathol. 1997;50(5):422–8.
19. Pollard K, Lunny D, Holgate CS, Jackson P, Bird CC. Fixation, processing, and immunochemical reagent effects on preservation of T-lymphocyte surface membrane antigens in paraffin-embedded tissue. J Histochem Cytochem. 1987;35(11):1329–38.
20. Petersen B, Sørensen M, Pedersen S, Rasmussen M. Fluorescence in situ hybridization on formalin-fixed and paraffin-embedded tissue. Appl Immunohistochem Mol Morphol. 2004;12(3):259–65.
21. O'Leary J, Browne G, Landers R, Crowley M, Healy I, Street J, et al. The importance of fixation procedures on DNA template and its suitability for solution-phase polymerase chain reaction and PCR in situ hybridization. Histochem J. 1994;26(4):337–46.
22. Jackson D, Lewis F, Taylor G, Boylston A, Quirke P. Tissue extraction of DNA and RNA and analysis by the polymerase chain reaction. J Clin Pathol. 1990;43(6):499–504.
23. Noguchi M, Furuya J, Takeuchi T, Hirohashi S. Modified formalin and methanol fixation methods for molecular biological and morphological analyses. Pathol Int. 1997;47(10):685–91.
24. Hey-Chi H, Shian-Yang P, Chia-Tung S. High quality of DNA retrieved for Southern blot hybridization from microwave-fixed, paraffin-embedded liver tissues. J Virol Methods. 1991;31(2–3):251–61.
25. Ruijter E, Miller G, Aalders T, Van De Kaa C, Schalken J, Debruyne F, et al. Rapid microwave-stimulated fixation of entire prostatectomy specimens. J Pathol. 1997;183(3):369–75.
26. Bödör C, Schmidt O, Csernus B, Rajnai H, Szende B. DNA and RNA isolated from tissues processed by microwave-accelerated apparatus MFX-800-3 are suitable for subsequent PCR and Q-RT-PCR amplification. Pathol Oncol Res. 2007;13(2):149–52.
27. Chu W, Liang Q, Tang Y, King R, Wong K, Gong M, et al. Ultrasound-accelerated tissue fixation/processing achieves superior morphology and macromolecule integrity with storage stability. J Histochem Cytochem. 2006;54(5):503–13.
28. Fracasso T, Heinrich M, Hohoff C, Brinkmann B, Pfeiffer H. Ultrasound-accelerated formalin fixation improves the preservation of nucleic acids extraction in histological sections. Int J Leg Med. 2009;123(6):521–5.
29. Brown R, Edwards J, Bartlett J, Jones C, Dogan A. Routine acid decalcification of bone marrow samples can preserve DNA for FISH and CGH studies in metastatic prostate cancer. J Histochem Cytochem. 2002;50(1):113–5.
30. Wickham C, Sarsfield P, Joyner M, Jones D, Ellard S, Wilkins B. Formic acid decalcification of bone marrow trephines degrades DNA: alternative use of EDTA allows the amplification and sequencing of relatively long PCR products. Mol Pathol. 2000;53(6):336.
31. Alers J, Krijtenburg P, Vissers K, van Dekken H. Effect of bone decalcification procedures on DNA in situ hybridization and comparative genomic hybridization: EDTA is highly preferable to a routinely used acid decalcifier. J Histochem Cytochem. 1999;47(5):703–9.
32. Babic A, Loftin I, Stanislaw S, Wang M, Miller R, Warren S, et al. The impact of pre-analytical processing on staining quality for H&E, dual hapten, dual color in situ hybridization and fluorescent in situ hybridization assays. Methods. 2010;52(4):287–300.
33. Reineke T, Jenni B, Abdou M, Frigerio S, Zubler P, Moch H, et al. Ultrasonic decalcification offers new perspectives for rapid FISH, DNA, and RT-PCR analysis in bone marrow trephines. Am J Surg Pathol. 2006;30(7):892–6.
34. Beaulieu M, Desaulniers M, Bertrand N, Deschesnes R, Beaudry G, Garon G, et al. Analytical performance of a qRT-PCR assay to detect guanylyl cyclase C in FFPE lymph nodes of patients with colon cancer. Diagn Mol Pathol. 2010;19(1):20–7.
35. Ribeiro-Silva A, Zhang H, Jeffrey S. RNA extraction from ten year old formalin-fixed paraffin-embedded breast cancer samples: a comparison of column purification and magnetic bead-based technologies. BMC Mol Biol. 2007;8(1):118.
36. Austin M, Smith C, Pritchard C, Tait J. DNA yield from tissue samples in surgical pathology and minimum tissue requirements for molecular testing. Arch Pathol Lab Med. 2016;140(2):130–3.

37. Elloumi F, Hu Z, Li Y, Parker J, Gulley M, Amos K, et al. Systematic bias in genomic classification due to contaminating non-neoplastic tissue in breast tumor samples. BMC Med Genet. 2011;4(1):54.
38. Kotoula V, Kalogeras K, Kouvatseas G, Televantou D, Kronenwett R, Wirtz R, et al. Sample parameters affecting the clinical relevance of RNA biomarkers in translational breast cancer research. Virchows Arch. 2012;462(2):141–54.
39. Poremba C, Uhlendorff J, Pfitzner B, Hennig G, Bohmann K, Bojar H, et al. Preanalytical variables and performance of diagnostic RNA-based gene expression analysis in breast cancer. Virchows Arch. 2014;465(4):409–17.
40. Mehrotra M, Singh R, Chen W, Huang R, Almohammedsalim A, Barkoh B, et al. Study of preanalytic and analytic variables for clinical next-generation sequencing of circulating cell-free nucleic acid. J Mol Diagn. 2017;19(4):514–24.
41. Bettegowda C, Sausen M, Leary R, Kinde I, Wang Y, Agrawal N, et al. Detection of circulating tumor DNA in early- and late-stage human malignancies. Sci Transl Med. 2014;6(224):224ra24.
42. Frenel J, Carreira S, Goodall J, Roda D, Perez-Lopez R, Tunariu N, et al. Serial next-generation sequencing of circulating cell-free DNA evaluating tumor clone response to molecularly targeted drug administration. Clin Cancer Res. 2015;21(20):4586–96.
43. El Messaoudi S, Mouliere F, Du Manoir S, Bascoul-Mollevi C, Gillet B, Nouaille M, et al. Circulating DNA as a strong multimarker prognostic tool for metastatic colorectal cancer patient management care. Clin Cancer Res. 2016;22(12):3067–77.
44. Nikolaev S, Lemmens L, Koessler T, Blouin J, Nouspikel T. Circulating tumoral DNA: preanalytical validation and quality control in a diagnostic laboratory. Anal Biochem. 2018;542:34–9.
45. Garcia J, Dusserre E, Cheynet V, Bringuier P, Brengle-Pesce K, Wozny AS, et al. Evaluation of pre-analytical conditions and comparison of the performance of several digital PCR assays for the detection of major EGFR mutations in circulating DNA from non-small cell lung cancers: the CIRCAN_0 study. Oncotarget. 2017;8(50):87890–996.
46. Bridge J. Advantages and limitations of cytogenetic, molecular cytogenetic, and molecular diagnostic testing in mesenchymal neoplasms. J Orthop Sci. 2008;13(3):273–82. PMID:18528664.
47. Tanas M, Goldblum J. Fluorescence in situ hybridization in the diagnosis of soft tissue neoplasms: a review. Adv Anat Pathol. 2009;16(6):383–91. PMID: 19851129.
48. Kallioniemi O, Kallioniemi A, Piper J, Isola J, Waldman F, Gray J, et al. Optimizing comparative genomic hybridization for analysis of DNA sequence copy number changes in solid tumors. Genes Chromosomes Cancer. 1994;10(4):231–43. PMID: 7522536.
49. Hömig-Hölzel C, Savola S. Multiplex ligation-dependent probe amplification (MLPA) in tumor diagnostics and prognostics. Diagn Mol Pathol. 2012;21(4):189–206. PMID: 23111197.
50. Drets M, Shaw M. Specific banding patterns of human chromosomes. Proc Natl Acad Sci U S A. 1971;68(9):2073–7. PMID: 4109065.
51. Yunis J. New chromosome techniques in the study of human neoplasia. Hum Pathol. 1981;12(6):540–9. PMID: 7275094
52. Philip P, Drivsholm A. G-banding analysis of complex aneuploidy in multiple myeloma bone marrow cells. Blood. 1976;47(1):69–77. PMID: 1244914.
53. Hastings R, Bown N, Tibiletti M, Debiec-Rychter M, Vanni R, Espinet B, et al. Guidelines for cytogenetic investigations in tumours. Eur J Hum Genet. 2015;24(1):6–13. PMID: 25804401.
54. Sorensen P, Liu X, Delattre O, Biggs C, Thomas G, Triche T. Reverse transcriptase PCR amplification of EWS/FLI-1 fusion transcripts as a diagnostic test for peripheral primitive neuroectodermal tumors of childhood. Diagn Mol Pathol. 1993;2(3):147–57. PMID: 7506981.
55. de Alva E, Ladanyi M, Rosai J, Gerald W. Detection of chimeric transcripts in desmoplastic small round cell tumor and related developmental tumors by reverse transcriptase polymerase chain reaction. A specific diagnostic assay. Am J Pathol. 1995;147(6):1584–91. PMID: 7495283.
56. Frohman M, Dush M, Martin G. Rapid production of full-length cDNAs from rare transcripts: amplification using a single gene-specific oligonucleotide primer. Proc Natl Acad Sci U S A. 1988;85(23):8998–9002. PMID: 2461560.

57. Chang K, Lu J, Wang G, Trujillo M, Estey E, Cork A, et al. The t(15;17) breakpoint in acute promyelocytic leukemia cluster within two different sites of the myl gene: targets for the detection of minimal residual disease by the polymerase chain reaction. Blood. 1992;79(3):554–8. PMID: 1310060.
58. Cassinat B, Zassadowski F, Balitrand N, Barbey C, Rain J, Fenaux P, et al. Quantitation of minimal residual disease in acute promyelocytic leukemia patients with t(15;17) translocation using real-time RT-PCR. Leukemia. 2000;14(2):324–8. PMID: 10673752.
59. Schouten J, McElgunn C, Waaijer R, Zwijnenburg D, Depvens F, Pals G. Relative quantification of 40 nucleic acid sequences by multiplex ligation-dependent probe amplification. Nucleic Acids Res. 2002;30(12):e57. PMID: 12060695.
60. Stuppia L, Antonucci I, Palka G, Gatta V. Use of the MLPA assay in the molecular diagnosis of gene copy number alterations in human genetic diseases. Int J Mol Sci. 2012;13(3):3245–76. PMID: 22489151.
61. Solinas-Toldo S, Lampel S, Stilgenbauer S, Nickolenko J, Benner A, Döhner H, et al. Matrix-based comparative genomic hybridization: biochips to screen for genomic imbalances. Genes Chromosomes Cancer. 1997;20(4):399–407. PMID: 9408757.
62. Pinkel D, Segraves R, Sudar D, Clark S, Poole I, Kowbel D, et al. High resolution analysis of DNA copy number variation using comparative genomic hybridization to microarrays. Nat Genet. 1998;20(2):207–11. PMID: 9771718.
63. Tsiatis A, Norris-Kirby A, Rich R, Hafez M, Gocke C, Eshleman J, et al. Comparison of sanger sequencing, pyrosequencing, and melting curve analysis for the detection of KRAS mutations. J Mol Diagn. 2010;12(4):425–32. PMID: 20431034.
64. Harrington C, Lin E, Olson M, Eshleman J. Fundamentals of pyrosequencing. Arch Pathol Lab Med. 2013;137(9):1296–303. PMID: 23991743.
65. Arcila M, Lau C, Nafa K, Ladanyi M. Detection of KRAS and BRAF mutations in colorectal carcinoma. J Mol Diagn. 2011;13(1):64–73. PMID: 21227396.
66. Hyman E. A new method of sequencing DNA. Anal Biochem. 1988;174(2):423–36. PMID: 2853582.
67. Liang Q, Wei M, Hodge L, Fanburg-Smith J, Nelson A, Miettinen M, et al. Quantitative analysis of activating alpha subunit of the G protein (Gsα) mutation by pyrosequencing in fibrous dysplasia and other bone lesions. J Mol Diagn. 2011;13(2):137–42. PMID: 21354047.
68. Lyon E. Mutation detection using fluorescent hybridization probes and melting curve analysis. Expert Rev Mol Diagn. 2001;1(1):92–101. PMID: 11901805.
69. Lorente A, Mueller W, Urdangarín E, Lázcoz P, von Deimling A, Castresana J. Detection of methylation in promoter sequences by melting curve analysis-based semiquantitative real time PCR. BMC Cancer. 2008;8(1). PMID: 18298842.
70. Quail M, Smith M, Coupland P, Otto T, Harris S, Connor T, et al. A tale of three next generation sequencing platforms: comparison of ion torrent, pacific biosciences and illumina MiSeq sequencers. BMC Genomics. 2012;13(1):341. PMID: 22827831.
71. Loman N, Misra R, Dallman T, Constantinidou C, Gharbia S, Wain J, et al. Performance comparison of benchtop high-throughput sequencing platforms. Nat Biotechnol. 2012;30(5):434–9. PMID: 22522955.
72. Samorodnitsky E, Jewell B, Hagopian R, Miya J, Wing M, Lyon E, et al. Evaluation of hybridization capture versus amplicon-based methods for whole-exome sequencing. Hum Mutat. 2015;36(9):903–14. PMID: 26110913.
73. Sipos B, Massingham T, Stütz A, Goldman N. An improved protocol for sequencing of repetitive genomic regions and structural variations using mutagenesis and next generation sequencing. PLoS One. 2012;7(8):e43359. PMID: 22912860.
74. Mandelker D, Amr S, Pugh T, Gowrisankar S, Shakhbatyan R, Duffy E, et al. Comprehensive diagnostic testing for stereocilin. J Mol Diagn. 2014;16(6):639–47. PMID: 25157971.

75. Minoche A, Dohm J, Himmelbauer H. Evaluation of genomic high-throughput sequencing data generated on Illumina HiSeq and genome analyzer systems. Genome Biol. 2011;12(11):R112. PMID: 28782984.
76. Yohe S, Thyagarajan B. Review of clinical next-generation sequencing. Arch Pathol Lab Med. 2017;141(11):1544–57. PMID: 28782984.
77. Shin S, Park J. Characterization of sequence-specific errors in various next-generation sequencing systems. Mol Biosyst. 2016;12(3):914–22. PMID: 26790373.
78. Yohe S, Carter A, Pfeifer J, Crawford J, Cushman-Vokoun A, Caughron S, et al. Standards for clinical grade genomic databases. Arch Pathol Lab Med. 2015;139(11):1400–12. PMID: 26516938.
79. Bhutiani N, Egger M, Ajkay N, Scoggins C, Martin R, McMasters K. Multigene signature panels and breast cancer therapy: patterns of use and impact on clinical decision making. J Am Coll Surg. 2018;226(4):406–412.e1.

Chapter 2
Next-Generation Sequencing

Alanna J. Church

Key Points

- Nucleic acids are prepared for sequencing by "library preparation," including fragmentation, adapter ligation, and target enrichment.
- Several types of sequencers exist, each one assessing the genetic sequence of the library in thousands or millions of parallel reactions.
- The informatics process of analyzing data is critical, including sequence alignment, variant calling, and variant annotation.
- There are many clinical applications for next-generation sequencing.

Key Online Resources

- Introduction to Genomic Technologies: https://www.coursera.org/learn/introduction-genomics
- Genetic Testing Methods: https://www.jax.org/education-and-learning/clinical-and-continuing-education/ccep-non-cancer-resources/genetic-testing-methods#
- Training Residents in Genomics: http://s3.amazonaws.com/ascpcdn/static/TRIG/OnlineModules/Introduction/story_html5.html

A. J. Church (✉)
Laboratory for Molecular Pediatric Pathology (LaMPP), Boston Children's Hospital and Harvard Medical School, Boston, MA, USA
e-mail: Alanna.Church@childrens.harvard.edu

L. J. Tafe, M. E. Arcila (eds.), *Genomic Medicine*,
https://doi.org/10.1007/978-3-030-22922-1_2

Introduction

Next-generation sequencing (NGS) has revolutionized the field of genomics. This powerful technology allows massive parallel sequencing, with up to 50,000 simultaneous reactions. The data is generated at a fraction of the prior cost, making it more accessible to research and clinical centers. The primary challenge now is harnessing this powerful technology to make the best use of it – how to test, what to look for, and what to do with the massive amounts of data. The uptake of NGS is exploding across research space, with innovative new applications being developed. This chapter focuses on the well-established techniques used in clinical laboratories.

Library Preparation

Depending on the assay design, almost any type of nucleic acid can be sequenced. Assays for analysis of DNA and RNA are widely used. Newer technologies like ChipSeq, which uses NGS to analyze protein interactions with DNA, will not be discussed in detail in this chapter, although it is important to note that newer-generation assays are in development.

The role of sample and library preparation is to create the substrate that will be sequenced: high-quality nucleic acid, of the appropriate size and type, with adapters.

Assay design should be thoughtful and well suited to the appropriate substrate. For example, long double-stranded DNA is very stable and allows for longer-read lengths, but fragmented processed nucleic acid is more common in clinical settings, with formalin-fixed paraffin-embedded tissue being a prime example of widely available degraded nucleic acid.

The basic steps of sample preparation are described below, although depending on the assay, the order of steps may be modified.

Nucleic Acid Isolation

DNA and mRNA are the most common substrates for sequencing in clinical laboratories, although it is possible to sequence other nucleic acids, like regulatory RNAs.

Cells are lysed with chaotropic salts and enzymes like proteinase K, depending on the sample type.

Nucleic acid extraction methods include column- and bead-based methods. In column-based extractions, nucleic acid binds to a column, is washed, and is then eluted. In bead-based extractions, nucleic acids are bound to magnetic beads, the solution is washed, and the nucleic acid is eluted.

Isolated nucleic acid is quantified, and often a quality assessment is performed before proceeding with library preparation with either spectrophotometric, fluorimetric, or gel electrophoretic methods.

Fragmentation

The optimal length of nucleic acid strands is determined by the platform and assay design.

Nucleic acids can be fragmented by a variety of methods:

- Acoustic shearing using focused short-wavelength, high-frequency energy
- Sonication using unfocused long-wavelength sonicators
- Enzymatic shearing by digesting both strands of DNA, or by generating nicks on each strand of double-stranded DNA (dsDNA); because the enzymes are directed as specific sequences, this method is known to introduce bias
- Mechanical shearing, either by centrifugal force, hydrodynamics, or needle shearing
- Nebulization

End Repair

Nucleic acid is often fragmented and degraded, with overhang of either the 5′ or 3′ strand. End repair removes or complements overhangs, ensuring that each molecule contains 5′ phosphate and 3′ hydroxyl groups.

Some libraries require blunt-ended adaptor ligation, and others incorporate dA-tails, in which a non-templated deoxyadenosine 5′-monophasphate (dAMP) is added onto the 3′ end. dA-tailing prevents the formation of concatemers, in which separate fragments are ligated together. dA-tails are then ligated to adapters with corresponding dT-overhangs.

Adapter Ligation

Adapters are complementary to the sequencing platform and must be ligated to each fragment of nucleic acid that is to be sequenced.

The functions of the adapters are to interact with the sequencing platform and to identify the origin of the fragment. Molecular barcodes differentiate one sample from another, which is important in library pooling (see below), and informatics analysis. Unique molecular identifiers can be used to identify individual molecules, which can facilitate analysis by recognizing duplicate reads.

Clever adaptations of the adapter include Y-shaped adapters and mate pair sequencing techniques.

Careful calibration of the amount of adapters being added to the ligation mix is important in avoiding contamination with adapter dimers.

Size Selection

The optimal size, or length, of the nucleic acid strands is determined by the assay design and largely by the specific sequencer. Material provided by the manufacturers of each sequencer will specify the optimum size selection.

Short-read sequencers are most efficient when provided with a library of similarly sized sequences. In contrast, long-read sequencers are more efficient with elimination of shorter fragments.

Size selection also facilitates efficient informatics analysis, particularly for paired-end libraries, mate pair sequencing, and double-digest restriction site-associated DNA sequencing (ddRADseq).

The size selection step is important at removing adapter dimers, which can contaminate the libraries.

Techniques for size selection include the following:

- Gel electrophoresis, in which adapted library fragments are run out on a gel and the band with the ideal fragment size is collected.
- Bead-based, in which paramagnetic beads are bound to nucleic acid fragments. Concentration of the buffer in the solution will affect which sizes of fragments bind to and elute from the beads.

Target Enrichment

Also known as sequence enrichment, this is a critical step in library construction. Ideally, a complex library is assembled with high coverage of target regions and a low quantity of off-target reads.

Uniformity of enrichment means that all targeted regions are represented equally and is a key measure of quality and performance.

Techniques for sequence enrichment include hybrid capture or amplicon-based techniques. See Fig. 2.1 for an overview of these two approaches.

1. Hybrid capture, in which long oligonucleotide baits hybridize to regions of interest. Bait design is critical, with careful positioning across target regions, with particular attention to challenging regions, such as GC-rich regions or internal tandem repeats. Hybrid capture methods include the following:

    - Array based: an immobilized probe captures targets. Nonspecific hybrids are washed away and hybridized probes are eluted.

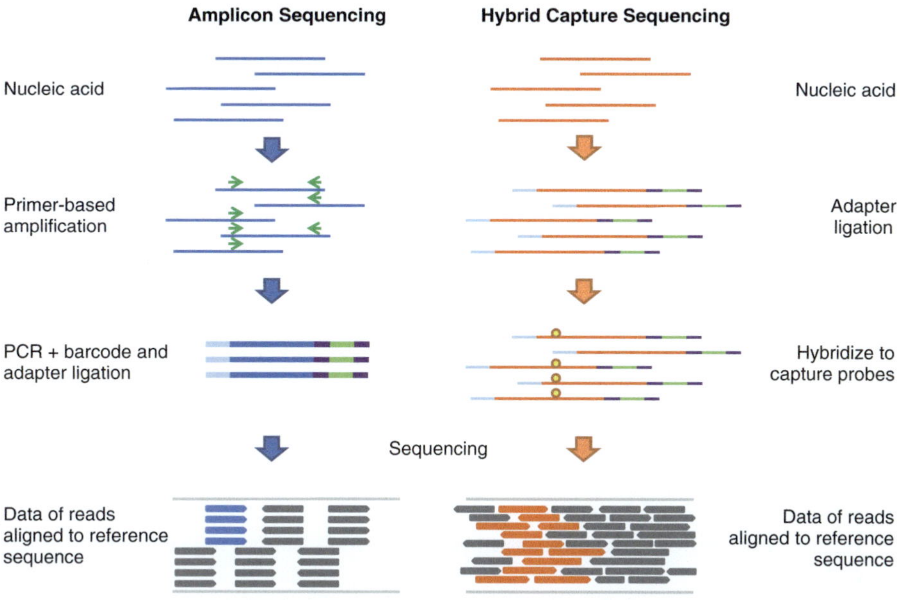

Fig. 2.1 Overview of target enrichment for amplicon and hybrid capture NGS assays. For amplification-based assays (left in blue): primer-based amplification selects regions of interest, followed by PCR with barcode and adapter ligation. Due to dual primer amplification, reads have the same start and stop coordinates. Overlapping or tiling of primer targets allows for complete coverage. For hybrid capture assays (right in orange): adapter ligation is followed by hybridization of capture probes. Target reads are aligned with variable start and stop sites. Tiling of capture probes allows for complete coverage of the region of interest

- Solution based: biotinylated oligonucleotide probes are added to the solution containing adapter-ligated sequences. Magnetic beads are used to capture and purify hybridized probes.

Advantages of the hybrid capture approach over amplicon enrichment include the following:

- Applicable for large assays
- Easy informatic removal of duplicates due to staggered start sites
- Capture of different lengths of sequences
- Greater tolerance to sequence variation of rearrangements and indels due to having only one part of the target hybridized, compared to binding of two flanking primers in amplicon sequencing
- Greater tolerance to sequence variation of single-nucleotide variants that lie under primer binding sites, which can lead to strand bias or allele dropout
- Easy to update a panel with additional targets without having to consider the complex interaction of many primers
- Overall, more uniform and complex coverage, and less likely to miss variants [1–4]

Disadvantages of hybrid capture compared to amplicon sequencing include the following:

- Longer library preparation time
- Requires more nucleic acid input for the same target set
- Highly sensitive to assay design

2. Amplicon-based enrichment, in which multiplexed polymerase chain reactions (PCR) target regions of interest
   Advantages of amplicon enrichment over hybrid capture are as follows:

- Efficient for use in small panels
- Short laboratory processing time (hours instead of days)
- Less nucleic acid input required
- Lower cost

Disadvantages of amplicon enrichment compared to hybrid capture are as follows:

- Presence of PCR artifacts
- Primer competition and nonuniform amplification of target regions due to varied GC content
- Overrepresentation of short sequences due to deletion and underrepresentation of longer sequences due to insertion
- Difficult to distinguish PCR duplicates on analysis without the use of unique molecular identifiers

Note that some of the variation in amplification efficiency can be mitigated by techniques that combine thousands of single-plex reactions.

Overall, amplicon target enrichment is generally preferred for smaller panels and hybrid capture for larger panels.

Note that repeat regions and pseudogenes are challenging regardless of target enrichment technique.

Amplification

Amplification of the library is often done with PCR-based techniques and may be incorporated into the PCR reactions for amplicon sequencing described above.

Quantitation and Quality Assessment

A quantity and quality assessment of each sample is made prior to sequencing, with the technique tailored to the type of library. Standard techniques include gel electrophoresis, spectrophotometry, real-time PCR (qPCR), or digital PCR.

Library Pooling

Typically, multiple samples are "pooled" together in the same sequencing run. Molecular barcodes on the adapters differentiate samples from one another during analysis.

Additional Steps

Depending on the type of library that is being constructed, additional steps may be required. For example, in mRNA sequencing, the mRNA sequences are typically converted to double-stranded cDNA sequences, which can be combined with the sequence selection step.

Sequencing

There are several types of sequencers available, which can be broadly grouped into short-read and long-read sequencers. For an overview, see Table 2.1.

Short-Read Sequencers (<1000 Nucleotides)

1. Sequencing by synthesis: Target strands are sequenced by DNA polymerase, creating a complementary strand. With the addition of each nucleotide, a signal is released and detected. One common method uses the flow of hydrogen ions through a semiconductor, which provides information about how many nucleotides have been added (Ion Torrent). Another technique uses fluorophore-labeled probes, with the fluorescence detected by a charged coupled device camera (Illumina).
2. Sequencing by ligation: This technique uses DNA ligase, which is sensitive to mismatches. Hybridization of fluorescent-labeled oligonucleotides generates fluorescence, which is captured and recorded (SOLiD). The primary limitation of this technology is very short reads (50 nt).

Long-Read Sequencing (>1000 Nucleotides)

1. Sequencing by synthesis: nano-chambers, each housing a single polymerase, synthesize DNA complementary to the target. Phospho-linked nucleotides are sequentially added, with a signal released with each reaction (Pacific Biosciences).
2. Protein nanopores allow single molecules to pass through, generating a characteristic disruption in the electric current with the passage of each nucleotide (Nanopore).

Table 2.1 Common sequencing techniques are described, highlighting read length, general techniques, reads generated, and time per run

Sequencer type	Read length (bp)	Sequencing technique	Signal detection	Other notes on technology	Reads per run	Time per run
Sequencing by synthesis (Illumina)	50–300	Synthesis	Fluorescence	Clusters are generated on a flow cell via bridge amplification with reversible terminator bases	Up to 3 billion	1–11 days
Ion semiconductor (Ion Torrent)	Up to 600	Synthesis	Ion flow through semiconductor	Targets sit in a microwell. Nucleotides are flooded in and incorporated via polymerase. The addition of each nucleotide generates a hydrogen ion which is detected by the semiconductor	Up to 80 million	2–5 hours
Sequencing by ligation (SOLiD)	50	Ligation	Fluorescence	DNA fragments are amplified on the surface of magnetic beads using DNA ligase	Up to 1.4 billion	1–2 weeks
Single-molecule real-time sequencing (Pacific Biosciences)	>100,000	Synthesis	Fluorescence	Single long oligonucleotides are sequenced in a nano-chamber housing a polymerase, using phospho-linked nucleotides	Up to 500,000 per well	1–9 days
Nanopore (Nanopore)	Up to 500 kb	Direct observation, passing through nanopore	Electric conductance through nanopore	Single long oligonucleotides pass through a nanopore, which measures the change in electric conductance for each nucleotide	User dependent, no upper limit	1 minute to 48 hours (sequencing can be stopped once satisfactory results are observed)

Informatics Process

The process or "pipeline" for the analysis of sequencing data is complex. The core components of common analysis methods are described below, with a focus on fundamental concepts and key quality metrics. See Fig. 2.2 for an overview. It is important to note that analytic algorithms are in constant flux and are changing more rapidly than any of the wet lab techniques described above. Although the individual components of the pipeline are described below in series, in practice many analytic steps happen in parallel.

Base Calls

The analytic pipeline begins with raw data generated from the sequencer. Depending on the type of sequencer (described above), the data exists as a series of signals, for example, a sequencer that generates fluorescent signals from clusters of oligonucleotides. Quality data is available at small and large scale for each component of the data file(s).

Each base call represents a nucleotide: A, G, C, or T. Typically another character is used for an indeterminate base call, often the character "N."

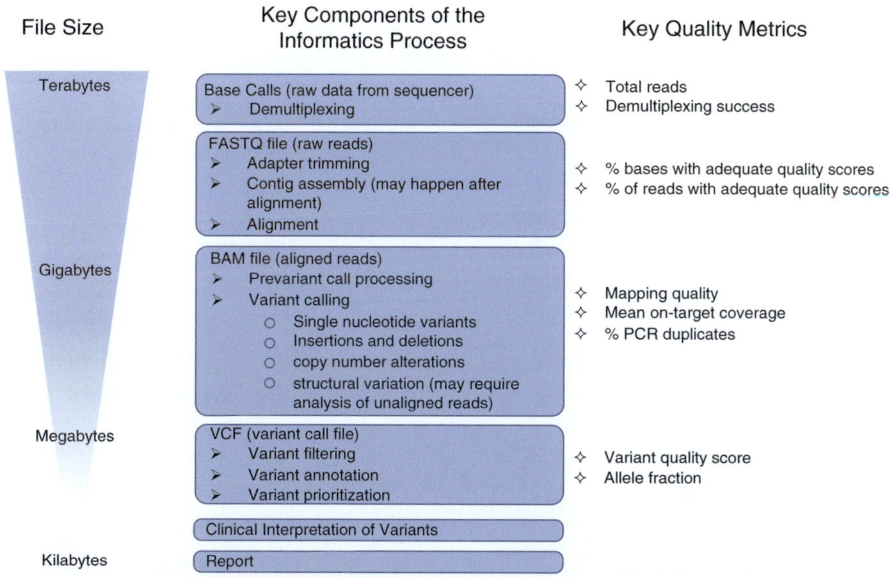

Fig. 2.2 Key components of the NGS informatics process from base calling to clinical reporting, annotated with file size and key quality metrics

Demultiplexing

In practice, sequencer runs typically consist of pooled samples, with each individual sample identified by a molecular barcode. In order to analyze data at a sample level, the base calls for each sample must be separated.

Demultiplexing success, in which all molecular identifiers are present and no unexpected molecular identifiers are detected, is a key quality metric.

FASTQ Files

After demultiplexing, each sample is associated with a file describing the sequence reads. The FASTQ format is a de facto standard and includes both the base call and a quality score for each base call, the Phred score:

Phred scores are a common technique for evaluating and annotating the quality of each individual signal. Originally developed for Sanger sequencing, the Phred score uses features like the signal peak shape and resolution in reference to datasets in which truth of the base call is known. The resulting quality metric describes the likelihood that a base call is incorrect, according the equation below in which Q is the quality score and P is the base calling error probability [5]:

$$Q = -10 \log_{10} P$$

The logarithmic relationship between these values is shown with examples below:

Phred quality score	Probability of incorrect base call	Base call accuracy
10	1 in 10	90%
20	1 in 100	99%
30	1 in 1000	99.9%
40	1 in 10,000	99.99%
50	1 in 100,000	99.999%

The quality score is associated with each signal and encoded using American Standard Code for Information Interchange (ASCII) characters, with an example below:

Identifier > @label

Sequence > AGTCCTGTTCGAACTGCTAGTC

+

Quality score > <>;##=><9=AAAAAAAAAA9#

FASTQ files need to be processed to informatically remove the adapter sequences.

Sequence Assembly

A sequence contig is an assembly of overlapping sequences representing a consensus region [6]. This assembly is particularly important for short-read sequencing technologies, in which the fragmented sequences are stitched back together to form longer consensus sequences, also known as "bottom-up sequencing."

In paired-end sequencing, the two ends of an oligonucleotide are sequenced, and the middle region may not be sequenced. Since the length of the fragment is known (a function of the library preparation technique), a contig can be constructed in which unsequenced fragments of known lengths are included. This technique is known as scaffolding.

The order of sequence assembly relative to alignment is variable and depends on the goals of the overall analysis. There are two general methods of alignment:

1. Primary alignment to reference genome with concurrent contig assembly
2. De novo sequence assembly, which is done without the use of a template, followed by either:

    (a) Alignment to reference genome: This technique is particularly helpful in identifying complex variations, including structural rearrangements, which may not align well to the reference genome.

    (b) OR creation of a de novo reference genome. This technique is particularly useful for analysis of data of genomes which do not have an established reference genome, like microorganisms.

Alignment

Also known as mapping, individual reads or contigs are aligned to a template or reference genome or transcriptome.

Broadly, techniques for alignment include either global or local alignment. Global alignment requires that the entire length of the read aligns to the reference, whereas a local alignment allows for mapping of parts of reads. Local alignment is generally preferred [7].

Important parameters of any pipeline include the general approach to alignment and the stringency applied to matching. A high stringency means that variants may be missed, whereas a low stringency may result in misalignment.

Local realignment around areas of potential insertions and deletions is helpful in identifying those alterations.

Alignment of short-read sequencing data is a challenging part of the informatics pipeline. Common pitfalls include misalignment of reads to homologous regions of the genome. The human genome has many regions of sequence homology, including 11,216 pseudogenes [8]. In a comprehensive analysis of homology, 2.2% of entire exons or large contiguous portions of exons have 100% identity to other loci. These sequences are referred to as "NGS dead zones" since short-read sequencing (250 bp) cannot reliably align these sequences [9].

Repetitive sequences are also common, accounting for up to half of the human genome, depending on the precise definition [10]. Repetitive regions that are longer than the read length cannot be aligned [11]. For example, a trinucleotide repeat region of 1000 bp cannot be assessed by sequencing 250 bp reads, since there is no "anchor" to a specific region.

Paired-end sequencing may result in two ends of the same read aligning to different parts of the reference genome, also known as discordant reads. An analytic step that specifically looks for discordant reads is helpful in identifying complex alterations like large insertions or deletions, or structural rearrangements like translocations. This analysis can be done in parallel to other assembly and alignment steps.

Variant Calling

Variant calling is the process of calling out mismatches in alignment. The simplest example is a single-nucleotide variant, in which one nucleotide is mismatched compared to the reference in a read which otherwise matches perfectly.

The accuracy of variant calling is highly dependent on the quality of called bases and aligned reads.

Standards for gene nomenclature and description of variants are available [12, 13].

Variant Filtering

Variant filtering is defined here as the process of removing variants that are likely to be artifacts of the assay. Variants may be suppressed as clinically low priority, described in "variant prioritization" below.

The use of multiple reads allows for statistical confidence that the mismatch is a true representation of the biology of the sample, rather than an artifact of the library preparation or sequencing process. In a sample in which two alleles are expected, a single-nucleotide variant is expected at about 50% or 100% allele fraction (% of reads), although strand bias may skew the fraction. In samples with mixed cell types, which are typical in analysis of tumor samples, variants may be present at a low allele fraction, particularly if tumor content is low or if the tumor contains subclones. In those mixed sample types, more reads (depth) provide confidence in variants at a low allele fraction.

Data used for filtering variants due to low confidence include base quality, alignment quality, read depth, and allele fraction. Determining thresholds for these important filtration steps is a key decision in the establishment of the analysis pipeline.

Variant Annotation

Variants aligned to the reference genome are further annotated with information that provides context to the biologic relevance, including:

1. Predicted position with respect to known genes and amino acid consequence of the nucleotide variation. For example:

$$\text{Variant genomic location in reference genome} > \text{chr7}:140753336\text{T} > \text{A}\left(\text{GRCh38}\right)$$
$$\text{Gene with cDNA annotation}\left(\text{transcript ID}\right) > \text{BRAF}\,\text{c.1799T} > \text{A}\left(\text{NM}\_004333.4\right)$$
$$\text{Gene with amino acid annotation}\left(\text{protein ID}\right) > \text{BRAF}\,\text{p.V600E}\left(\text{NP}\_004324.2\right)$$

Predicted amino acid sequence alterations allow for variants to be grouped into those that are predicted to alter the sequence and how they alter the sequence (missense, nonsense, silent, frameshift, splice site, intronic, etc.). The BRAF V600E example above would be classified as a missense variant.

This gene annotation process is heavily dependent on the use of known gene transcripts, included in the example above. Selection of transcripts for use in the pipeline has significant consequences for annotation.

2. Prevalence of the variant in the population. A variant is defined as a difference from the reference standard, but does not necessarily imply association with disease. Polymorphisms are genetic differences between subjects and represent a large proportion of called variants.

   Databases of genomic information from large populations are now available, making this component of the annotation process increasingly reliable.

   Although databases are improving their diversity over time, there is still an overrepresentation of some populations and an underrepresentation of others. A known consequence of this skewed representation is that a sample from a subject of an ethnicity that is not well described in database will have more variants that are not recognized as polymorphisms.

Variant Prioritization

The decisions about which variants to include in the review process and report are a key part of the design of a clinical assay. Decisions include gene lists, regions within a gene (exons only, splice sites, introns), which types of variants (nonsense, missense, etc.), quality thresholds across the entire process, allele fraction, and population frequency cutoffs. More permissive thresholds mean that more variants will be reported, some of which may be false positives, or not clinically relevant; restrictive thresholds lead to a shorter list of variants, but may result in false negative of missed results. All thresholds should be made in the context of the greater clinical aim of the assay.

Clinical Reporting

The construction of the final report represents the final step in the assay. The prioritized variants are reviewed and typically tiered according to their clinical significance.

Guidelines exist for the interpretation of both germline and somatic variants [14, 15], although some labs continue to use their own tiering systems. These recommendations have been widely implemented, particularly for germline variants, and are useful in improving variant classification consistency [16–18].

Flow and Storage of Data

Abundant data is generated by a single NGS assay. The wet lab process generates quality metrics, which are similar to other molecular assays. The sequencing analysis and informatics process generate a huge volume of primary, intermediate, and reportable data, which is a challenge to process and store [19]. As an example, the raw sequencing data for a single run is measured in terabytes. Many laboratories store intermediate files like FASTQ or BAM, rather than the primary sequencing data. BAM files are significantly smaller than FASTQ files and include all of the same data except for unaligned and filtered reads. Data storage at each step of the process is an important consideration.

Because sequencing data includes sample identifiers and genetic data that is potentially identifiable, data security is an important responsibility of the clinical laboratory. Data security is needed for all temporary and longterm storage locations, and for each file transfer, including within a cloud computing environment.

Clinical Applications of NGS

The clinical implementation of NGS is still in early development. Targeted gene panels with short-read sequencers have been the first to be clinically validated, with whole-exome sequencing becoming increasingly available. Common clinical panels include germline panels for neurologic conditions, cardiac dysfunction, metabolic disorders, hearing loss, and cancer predisposition. Somatic cancer panels are widely available for sequencing tumor, providing information about diagnosis, prognosis, and treatment response.

The primary limitations of NGS at a technical level are related to read length, making it difficult to interrogate homologous or repeat regions. Much of the informatics process is dedicated to reassembling reads into their true biologic orientation, which is only necessary for short-read sequencing. As long-read sequencing technology improves and becomes more accessible over time, these limitations will shift and new challenges will emerge.

Several challenges exist in bringing NGS into a patient care setting, some of which have been described above. Generally, clinical programs with a need for genetic sequencing can decide to build a platform in-house, or send-out to a reference lab. Challenges in clinical implementation are described as follows:

1. Challenges in creating a clinical sequencing platform
    - The clinical laboratory regulatory environment is very challenging, with multiple agencies providing different guidance and oversight.
    - Reimbursement from payors is uncertain.
    - A team that can accommodate all the parts of testing and analysis must be assembled, with heavy emphasis on informatics support.
    - Data analysis and storage are far greater for NGS than for any traditional techniques.
2. Challenges in ordering tests for patients (in-house or as a send-out to a reference lab)
    - The cost of each assay is high compared to more traditional techniques (like karyotype or FISH), although the costs are diminishing over time.
    - Reimbursement from payors is uncertain.
    - So much data is generated that it is challenging to take it in and understand it.
    - Clinicians must be prepared to review results with their patients, including many variants of uncertain significance.

Conclusion

Next-generation sequencing is a powerful tool that has changed the landscape of genetic research and clinical genomics. Several challenges and opportunities exist in making use of the technology and adapting it for effective clinical use.

References

1. Wong SQ, Li J, Salemi R, Sheppard KE, Do H, Tothill RW, et al. Targeted-capture massively-parallel sequencing enables robust detection of clinically informative mutations from formalin-fixed tumours. Sci Rep. 2013;3:3494.
2. Samorodnitsky E, Jewell BM, Hagopian R, Miya J, Wing MR, Lyon E, et al. Evaluation of hybridization capture versus amplicon-based methods for whole-exome sequencing. Hum Mutat. 2015;36(9):903–14.
3. Wang J, Yu H, Zhang VW, Tian X, Feng Y, Wang G, et al. Capture-based high-coverage NGS: a powerful tool to uncover a wide spectrum of mutation types. Genet Med. 2016;18(5):513–21.
4. Hung SS, Meissner B, Chavez EA, Ben-Neriah S, Ennishi D, Jones MR, et al. Assessment of capture and amplicon-based approaches for the development of a targeted next-generation sequencing pipeline to personalize lymphoma management. J Mol Diagn. 2018;20(2):203–14.
5. Ewing B, Green P. Base-calling of automated sequencer traces using phred. II. Error probabilities. Genome Res. 1998;8(3):186–94.

6. Staden R. A strategy of DNA sequencing employing computer programs. Nucleic Acids Res. 1979;6(7):2601–10.
7. Polyanovsky VO, Roytberg MA, Tumanyan VG. Comparative analysis of the quality of a global algorithm and a local algorithm for alignment of two sequences. Algorithms Mol Biol. 2011;6(1):25.
8. Pei B, Sisu C, Frankish A, Howald C, Habegger L, Mu XJ, et al. The GENCODE pseudogene resource. Genome Biol. 2012;13(9).:R51-2012-13-9-r51.
9. Mandelker D, Schmidt RJ, Ankala A, McDonald Gibson K, Bowser M, Sharma H, et al. Navigating highly homologous genes in a molecular diagnostic setting: a resource for clinical next-generation sequencing. Genet Med. 2016;18(12):1282–9.
10. Batzer MA, Deininger PL. Alu repeats and human genomic diversity. Nat Rev Genet. 2002;3(5):370–9.
11. Alkan C, Coe BP, Eichler EE. Genome structural variation discovery and genotyping. Nat Rev Genet. 2011;12(5):363–76.
12. den Dunnen JT, Dalgleish R, Maglott DR, Hart RK, Greenblatt MS, McGowan-Jordan J, et al. HGVS recommendations for the description of sequence variants: 2016 update. Hum Mutat. 2016;37(6):564–9.
13. Braschi B, Denny P, Gray K, Jones T, Seal R, Tweedie S, et al. Genenames.org: the HGNC and VGNC resources in 2019. Nucleic Acids Res. 2019;47(D1):D786–92.
14. Richards S, Aziz N, Bale S, Bick D, Das S, Gastier-Foster J, et al. Standards and guidelines for the interpretation of sequence variants: a joint consensus recommendation of the American College of Medical Genetics and Genomics and the Association for Molecular Pathology. Genet Med. 2015;17(5):405–24.
15. Li MM, Datto M, Duncavage EJ, Kulkarni S, Lindeman NI, Roy S, et al. Standards and guidelines for the interpretation and reporting of sequence variants in cancer: a Joint Consensus Recommendation of the Association for Molecular Pathology, American Society of Clinical Oncology, and College of American Pathologists. J Mol Diagn. 2017;19(1):4–23.
16. Amendola LM, Jarvik GP, Leo MC, McLaughlin HM, Akkari Y, Amaral MD, et al. Performance of ACMG-AMP Variant-Interpretation Guidelines among Nine Laboratories in the Clinical Sequencing Exploratory Research Consortium. Am J Hum Genet. 2016;99(1):247.
17. Harrison SM, Dolinsky JS, Knight Johnson AE, Pesaran T, Azzariti DR, Bale S, et al. Clinical laboratories collaborate to resolve differences in variant interpretations submitted to ClinVar. Genet Med. 2017;19(10):1096–104.
18. Nykamp K, Anderson M, Powers M, Garcia J, Herrera B, Ho YY, et al. Sherloc: a comprehensive refinement of the ACMG-AMP variant classification criteria. Genet Med. 2017;19(10):1105–17.
19. Roy S, LaFramboise WA, Nikiforov YE, Nikiforova MN, Routbort MJ, Pfeifer J, et al. Next-generation sequencing informatics: challenges and strategies for implementation in a clinical environment. Arch Pathol Lab Med. 2016;140(9):958–75.

Chapter 3
Cell-Free DNA Testing

Brennan Decker and Lynette M. Sholl

Key Points

- Cell-free DNA (cfDNA) is currently in clinical use for noninvasive prenatal testing, for monitoring of solid organ transplantation, and as a predictive biomarker for treatment selection in non-small cell lung cancer.
- Pre-analytical assay optimization strategies are driven by the unique biology of cfDNA and include specimen type, collection method, storage, and extraction techniques.
- Assays in use for analysis of cfDNA are broadly based either on polymerase chain reaction or next-generation sequencing technologies that may be employed based on clinical requirements for sensitivity versus breadth of target detection.
- Rapid evolution in chemistry, informatics, and sequencing technology will drive further expansion of clinical applications of cfDNA testing to include disease monitoring and screening.

Key Online Resources

- AMP Liquid Biopsy Webinar Series: https://educate.amp.org/store/seminar/seminar.php?seminar=128701
- Liquid biopsies come of age: towards implementation of circulating tumour DNA. Wan, et al.: https://www.ncbi.nlm.nih.gov/pubmed/28233803

B. Decker · L. M. Sholl (✉)
Department of Pathology, Brigham and Women's Hospital, Boston, MA, USA
e-mail: bdecker@bwh.harvard.edu; lmsholl@bwh.harvard.edu

L. J. Tafe, M. E. Arcila (eds.), *Genomic Medicine*,
https://doi.org/10.1007/978-3-030-22922-1_3

Introduction

Cell-free DNA (cfDNA) is genetic material that is within the body but found outside of viable cells. Cell-free DNA is released from tumor cells by a variety of mechanisms [1]. The majority of cell-free genetic material is thought to derive from nuclear breakdown in the setting of apoptosis or necrosis. DNA can also be secreted frolm cells in the form of exosomes. When cfDNA diffuses from the site of origin, it can become a solute in proximate body fluids, such as sputum, cerebrospinal fluid, urine, or stool. Cell-free nucleic acids can also enter the bloodstream, where they become circulating cfDNA. Once in a compartment amenable to collection, purification, and evaluation, cfDNA can be quantified and characterized as a measure of health and disease.

Circulating nucleic acids were first discovered in the bloodstream in 1948 [1]. It was subsequently noted that the quantity of cfDNA varies from one healthy individual to another. Furthermore, it was found that cfDNA changes are also observable in the setting of numerous physiologic or pathologic conditions, including trauma, myocardial infarction, stroke, transplantation, pregnancy, and cancer (Table 3.1).

In traumatic or ischemic events, the raw quantity of cfDNA may correlate with the extent of injury [2]. Posttransplant quantification of donor-derived cfDNA correlates with acute and chronic rejection of transplanted organs [3–6]. In pregnancy, the FDA has approved cfDNA as a biomarker in noninvasive prenatal testing, wherein relative quantification of cfDNA mapped to their origin in the reference genome identifies chromosomal aneuploidy, as in Down syndrome [7].

Cancer is one of the most complex, yet potentially most clinically impactful, applications of cfDNA testing. All malignancies are caused by genomic alterations that dysregulate cell biology. These genetic changes include single-nucleotide

Table 3.1 Selected clinical applications of cfDNA testing

Application	Aim	Technology	References
Trauma	Quantification of total cfDNA	Quantitative PCR	[2]
Noninvasive prenatal testing	Detection of fetal aneuploidy in the maternal circulation	Random whole-genome sequencing Targeted SNP profiling	[7]
Solid organ transplantation	Evaluation of graft rejection	Y-chromosome gene PCR (sex-mismatched transplants) HLA-mismatched PCR SNP genotyping	[3] [4] [5] [6]
Solid tumor biomarker testing	Predictive biomarker testing Diagnostics Monitoring Screening	Allele-specific quantitative PCR Digital PCR BEAMing Targeted hybrid capture panel NGS Targeted amplicon NGS Whole-exome sequencing Ultralow-pass whole-genome sequencing	[17]

mutations, small insertion/deletion mutations, larger copy number changes, structural rearrangements, and epigenetic alterations, all of which are specific to neoplastic cells and drive the aberrant growth of the tumor. The ubiquity of these genetic changes across all cancer types facilitates their use as biomarkers specific to the oncogenic forces at work within an individual patient's tumor.

Current Applications: Noninvasive Prenatal Testing

Noninvasive prenatal testing (NIPT) represents the first widespread clinical application of cfDNA. NIPT exploits the fact that cfDNA, which is generally representative of the fetal genome, is released from placental trophoblasts into the maternal circulation. NIPT has largely replaced maternal serum biochemical screening and fetal ultrasound for detection of fetal aneuploidies. The high specificity and positive predictive value of cfDNA testing for detection of fetal aneuploidy have enabled a substantial drop in the rates of false positive results as compared to multiple-marker screening. As a consequence, the routine use of NIPT in high-risk maternal populations in the last decade is estimated to have halved the frequency of invasive confirmatory testing including amniocentesis and chorionic villous sampling [7].

The most common NIPT assays examine fetal sex and trisomies 13, 18, and 21. Dominant methods for quantifying fetal chromosomes include random whole-genome and targeted sequencing. In random whole-genome sequencing, representative random cfDNA fragments derived from fetal and maternal genomes are sequenced, mapped, and counted; proportionally higher numbers of sequencing reads from one chromosome will point to a fetal trisomy [8]. In targeted sequencing, characterized SNPs are amplified and sequenced; skewing of SNP allelic ratios may indicate the presence of aneuploidy [9].

NIPT is feasible starting at week 10 of gestation; before this, the levels of fetal DNA are typically too low to generate informative results. After 10 weeks, low fetal fraction may occur in a variety of scenarios, including high maternal body mass index, pregnancies resulting from assisted reproductive technologies, or as a result of some aneuploidies. Low fetal fraction may lead to false negative results; therefore, a testing step that evaluates the fraction of placental versus total cfDNA is recommended [10]. False positive results may occur in the context of confined placental mosaicism, particularly for chromosomes 18 and 21. Other reasons for false positivity include autosomal trisomies, vanishing twin syndrome, or maternal factors, such as copy number variants, prior transplant, or subclinical neoplasm.

Although assessment of fetal aneuploidies is the dominant indication for NIPT, this technology has been extended to assess micro-deletions and micro-duplications as well as noninvasive detection of fetal single-gene disorders. The use of NIPT has been reported for the prenatal detection and management of a variety of inherited disorders including blood group incompatibility, skeletal dysplasias, congenital adrenal hyperplasia, and hemoglobinopathies [7].

Current Applications: Solid Organ Transplantation

Periodic rejection surveillance of transplanted solid organs is used to titrate immunosuppressive regimens in order to prevent or slow graft failure. Traditional surveillance approaches employ invasive biopsy sampling of the engrafted organ and histopathologic evaluation; this process is prone to sampling bias and pathologist variability, as well as morbidity related to invasive biopsies. Donor-derived cfDNA is detectable in transplant recipients and has been exploited as a biomarker of graft rejection in a variety of organ contexts. Donor-derived cfDNA increases as a fraction of total cfDNA in the setting of acute rejection following heart, liver, kidney, and lung transplantation, and levels correlate with biopsy-proven rejection. The fraction of donor-derived cfDNA can be determined using Y-chromosome measurements in sex-mismatched transplants, SNP genotyping, human leukocyte antigen mismatch, or comparison of copy number polymorphisms. Many approaches rely on a priori knowledge of donor and recipient genotypes; however, SNP-panel NGS tests that exploit bioinformatics tools to assign recipient and donor status have also been validated for detection of rejection in cardiac and kidney allograft patients [6, 11].

The positive predictive value of elevated donor-derived cfNDA for rejection is relatively low, as cfDNA can be released due to a variety of pathologies affecting the graft, such as infection or inflammatory conditions [5]. Therefore, current assays are unlikely to replace tissue biopsy as a gold standard for rejection evaluation, but may have value as a noninvasive monitoring tool to inform the timing and/or interpretation of posttransplant biopsies.

Current Applications: Cancer

In the setting of malignancy, the subset of cfDNA in the systemic circulation that is derived from tumor cells is called circulating tumor DNA (ctDNA). Qualitative or quantitative assays designed to query ctDNA is one type of "liquid biopsy," a concept that has long been considered a "holy grail" of cancer testing, because a fully optimized, targeted test could minimize the risk and invasiveness of diagnostic procedures for some cancer types.

Assays targeting ctDNA have numerous potential advantages. Many studies have demonstrated significant genetic heterogeneity both within a primary tumor, as well as between the primary tumor and metastatic site(s). For example, in lung cancers, mutations associated with treatment resistance have been identified in some tumor cell populations, but not in others. Stochastic and sampling factors inherent to tissue biopsy can inhibit full characterization of system-wide disease. This missing information can adversely affect clinical management. In contrast, a liquid biopsy represents multiple tumor sites in proportion to the amount of ctDNA produced by each focus, potentially yielding a more complete account of the patient's cancer genome.

The absolute and relative quantity of ctDNA is highly variable and depends on the tissue of origin, disease burden, exposure to therapy, extent of treatment response, and other aspects of tumor biology [12]. Plasma cfDNA originates from increased cell death, via both apoptosis and necrosis, of tumor tissue, and circulating tumor DNA (ctDNA) typically represents a minor fraction of overall cfDNA. Nevertheless, there is a reproducible correlation between cancer burden and levels of cfDNA [13, 14]. In non-small cell lung cancer (NSCLC), patients with disease confined to the lungs tend to have very low levels of ctDNA – often undetectable using standard clinical techniques, such as droplet digital PCR or targeted NGS – whereas those with metastatic disease have detectable ctDNA in 60–100% of cases [14]. The prevalence of ctDNA in patients with metastatic cancer enables the use of cfDNA for detection of cancer-specific molecular biomarkers, such as oncogene single-nucleotide or indel variants, including a subset that can be used for treatment selection and monitoring, via targeted PCR-based assays. Detection of a broader array of variants, as well as amplifications and rearrangements, can be accomplished by use of NGS-based technologies [13, 15, 16].

Ultrasensitive assays, such as allele-specific quantitative PCR or bespoke amplicon sequencing, can be used to detect ctDNA even in those patients with early stage/organ-confined disease [17]. Pathologic features that predict the presence of detectable ctDNA in surgically resectable NSCLC include squamous morphology, high tumor cell proliferation rate, and lymphovascular invasion [18]. These exceptionally sensitive assays could be used for detection of tumor-specific cfDNA alterations following surgery or other definitive therapy, enabling longitudinal monitoring for disease recurrence prior to development of radiographic or clinical evidence of relapse [18, 19].

As of 2018, only one cfDNA assay for predictive molecular biomarkers was approved in the United States by the Food and Drug Administration; the approved assay assesses *EGFR* hot spot activating mutations (exon 19 deletion mutation and L858R) as well as the resistance mutation T790M in patients with advanced NSCLC. As such, it may be used in patients with an established NSCLC diagnosis to guide choice of therapy when tissue is insufficient or unavailable for molecular profiling or in the setting of relapse to detect the T790M variant [20]. In either setting, a negative result should prompt follow-up tissue testing prior to therapy decisions, because of the lower sensitivity of cfDNA-based profiling relative to tumor tissue [21]. While ctDNA profiling has gained the most traction in the context of biomarker assessment in NSCLC, applications have been described in numerous other tumor types (Table 3.2).

Pre-analytical Considerations

Specimen collection and handling are critical for cfDNA assays. Factors that accelerate cfDNA degradation or dilute cfDNA concentration can decrease assay sensitivity. Pre-analytical variables including cfDNA biology, specimen type, collection and processing protocols, and DNA purification strategies can all affect the quality and quantity of starting material [22, 23].

Table 3.2 Applications for cfDNA testing in solid tumors

Diagnosis	Molecular target(s)	Clinical implications	Reference
Bladder cancer	*ERBB2*, TSC genes, *PIK3CA*, and others	Targeted therapy selection/ clinical trials	[39]
Breast and ovarian cancer	BRCA reversion events	Selection of PARP inhibitors	[40]
Gastric cancer	*ERBB2* amplification, others	HER2-targeted therapy, surveillance, identification of mechanisms of relapse	[41]
Hepatocellular carcinoma	Methylation marker panel	Diagnosis, prognosis	[42]
Melanoma	*BRAF* codon V600	BRAF targeted therapy	[43]
Oropharyngeal cancer	HPV	Disease monitoring	[44]
Pancreatic adenocarcinoma	*KRAS* mutation	Prognosis in surgically resected patients	[45]
Prostate cancer (relapse)	*BRCA2* reversion, *AR* mutations	PARP inhibitor resistance, androgen blockade resistance	[46–48]
Sarcoma	*EWSR1* fusions, *TP53* mutations, others	Disease monitoring, prognosis	[49, 50]
Small cell lung carcinoma	*TP53*, *RB1*, *PTEN*, *NOTCH* genes, MYC genes, others	Response assessment, disease monitoring	[51]

cfDNA Biology

cfDNA is rapidly removed from the bloodstream, via both nuclease degradation and renal clearance, with a half-life of approximately 16 minutes to 2 hours [24, 25]. In one study, quantification of ctDNA before and at time points following surgical resection show that the concentration decreases by 96.7% at 24 hours following surgery, with the drop in ctDNA concentration preceding decreases in protein biomarker levels [24]. This turnover and the possibility of early, high-sensitivity interpretation suggest that ctDNA may represent a multi-cancer posttreatment biomarker for minimal residual disease and disease recurrence.

Because cfDNA is derived from apoptotic and necrotic cells and is subsequently exposed to unfavorable extracellular conditions, the fragment length of cfDNA is generally shorter than DNA isolated from tissue or whole blood. DNA harvested from lymphocytes or fresh tissue can extend to the tens or hundreds of kilobases in length. DNA extracted from formalin-fixed, paraffin-embedded tissue degrades with storage time, but tissue archived within months to several years has been shown to yield DNA fragment sizes in the kilobases [26]. While these other sources of genetic material generally conform to a normal distribution of fragment length, cfDNA exhibits a multimodal length distribution with peaks at approximately 150, 300, and 450 bp. This ~150 bp fragment length periodicity reflects the number of bases wrapped around, and thereby protected from degradation, by a single nucleosome or chromatosome [27]. The ~300 bp and ~450 bp peaks represent cfDNA fragments wound around two and three nucleosomes, respectively. In samples from most cancer types, ~90% of ctCNA falls in the ~150 bp band, with decreasing representation of sequentially larger fragment size peaks [28].

Assays must be consciously designed to account for the short fragment length of cfDNA. In particular, PCR-based assays must utilize small amplicons in order to produce sufficient amplification for detection.

Specimen Type

Whole blood samples contain nucleated white blood cells (WBCs). If these WBCs are lysed prior to cfDNA extraction, released enzymes may accelerate cfDNA degradation. Furthermore, WBC lysis results in the liberation of cellular non-tumor DNA, diluting the ctDNA and reducing assay sensitivity. Quantification of unique Y-chromosome sequences in cfDNA from sex-mismatched bone marrow transplant recipients demonstrates that this process is a major source of cfDNA [29, 30].

Serum and plasma are acellular subsets of whole blood, with serum representing plasma that has been depleted of clotting factors. In practice, plasma is derived via centrifugation, whereas serum isolation is accomplished via in vitro induction of clotting prior to centrifugation. The clotting step intrinsic to serum collection induces greater release of WBC-derived cfDNA compared to centrifugation alone, resulting in a higher total cfDNA concentration in serum than plasma [30]. However, due to the dilution effect, the ctDNA:cfDNA ratio is greater in plasma. Therefore, consensus recommendations favor the use of plasma as the source material for ctDNA testing [21, 31].

Collection and Processing

Collection tube type, time to centrifugation, storage, and DNA isolation approaches can also affect the degradation and relative concentration of ctDNA.

Current ctDNA assay technologies use PCR to amplify, and in some cases analyze, genetic material. Heparin is widely used to prevent coagulation in blood collection tubes, but this drug has been shown to interfere with the biochemistry of the PCR reaction [32], and, accordingly, heparin-containing tubes should not be used to collect material for ctDNA testing. Instead, tubes with alternative anticoagulants, such as EDTA, standard lavender-top tubes, or tubes with leukocyte stabilization compounds are preferred for downstream ctDNA analysis. One study directly compared ctDNA yield for EDTA, Streck (Streck, Inc., La Vista, NE), and CellSave (Menarini Silicon Biosystems, Inc., Huntington Valley, PA) tubes, including with different post-collection handling protocols [33]. The authors found that these tube types had similar ctDNA yields when plasma was isolated within 6 hours of collection. By 48 hours, however, the yield from EDTA tubes was less reliable, whereas the CellSave and Streck tubes did not show a significant decrease in harvested ctDNA. Thus, plasma should be produced within hours of collection for EDTA tube samples. The use of leukocyte stabilization tubes can extend the plasma isolation window to days; there are now numerous commercially available options, and optimal protocols are highly dependent on the properties of each tube type [34].

Short-term storage at 4 °C versus room temperature has been shown to have negligible effect on ctDNA harvest [33]. However, depending on the tube type, higher temperatures and longer intervals can increase contamination with leukocyte-derived DNA. In general, it is ideal to refrigerate samples as soon as possible until plasma is isolated. Freezing of plasma prior to cfDNA isolation does not affect the quantity or analytical quality of the genetic material. However, as with all types of DNA samples, multiple freeze-thaw cycles cause degradation, so plasma or isolated cfDNA should be stored as aliquots in order to avoid this problem.

The need for additional and/or specialized blood collection tubes, specific sample handling, and rapid DNA isolation requires equipment, education, and, crucially, buy-in from institutions, clinicians, administration, and staff. In the inpatient or cancer center setting, it may be most economical to implement the use of already widely utilized EDTA tubes, followed by DNA isolation within 6 hours. However, stabilizing tubes may be more practical in outpatient settings where staffing and infrastructure for rapid DNA isolation are more challenging.

cfDNA Detection and Quantification Technologies

cfDNA detection and quantification assays fall into two general groups: sequencing based and PCR based. Sequencing-based assays enable discovery of the spectrum of circulating somatic alterations in the genome, exome, or targeted regions. In contrast, PCR-based tests specifically target hot spot or previously identified mutations, but generally have faster turnaround time and higher analytical sensitivity. For either approach, assay validation should be carried out via comparison against the appropriate gold standard based on the specific application (e.g., tumor tissue in cancer, donor tissue for transplant, karyotype for noninvasive prenatal diagnosis, etc.). A summary of technologies and their optimal cancer-related applications are found in Table 3.3.

Limitations

Clinical ctDNA testing has several potential limitations compared to direct tissue testing. The principal limitation is the low concentration of overall cfDNA, and ultimately the low level of ctDNA, present in most patients with solid tumors. On average, cfDNA is reportedly present at a concentration of 20–25 ng/mL (or 3000 genomic equivalents) in the plasma of patients with metastatic carcinoma [35]. For variants present at 0.1% allele fraction (1 in 1000 genomic equivalents) and input amount of 3000 genomic equivalents, there is an approximately 5% chance that this

Table 3.3 ctDNA detection and quantification technologies

Platform	Scope	Underlying technology	Example implementation	Detectable variant type(s)	Mutant allele sensitivity	Number of testable loci	Optimal applications
Sequencing based	Genome-wide	Whole-genome sequencing	Plasma-Seq [52]	Aneuploidy, structural variants	5–10%	Whole genome	ctDNA quantification, disease burden estimation, detection of aneuploidy or structural variants
		Tiled amplicon sequencing	Fast-SeqS [53]	Aneuploidy		Genome-wide targeted LINE-1 elements	
	Targeted panel	Hybrid capture	Exome sequencing [54, 55]	Aneuploidy, targeted structural variants, SNVs/indels	5%	Whole exome	ctDNA quantification, disease burden estimation, cancer gene profiling, identification of actionable mutations, monitoring treatment resistance mutations
			CAPP-Seq [16]	Targeted structural variants, SNVs/indels	0.1–0.5%	Targeted panel	
		Amplicon-based	TAm-Seq [56]	Aneuploidy, targeted structural variants, SNVs/indels	<0.5%	Targeted panel	
			Safe-SeqS [57]			Targeted panel	

(continued)

Table 3.3 (continued)

Platform	Scope	Underlying technology	Example implementation	Detectable variant type(s)	Mutant allele sensitivity	Number of testable loci	Optimal applications
PCR based	Single locus or multiplexed panel	Emulsion PCR	Digital PCR [58]	Targeted structural variants, SNVs/indels	<0.01%	Single locus or multiplexed panel	Disease burden estimation, identification of actionable mutations, quantification of hot spot mutations, monitoring treatment resistance mutations
			BEAMing [59]				
	FDA approved	Companion diagnostics	Therascreen EGFR (approved for cfDNA testing in EU only) [60]	Targeted structural variants, SNVs/indels	25–100 copies/mL	Multiplex panel in EGFR gene	Identification of actionable mutations, quantification of hot spot mutations, monitoring treatment resistance mutations, FDA-approved testing
			Cobas EGFR [20]		Variable, median 1.4%		

Table 3.4 Factors contributing to false positive or nonrepresentative results in ctDNA testing

Factor	Potential limitation (compared to tissue testing)	Mitigation strategies
Germ line variants	Mosaicism or some inherited variants could be interpreted as somatic mutations	Parallel testing of germ line DNA (at least once for each patient)
Multiple primary cancers	Difficult to determine tissue of origin of a specific somatic mutation	Parallel testing of tissue biopsy (at least once for each primary tumor)
Multifocal disease	Differential contribution to ctDNA of different tumor sites, obscuring diversity	Serial testing, selection of appropriately sensitive method
Contamination	Low-level contamination can mimic somatic mutations	Bioinformatics evaluation for evidence of contamination
PCR artifacts	Requires increase in lower limit of detection and decreased sensitivity	Use of unique molecular identifiers to identify strand-specific artifacts
Other clonal proliferations	Presence of mutant cfDNA arising from a source other than tumor cells of interest (e.g., *TP53* mutation in clonal hematopoiesis of indeterminate potential)	Parallel testing of buffy coat Future consideration: healthy baseline testing

variant will go undetected in 1 mL of tested plasma. Obviously, lower cfDNA concentrations elevate the possibility of false negative results, purely by chance. This limitation can be at least partially mitigated by testing for multiple variants, where feasible [1].

Additional challenges in the interpretation of detected variants derive from the fact that it is not possible to ascribe an origin to a specific fragment of cfDNA, and it is difficult to ascertain, a priori, the relative contribution of ctDNA to the overall cfDNA population. There is evidence, however, that the distribution of cfDNA fragment lengths shifts to the left in samples with high levels of ctDNA, with a peak length of less than 145 base pairs in samples with detectable tumor mutations [36]. These differential fragment length distributions may enable better assessment of the levels of ctDNA in a sample.

Factors that may contribute to false positive results or lead to incorrect attribution of a variant to patient's known cancer are summarized in Table 3.4.

Future Directions

Though few cfDNA tests currently have regulatory approval for general use, numerous novel analysis approaches are currently under development for clinical applications, such as generalized and tissue of origin-specific gene panel sequencing and bespoke, personalized testing. Advances in technology employing cost-effective, ultrasensitive detection of DNA variants are likely to shift clinical practice models to enable monitoring of patients with early stage disease; permit use of alternative body fluids, such as saliva, as a source of cfDNA; and ultimately allow for early cancer detection in high-risk populations [37, 38]. Application-oriented validation standards and reference materials, clinician buy-in, and comparative clinical studies will be required for these technologies to achieve wide use in a variety of practice settings.

References

1. Wan JCM, et al. Liquid biopsies come of age: towards implementation of circulating tumour DNA. Nat Rev Cancer. 2017;17:223–38.
2. Gögenur M, Burcharth J, Gögenur I. The role of total cell-free DNA in predicting outcomes among trauma patients in the intensive care unit: a systematic review. Crit Care. 2017;21:14.
3. García Moreira V, Prieto García B, Baltar Martín JM, Ortega Suárez F, Alvarez FV. Cell-free DNA as a noninvasive acute rejection marker in renal transplantation. Clin Chem. 2009;55:1958–66.
4. Gadi VK, Nelson JL, Boespflug ND, Guthrie KA, Kuhr CS. Soluble donor DNA concentrations in recipient serum correlate with pancreas-kidney rejection. Clin Chem. 2006;52:379–82.
5. De Vlaminck I, et al. Circulating cell-free DNA enables noninvasive diagnosis of heart transplant rejection. Sci Transl Med. 2014;6:241ra77.
6. Grskovic M, et al. Validation of a clinical-grade assay to measure donor-derived cell-free DNA in solid organ transplant recipients. J Mol Diagn. 2016;18:890–902.
7. Bianchi DW, Chiu RWK. Sequencing of circulating cell-free DNA during pregnancy. N Engl J Med. 2018;379:464–73.
8. Fan HC, Blumenfeld YJ, Chitkara U, Hudgins L, Quake SR. Noninvasive diagnosis of fetal aneuploidy by shotgun sequencing DNA from maternal blood. Proc Natl Acad Sci U S A. 2008;105:16266–71.
9. Vermeesch JR, Voet T, Devriendt K. Prenatal and pre-implantation genetic diagnosis. Nat Rev Genet. 2016;17:643–56.
10. Wou K, Chung WK, Wapner RJ. Laboratory considerations for prenatal genetic testing. Semin Perinatol. 2018;42:307–13.
11. Bloom RD, et al. Cell-free DNA and active rejection in kidney allografts. J Am Soc Nephrol. 2017;28:2221–32.
12. Hovelson DH, et al. Rapid, ultra low coverage copy number profiling of cell-free DNA as a precision oncology screening strategy. Oncotarget. 2017;8:89848–66.
13. Müller JN, et al. Concordance between comprehensive Cancer genome profiling in plasma and tumor specimens. J Thorac Oncol. 2017;12:1503–11.
14. Sacher AG, et al. Prospective validation of rapid plasma genotyping for the detection of EGFR and KRAS mutations in advanced lung Cancer. JAMA Oncol. 2016;2:1014–22.
15. Forshew T, et al. Noninvasive identification and monitoring of cancer mutations by targeted deep sequencing of plasma DNA. Sci Transl Med. 2012;4:136ra68.
16. Newman AM, et al. An ultrasensitive method for quantitating circulating tumor DNA with broad patient coverage. Nat Med. 2014;20:548–54.
17. Burgener JM, Rostami A, De Carvalho DD, Bratman SV. Cell-free DNA as a post-treatment surveillance strategy: current status. Semin Oncol. 2017;44:330–46.
18. Abbosh C, et al. Phylogenetic ctDNA analysis depicts early-stage lung cancer evolution. Nature. 2017;545:446–51.
19. Chabon JJ, et al. Circulating tumour DNA profiling reveals heterogeneity of EGFR inhibitor resistance mechanisms in lung cancer patients. Nat Commun. 2016;7:11815.

20. Premarket Approval (PMA): Cobas EGFR MUTATION TEST V2. Available at: https://www.accessdata.fda.gov/scripts/cdrh/cfdocs/cfpma/pma.cfm?id=P150047.
21. Lindeman NI, et al. Updated molecular testing guideline for the selection of lung cancer patients for treatment with targeted tyrosine kinase inhibitors: guideline from the College of American Pathologists, the International Association for the Study of Lung Cancer, and the Association for Molecular Pathology. J Mol Diagn. 2018;20:129–59.
22. El Messaoudi S, Rolet F, Mouliere F, Thierry AR. Circulating cell free DNA: preanalytical considerations. Clin Chim Acta. 2013;424:222–30.
23. Bronkhorst AJ, Aucamp J, Pretorius PJ. Cell-free DNA: preanalytical variables. Clin Chim Acta. 2015;450:243–53.
24. Diehl F, et al. Circulating mutant DNA to assess tumor dynamics. Nat Med. 2008;14:985–90.
25. Lo YM, et al. Rapid clearance of fetal DNA from maternal plasma. Am J Hum Genet. 1999;64:218–24.
26. Ludyga N, et al. Nucleic acids from long-term preserved FFPE tissues are suitable for downstream analyses. Virchows Arch. 2012;460:131–40.
27. Snyder MW, Kircher M, Hill AJ, Daza RM, Shendure J. Cell-free DNA comprises an in vivo nucleosome footprint that informs its tissues-of-origin. Cell. 2016;164:57–68.
28. Volik S, Alcaide M, Morin RD, Collins C. Cell-free DNA (cfDNA): clinical significance and utility in cancer shaped by emerging technologies. Mol Cancer Res. 2016;14:898–908.
29. Lui YYN, et al. Predominant hematopoietic origin of cell-free DNA in plasma and serum after sex-mismatched bone marrow transplantation. Clin Chem. 2002;48:421–7.
30. Lee TH, Montalvo L, Chrebtow V, Busch MP. Quantitation of genomic DNA in plasma and serum samples: higher concentrations of genomic DNA found in serum than in plasma. Transfusion. 2001;41:276–82.
31. Merker JD, et al. Circulating tumor DNA analysis in patients with cancer: American Society of Clinical Oncology and College of American Pathologists Joint Review. J Clin Oncol. 2017;867(2018):76. https://doi.org/10.1200/JCO.2017.76.8671.
32. Beutler E, Gelbart T, Kuhl W. Interference of heparin with the polymerase chain reaction. Biotechniques. 1990;9:166.
33. Kang Q, et al. Comparative analysis of circulating tumor DNA stability in K3EDTA, Streck, and CellSave blood collection tubes. Clin Biochem. 2016;49:1354–60.
34. Toro PV, et al. Comparison of cell stabilizing blood collection tubes for circulating plasma tumor DNA. Clin Biochem. 2015;48:993–8.
35. Mehrotra M, et al. Study of preanalytic and analytic variables for clinical next-generation sequencing of circulating cell-free nucleic acid. J Mol Diagn. 2017;19:514–24.
36. Yang N, et al. The characteristics of ctDNA reveal the high complexity in matching the corresponding tumor tissues. BMC Cancer. 2018;18:319.
37. Wei F, et al. Electric field-induced release and measurement liquid biopsy for noninvasive early lung cancer assessment. J Mol Diagn. 2018;20:738–42.
38. Wei F, et al. Noninvasive saliva-based EGFR gene mutation detection in patients with lung cancer. Am J Respir Crit Care Med. 2014;190:1117–26.
39. Vandekerkhove G, et al. Circulating tumor DNA reveals clinically actionable somatic genome of metastatic bladder cancer. Clin Cancer Res. 2017;23:6487–97.
40. Weigelt B, et al. Diverse BRCA1 and BRCA2 reversion mutations in circulating cell-free DNA of therapy-resistant breast or ovarian cancer. Clin Cancer Res. 2017;23:6708–20.
41. Kim ST, et al. Impact of genomic alterations on lapatinib treatment outcome and cell-free genomic landscape during HER2 therapy in HER2+ gastric cancer patients. Ann Oncol. 2018;29:1037–48.
42. Xu R-H, et al. Circulating tumour DNA methylation markers for diagnosis and prognosis of hepatocellular carcinoma. Nat Mater. 2017;16:1155–61.
43. Janku F, et al. BRAF mutation testing in cell-free DNA from the plasma of patients with advanced cancers using a rapid, automated molecular diagnostics system. Mol Cancer Ther. 2016;15:1397–404.

44. Hanna GJ, et al. Plasma HPV cell-free DNA monitoring in advanced HPV-associated oropharyngeal cancer. Ann Oncol. 2018;29:1980–6.
45. Kim MK, et al. Prognostic implications of multiplex detection of KRAS mutations in cell-free DNA from patients with pancreatic ductal adenocarcinoma. Clin Chem. 2018;64:726–34.
46. Quigley D, et al. Analysis of circulating cell-free DNA identifies multiclonal heterogeneity of BRCA2 reversion mutations associated with resistance to PARP inhibitors. Cancer Discov. 2017;7:999–1005.
47. Wyatt AW, et al. Genomic alterations in cell-free DNA and enzalutamide resistance in castration-resistant prostate cancer. JAMA Oncol. 2016;2:1598–606.
48. Azad AA, et al. Androgen receptor gene aberrations in circulating cell-free DNA: biomarkers of therapeutic resistance in castration-resistant prostate cancer. Clin Cancer Res. 2015;21:2315–24.
49. Shukla NN, et al. Plasma DNA-based molecular diagnosis, prognostication, and monitoring of patients with EWSR1 fusion-positive sarcomas. JCO Precis Oncol. 2017;2017:1–11.
50. Shulman DS, et al. Detection of circulating tumour DNA is associated with inferior outcomes in Ewing sarcoma and osteosarcoma: a report from the Children's Oncology Group. Br J Cancer. 2018;119:615–21.
51. Almodovar K, et al. Longitudinal cell-free DNA analysis in patients with small cell lung cancer reveals dynamic insights into treatment efficacy and disease relapse. J Thorac Oncol. 2018;13:112–23.
52. Farris C, Trimarchi JM. Plasma-seq: a novel strategy for metastatic prostate cancer analysis. Genome Med. 2013;5:35.
53. Belic J, et al. Rapid identification of plasma DNA samples with increased ctDNA levels by a modified FAST-SeqS approach. Clin Chem. 2015;61:838–49.
54. Murtaza M, et al. Non-invasive analysis of acquired resistance to cancer therapy by sequencing of plasma DNA. Nature. 2013;497:108–12.
55. Adalsteinsson VA, et al. Scalable whole-exome sequencing of cell-free DNA reveals high concordance with metastatic tumors. Nat Commun. 2017;8:1324.
56. Gale D, et al. Development of a highly sensitive liquid biopsy platform to detect clinically-relevant cancer mutations at low allele fractions in cell-free DNA. PLoS One. 2018;13:e0194630.
57. Kinde I, Wu J, Papadopoulos N, Kinzler KW, Vogelstein B. Detection and quantification of rare mutations with massively parallel sequencing. Proc Natl Acad Sci. 2011;108:9530–5.
58. Vogelstein B, Kinzler KW. Digital PCR. Proc Natl Acad Sci U S A. 1999;96:9236–41.
59. Dressman D, Yan H, Traverso G, Kinzler KW, Vogelstein B. Transforming single DNA molecules into fluorescent magnetic particles for detection and enumeration of genetic variations. Proc Natl Acad Sci. 2003;100:8817–22.
60. Quillien V, et al. Clinical validation of the CE-IVD marked Therascreen MGMT kit in a cohort of glioblastoma patients. Cancer Biomark. 2017;20:435–41.

Chapter 4
Role of Bioinformatics in Molecular Medicine

Chad Vanderbilt and Sumit Middha

Key Points

- Laboratories often choose to have internally customized bioinformatics tools developed by bioinformatics specialists.
- The process from raw data sequence to variant annotation is mostly standardized, but different open source tools are available for the key tasks which can be customized to meet the needs of the laboratory.
- The field of Clinical Informatics continues to evolve and develop tools for more complex variant analysis

Key Online Resources

- https://www.broadinstitute.org/genomics
- http://bioinformaticsonline.com/pages/view/26617/list-of-bioinformatics-software-tools-for-next-generation-sequencing

Introduction

The term bioinformatics has many diverse meanings and settings for applications in the biological sciences. Bioinformatics is best understood as a recognition that "information techniques" and "computational methods," well established

C. Vanderbilt (✉) · S. Middha
Department of Pathology, Memorial Sloan Kettering Cancer Center, New York, NY, USA
e-mail: vanderbc@mskcc.org; middhas@mskcc.org

L. J. Tafe, M. E. Arcila (eds.), *Genomic Medicine*,
https://doi.org/10.1007/978-3-030-22922-1_4

in computer science, can be broadly applied to better conceptualize and understand complex biological systems [1, 2]. Applications for bioinformatics can be found in topics as diverse as protein folding prediction, ecological interactions, and RNA expression profiling [3–5]. However, when framed within the context of next-generation sequencing (NGS) in the clinical laboratory, bioinformatics refers to computational processes that take raw DNA or RNA sequence files from the next-generation sequencing instrument and analyze these data to provide clinically informative results related to the nucleic acid sequence [6]. We add the modifier "clinical" to reinforce the important role the bioinformatics teams contribute to the clinical management of patients. The term "clinical bioinformatics" has also been used to describe a broad range of activities that bioinformatics expertise can play in other areas of clinical medicine [7]. Here we focus our discussion to the role of bioinformatics within the clinical NGS laboratory.

Because the field of bioinformatics is a confluence of the biological and computational sciences, both areas of knowledge and expertise are important to the development of effective and high-quality analyses. Many common terms from computer science begin to enter the common parlance in bioinformatics. As an example, the established phrase that refers collectively to the bioinformatics analyses processes is "bioinformatics pipeline." The term pipeline simply refers to unidirectional and sequential steps of data processing. This reflects the modular nature of bioinformatics pipelines that we will discuss in detail in this chapter. For simplification of language, unless otherwise indicated, "pipeline" will refer collectively to all of the data processing steps that occur from when sequencing completes to when the report is generated.

Due to the critical nature that bioinformatics pipelines play in accurately reporting variant calls, most NGS laboratories employ at least one clinical bioinformatics specialist who is trained in operating and overseeing the pipeline. The amount of bioinformatics expertise required to successfully operate an NGS laboratory depends on the amount of systems the laboratory develops internally. Many commercially available products are available to assist with deploying various components of the pipeline. However, even with the exclusive use of commercial products, it is advised to have an internal bioinformatics specialist who is available to troubleshoot problematic findings or failures identified during routine quality assurance procedures.

Many laboratories prefer to have the flexibility of a customizable bioinformatics pipeline that allows for implementation of new biomarker detection and for updates that improve the end user experience in working with NGS data. Laboratories that choose custom, laboratory-developed pipelines often have large teams of bioinformatics specialists. Some of the subfields within bioinformatics that are necessary for maintaining a robust pipeline include pipeline developers, NGS variant analysts, operations managers, and graphical user interface developers.

Along with NGS in the clinical laboratory, clinical bioinformatics is a rapidly evolving and maturing area of specialized expertise. We anticipate many innovations and updated techniques to evolve current understanding of best practices in clinical bioinformatics. To keep the content of the chapter reasonably up to date, we will refer to pipeline processes in general terms that have persisted in clinical practice and are likely to continue to contribute to bioinformatics pipelines going forward. We recognize a diversity of tools have been developed that are available for every step in the bioinformatics process. We do not intend to provide an exhaustive or prescriptive list of tools but will refer to most common tool sets that are up to date, as determined by our own clinical practice and in the literature.

Herein, we describe the standard file types and processes that contribute to a modern pipeline, which is the standard of care in clinical NGS laboratories. We discuss the theory behind these data processing steps and refer the reader to references for more granular discussions of the individual topics. Finally, we discuss the current regulatory environment for bioinformatics and discuss the emerging trends we believe will likely to become standard practice in the near future.

Central Dogma of NGS Bioinformatics

We recognize that a large proportion of the readers of this text will come to this chapter with very limited knowledge in computer science, but with a strong background in genetics, molecular biology, and biochemistry. Thus, we want to provide a familiar framework on which a knowledge base in bioinformatics can be built. We hope to accomplish this by providing a simplification that frames the core processes of the bioinformatics pipeline analogous to the well-known concept of the "Central Dogma of molecular biology" or simply the Central Dogma. As a brief refresher, the Central Dogma is the steps of transformation from DNA to protein that occurs in cells (Fig. 4.1).

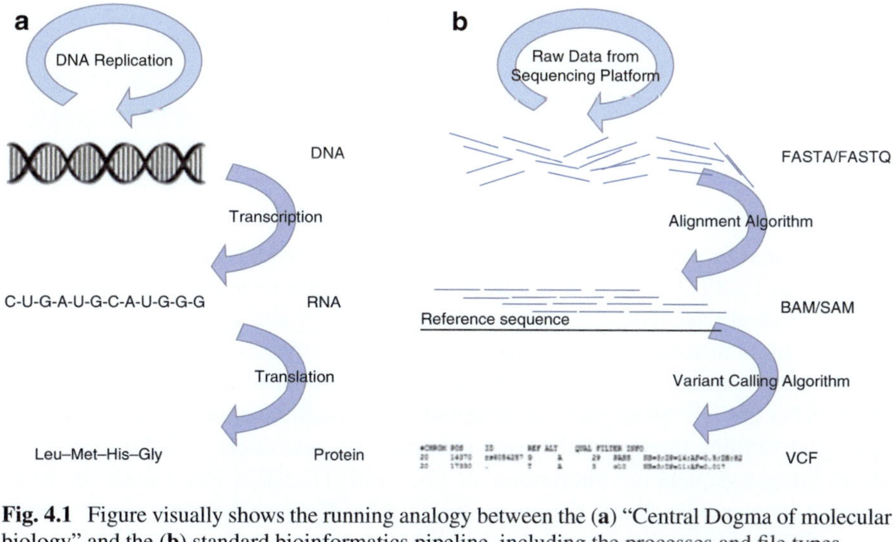

Fig. 4.1 Figure visually shows the running analogy between the (**a**) "Central Dogma of molecular biology" and the (**b**) standard bioinformatics pipeline, including the processes and file types

We recognize that the analogy between these two processes is not perfect, and we do not wish to infer precise correlation. However, we can think of both bioinformatics pipelines and DNA expression as unidirectional data processing, in which one form of data storage is transformed to another in sequential steps. Figure 4.1a,b shows the analogous steps along both processes, which can be referenced throughout this discussion.

FASTA/FASTQ

While the core chemistry of the different sequencing platforms varies, the raw data output after data processing can be generalized to the standard FASTA/FASTQ format. Like DNA in molecular biology, FASTA/FASTQ files are the raw material for the beginning of the process. As described throughout this textbook, NGS platforms generate millions of short reads (70–500 bp in length) for each sample and for each run.

For simplicity and interchangeability, FASTA/FASTQ files are written to disk as standard text files in structured format [8]. The FASTA file is the most basic format and can be quickly used for sequence alignment queries like BLAST [9] when troubleshooting pipeline problems.

The FASTA format consists of just two lines. The first line is a comment or title to describe the read and always begins with a greater-than sign (>). The comment sections can be used to identify the sample that the read belongs to, the locus on the chip, or any other purpose that allows for downstream processing or later clarification of derivation. The second line of a FASTA file is the entire sequence of bases represended by the read. No symbol is used to demarcate the sequence line.

Example of FASTA file format

```
> This is a FASTA file
TTGAACACAATGGAATTATCCTTCCTATGCCCAGCATACTCAGAAGAG
GCATAGGACAATGGTTTCTAAAGAAAAAAACCACGCTAGACAAAACT
GATGC
```

The format for a FASTQ file is similar to that of the FASTA file with the exception that the FASTQ file allows for incorporating the quality score corresponding to each individual base. FASTQ file format predates NGS and was originally derived for use with automated Sanger sequencing tracing analyzers, which were used for the Human Genome Project [10]. The now well-established quality component of the FASTQ file is derived from the original Phred quality score (Phred+33) developed to determine the probability that the base was accurately called during automated Sanger sequencing interpretation. The PHRED quality score scale has been retained for use with NGS. However, due to the difference between signal analysis for NGS compared to Sanger sequencing and the variation among NGS instruments, the quality score must be recalibrated for specific instruments. Regardless of the sequencing technique, the PHRED quality score allows for a wide range of probability predictions, over 94 orders of magnitude, for the accuracy of a base call [10–12]. The information is subsequently utilized by downstream processes.

The structure of the FASTQ file, like the FASTA, is plain text. In the case of the FASTQ, four lines are used instead of two. Lines 1 and 2 are perfectly analogous to the FASTA file with the only exception being that the line 1 begins with the "at" sign "@." The third line in FASTQ is another comment or title line that often matches line 1 for the same file. Instead of an "@" to begin the line, the third line starts with a plus sign "+." Line 4 is the Phred score for each individual base. Thus, the length of line 4 will always match the length of line 2. The symbols used for line 4 are single symbol representations for a number from 0 to 93 using the American Standard Code for Information Interchange (ACSII) symbols 33 to 126, which is a standardized way of representing numeric data with one character per number.

Example of FASTQ file format

```
  @ This is a FASTQ file
  TTGAACACAATGGAATTATCCTTCCTATGCCCAGCATACTCAGAAGAG
GCATAGGACAATGGTTTCTAAAGAAAAAAACCACGCTAGACAAAACT
GATGC
  +Below is the quality of the bases above
  efcfffffcfeefffcffffffddf`feed]`]_Ba_^__
[YBBBBBBBBBBRTT\]][]dddd`ddd^dddadd^BBBBBBBBBBBBBB
BBBBBBBBB
```

Each FASTQ file represents a set of individual reads sequenced on an NGS run. All reads for a sample are merged (concatenated) into a single file to represent millions of individual reads. This concatenated file is the raw file that enters the pipeline for analysis in almost all modern clinical NGS sequencing operations.

Alignment

Once a FASTQ file is generated, the next major step is to align each individual read to a reference genome. Alignment, or converting random assortments of FASTQ files to reads that are fully aligned to a reference genome, corresponds to transcription of DNA to RNA in our analogy to the Central Dogma. The alignment process transforms one data structure into another. When the reference sequence is unknown, a complutationally intensive process known as 'de novo assembly' can be used to convert short sequence reads to larger genomic sequences [13].

The alignment process of the pipeline is one of the most computationally "expensive" components of most pipelines. To conceptualize the complexity of sequence alignment, imagine that you have a random sequence of numbers that is 3.1 billion numbers long. You then have several million short sequences of numbers about 100 numbers long that you must match somewhere in the 3.1 billion numbers. You must search for the location where these short sequences match and repeat this each time for each short sequence. What makes it even more complicated is that the short sequences do not always have an exact place in the larger sequence. Even worse is that some of the smaller sequences are split and one-half matches one part of the large sequence and the other half matches another area, and one must consider that some of the numbers may not be accurate. It would take several lifetimes for one person to complete this task just once.

Fortunately, this is a class of problems that had previously been considered in computer science long before NGS was invented, and several robust solutions emerged early on in the development of NGS [14–18]. The Burrows-Wheeler Alignment (BWA) tool, an open source tool, has withstood the test of time and remains among the most popular and robust alignment algorithms used in large-scale clinical sequencing operations [19–21]. Many additional strategies for aligning reads to the reference genome exist and are in development that employ different strategies for alignment that optimize for different sizes of reads or for speed of alignment [22]. The bioinformatics specialist and laboratory director should consider the specific needs of the laboratory to choose the preferred alignment algorithm.

BAM/SAM

The standard output file of an alignment algorithm is the Sequence Alignment/Map (SAM), almost always transformed to the binary format Binary Alignment/Map (BAM) [23]. Other alignment file formats are being considered but have not had wide adoption. The SAM/BAM, like mRNA in molecular biology, is the intermediate data step in pathway to completion of the bioinformatics pipeline. The BAM file is most well-known to the non-bioinformatician as the file type that allows for aligned visualization of NGS data in genome browsers like the Integrative Genomics Viewer (IGV) [24]. Thus, the BAM file is the first data output that allows for manual human interpretation.

The data structure of the SAM/BAM file is written to disk as a standardized text file format. Instead of each data element being separated by individual lines, the text is tab delimited. The first portion of the SAM/BAM file is called the header. The header contains important information about the data in the file, such as the version of the format, information about the reference sequence used, information about the software that was used, etc. None of these fields are required, and each section is identified by an "at" sign (@), and a series of standardized two-letter codes are used to inform of the data type being entered (e.g., PN for program name).

The second and much larger component of the SAM/BAM file is the alignment section. Each line of the alignment section refers to an individual mapped read, and specific fields are required for each mapped read. The most updated information about SAM/BAM files can be found at http://samtools.github.io/hts-specs/SAMv1.pdf (last accessed June 2018). Additional, nonstandard SAM/BAM fields can be added to a standard SAM/BAM if required by the laboratory's pipeline.

We will focus on a few of the granular details to illustrate the flexibility of the SAM/BAM format. First, it is important to remember that the essential information from the FASTQ file of each read is retained in the SAM/BAM file such that the sequence and Phred base quality score can be extracted from a SAM/BAM file and is stored in fields 10 and 11, respectively. The remaining additional information contained within the SAM/BAM file is related to the metrics determined by the alignment algorithm, including the position in the reference sequence that the read is aligned to (field 4) and the mapping quality score (field 5). The mapping quality score is also measured on the same Phred scale as the base calling quality score. It is important to distinguish between these two quality scores because the two different quality scores play markedly different roles in variant calling.

The other important element within a SAM/BAM file is the CIGAR string (field 6). CIGAR is a compact notation to allow representation of multiple possible outcomes for a sequence as a relationship to the reference sequence. The code embedded within the CIGAR string informs any variations from reference, including insertions, deletions, mismatches, and soft-clipped bases. Briefly, soft-clipped bases are bases that are present at the end of a read but are not present in the reference. Soft-clipped bases can represent base calling error from the sequencer at the end of the read or can also represent a structural variant where a portion of the read aligns to the reference in two separate parts of the genome.

Variant Calling

Variant calling is the ultimate goal of the bioinformatics pipeline, much like protein generation is the end goal in the Central Dogma. As the field of NGS bioinformatics analysis has matured, greater emphasis has been laid on the downstream steps of pipeline including variant calling and efficient annotation. These variant callers utilize different underlying statistical algorithms like Bayesian or Hidden Markov models. Sorted and indexed BAM files are the most common input file for variant callers. As we will discuss in the final section of this chapter, NGS allows for a wide array of DNA and RNA variant type detection from a BAM file. However, the current standard for clinical NGS is that clinical laboratories have robust pipelines for the detection of single-nucleotide variants (SNVs) and small insertion/deletion events (indels) that are 21 base pairs or less in length.

Before a BAM file can be utilized for variant calling, the file must be processed. Several BAM file processing packages exist that are open access. The most commonly used packages in clinical sequencing are SAMTools, Picard, and GATK [23, 25]. These packages also have variant calling components, which we will discuss separately. Various quality metrics, such as average coverage and sample-level base quality assessments, are calculated and documented prior to variant calling. These tools also ensure that the reads are consistently reflecting the correct base pair throughout the entire genomic region of interest. Most modern pipelines employ a realignment tool before variant calling to correct any minor errors the alignment algorithm did not resolve, particularly in areas where indels or complex variants exist [26]. Variant calling is typically performed on individual samples. In pipelines that incorporate a paired tumor-normal sample for somatic variant detection, the variants called on each sample are compared, and presumed germline variants are dropped in the annotation phase. The utilization of a matched normal sample allows identification of true somatic variants present only in the tumor sample with confirmed absence in the normal.

The most common strategy for SNV and indel variant calling is to traverse the genomic regions of interest, "walking" the algorithm in a single direction documenting the pileup (all documented base calls from all reads that represent a genomic base pair) at each genomic base position. The threshold for calling a variant is user determined and generally optimized such that the variant caller does not report every bit of sequencing noise. Noise refers to the inherent amount of incorrect base calls that will be called when sequencing many reads at a high depth of coverage.

Clinical NGS platforms have required Phred base quality score to be greater than 30. At a Phred score of 30, we expect the sequencer to incorrectly call a base every 1000 attempts. When we sequence to a depth of coverage (DOC) of 500–1000 reads, which is standard for most somatic NGS laboratories, we expect that, on average, we will have an inaccurate base at nearly every genomic position. It would be very inefficient if the variant caller documented every genomic position with 1–5 reads that do not match reference, because we expect this to occur just by chance. These randomly occurring variations from reference are often well below the variant allele fraction (VAF) that clinical assays are validated to detect variants. It is far more efficient to allow the variant caller to ignore these random errors and focus on genomic regions with many reads that deviate from reference.

We have included a semi-comprehensive list of SNV and indel variant calling algorithms that are available for open-source use (Table 4.1). It is important to note that each of these algorithms have their own strengths and weaknesses. This makes choosing an appropriate variant calling algorithm challenging [27]. A common strategy that has emerged to overcome this problem is to use multiple separate algorithms and allow the outputs of the individual algorithms to converge in one Variant Call Format (VCF) file. Any major discrepancies among the variant calling algorithms can then be resolved by a bioinformatics analyst or molecular pathologist at the time of sign out. This strategy assures that the pipeline does not miss variants due to idiosyncrasies of the individual variant calling algorithm.

Variant Call Format (VCF) File

The VCF file is the end product of the bioinformatics pipeline and thus represents the end product (protein in our analogy to the Central Dogma). The VCF file was initially developed to support the 1000 genomes project [28], allowing for a

Table 4.1 List of common algorithms with online resources and source code repositories for the most common bioinformatic components of a standard clinical bioinformatics pipeline

Alignment algorithms		
Burrows-Wheeler Alignment tool (BWA)	https://github.com/lh3/bwa	[19–21]
Bowtie	https://github.com/BenLangmead/bowtie	
Novalign	http://www.novocraft.com/products/novoalign/	
SOAP2	http://soap.genomics.org.cn/soapaligner.html	
ABRA	https://github.com/mozack/abra	[26]
BAM/SAM analysis and editing software		
SamTools	http://samtools.github.io/	[23]
GATK	https://github.com/broadinstitute/gatk	[25]
Picard	https://github.com/broadinstitute/picard	
FreeBayes	https://github.com/ekg/freebayes	
Integrated Genomic Viewer	http://software.broadinstitute.org/software/igv/	[24]
Variant Calling Software		
MuTect	https://github.com/broadinstitute/mutect	
Vardict	https://github.com/AstraZeneca-NGS/VarDict	
Pindel	https://github.com/genome/pindel	
SamTools	http://samtools.github.io/	[23]
GATK	https://github.com/broadinstitute/gatk	[25]
Picard	https://github.com/broadinstitute/picard	
FreeBayes	https://github.com/ekg/freebayes	

standardized format of documenting human genome polymorphisms. The VCF format has evolved and is now the standard format for all NGS sequencing, including germline and somatic testing. Compared to the FASTQ and BAM files, the VCF is a much more manageable size (generally megabytes instead of gigabytes) and allows for documentation of single-nucleotide variants, insertion/deletion event, and structural variants.

The VCF, like the other formats, is standardized as a text file. The format of the text file allows the conversion of the generated VCF file to be efficiently incorporated into the database of the laboratory [29]. Indexing the data into a database allows for efficient storage and retrieval of the variant information for purposes of representing the data for clinical sign-out, quality control, or data mining.

Like the FASTA/FASTQ and BAM files, the first component of the file is a label that contains information related to the sample specimen, sequencing run, and software used to generate the file. In the VCF file, the label is referred to as the "header," and each line representing the header starts with the symbols double-hash sign (##). The final line of the header is demarcated by single-hash sign (#). This line is tab delimited with the essential components for identifying the various forms of variation. Essential elements included in all VCF files are the chromosome position and reference base(s) adjacent to the variant being described. The VCF file also has the capability of incorporating information from public databases, such as dbSNP or COSMIC, that allow for determining the potential clinical significance of variants. A complete list of standard/common fields for VCF files is provided. The remainder of the VCF file is referred to as the "body." The body consists of the date from the samples with respect to the variants identified by the variant calling algorithm(s). Each line represents a single unique event.

Variant Annotation and Prioritization

While the generation of the VCF file is the formal end of the standard bioinformatics pipeline, like with protein translation, most laboratories incorporate post pipeline processing of the variants included in the VCF file. These steps vary widely by laboratory but often include steps to suppress recurrent, expected, or predictable sequencing artifacts and incorporate annotations of clinically relevant details and therapy-related recommendation. A commonly used, open-source algorithm employed for this purpose is ANNOVAR. ANNOVAR can incorporate multiple annotation databases to exclude variants not implicated in changes in coding sequence or that are common germline single-nucleotide polymorphism. ANNOVAR remains fully supported and regular updates are available for download [30].

Often laboratories will save variant annotations from prior cases for common variants that are modifiable depending on the tumor type or clinical situation. As an example, the *BRAF* p.V600E variant has an FDA-approved therapy for melanoma, but, when the variant occurs in colon cancer, the variant does not have a specific, FDA-approved targeted therapy. Thus, annotations must rely on curated clinical inputs, such as tumor type, to maintain robust clinical accuracy. In the germline setting, ClinVar is commonly used for variant annotation data from the database which can be automatically incorporated into report [31]. Publicly available curated annotations for somatic mutations are also available [32, 33].

Beyond annotation, tools to predict putative effect of genomic mutations are also frequently used to prioritize results. Common among those are SIFT, PolyPhen, and aggregator tools like REVEL and MetaSVM that facilitate seamless prioritization of genomic mutations to ascertain pathogenicity or disruption of protein function. These are critical to optimize review time.

Regulatory Considerations

NGS was rapidly adopted into the clinical laboratory at a time when the bioinformatics techniques were not fully mature or standardized. The data size and complexity employed with NGS had never previously been utilized for routine clinical reporting [34]. For many laboratories, the pipelines that were used for nonclinical research tests were repurposed for the clinical laboratory. The rigor required for proper validation of diverse software application was not initially appreciated. While many laboratories completed complex and comprehensive validations, systematic studies of bioinformatics pipelines showed that interlaboratory variant calling agreement was poor for specific variant types [35].

Over time clinical guidelines for clinical testing have been established for the entire NGS process, including bioinformatics [36, 37]. Subsequently, The Association for Molecular Pathology (AMP), American Medical Informatics Association (AMIA), and the College of American Pathologists (CAP) collaborated to recommend a list of best practices that are specific to the bioinformatic component of the NGS assay [38]. All of these reference documents are valuable to the practitioner looking to establish or improve the bioinformatics processes in the NGS laboratory but are not currently binding from a regulatory perspective.

These guidelines can be read in more detail, but we will summarize here. Bioinformatics analysis should be considered a component of the laboratory test and be implemented and validated as one would consider any "wet lab" component of a laboratory test. The laboratory director is ultimately responsible for the results that are generated by the bioinformatics pipeline and should evaluate and approve all components of the process. If the laboratory director does not have the requisite training or knowledge to adequately evaluate the robustness of the pipeline, she/he can appoint a trained bioinformatics specialist. Validation should be performed in the same computational environment that clinical testing will be performed on. The laboratory director should consider and comply with patient privacy laws relevant to local and national regulatory environment. Each individual file in the pipeline (FASTQ, BAM, VCF) should have appropriate patient labeling to ensure that data does not get lost or confused among other patient samples. Steps should be put in place to ensure that whenever files are transferred or compressed, those files are not truncated, which could result in inaccurate results. It should be kept in mind that these guidelines represent only expert opinion as the authors were not able to identify enough relevant published data to make recommendations based on empiric research. These guidelines will likely undergo modifications in the years to come.

CAP, which is the most commonly used "deemed agency" for fulfilling the requirements of Clinical Laboratory Improvement Amendments (CLIA) in the United States, understanding the specific challenges of bioinformatics, have established in silico proficiency testing (PT), which is now a standard component of PT that NGS laboratories subscribe to as part of compliance with CLIA. In silico PT consists of FASTQ files that have been manually constructed to simulate mutations in the data. The files are distributed to individual laboratories and are to be treated as biological PT material. Laboratories must have the knowledge and capability to download the FASTQ files provided by CAP and allow for the pipeline to analyze the files in the same way that FASTQ files exported from the sequencing machine are analyzed. In silico PT allows regulatory agencies to customize challenges for pipelines that does not require the cost of obtaining biologic material with a specific profile and having to generate large batches for many laboratories [39, 40].

Advanced Applications

Copy Number Alterations

Copy number alterations (CNA) are known to cause disease, and NGS allows finer granularity in detection of such abnormal number of copies of large genomic regions within a cell. Five distinct bioinformatics approaches to detect CNA have been previously summarized – paired-end mapping, split-read mapping, read depth, and assembly-based and combinatorial approaches [41]. NGS bioinformatics tools use different statistical models and thresholds based on one or more of these approaches to detect CNA. An additional feature utilizing variant allele fraction allows for much more efficient analysis of allele-specific copy number event from NGS data [42]. This bioinformatics algorithm allows for precise annotation of homozygous/heterozygous deletions, copy-neutral loss of heterozygosity, and allele-specific gains/amplifications with standard hybridization capture NGS BAM files.

Structural Variants

Structural variants (SV), or genomic rearrangements larger than 50 bp, play an important role in various diseases. However, identification and characterization of these variants remain challenging from NGS data, especially targeted sequencing panels. The complexity in calling SV is amplified in the poorly characterized human genomic regions like repeat regions and pseudogenes [43]. Similar to CNA, read-pairs, split-reads and assembly-based bioinformatics approaches are utilized for SV detection. Beyond automated analysis to identify SV, manual review of these events remains critical for confident vetting of these genomic events. Manual confirmation of SV is performed using visualization tools like Integrated Genomics Viewer (IGV) to confirm presence of split and paired reads supporting the genomic alteration.

Microsatellite Instability

The ability to detect microsatellite instability (MSI) or mismatch repair-deficient (MMR-d) status using NGS data has recently been established. Essentially, the BAM files from aligned sequence reads from tumor and matched non-tumor samples are compared to identify statistically different alignments in microsatellite regions. The proportion of such microsatellite loci which deviate in the tumor is an indication of MSI. Clinical validations of NGS-based methods have been shown to perform similarly to standard PCR-based approaches [44].

References

1. Hogeweg P. The roots of bioinformatics in theoretical biology. PLoS Comput Biol. 2011;7:e1002021.
2. Luscombe NM, Greenbaum D, Gerstein M. What is bioinformatics? A proposed definition and overview of the field. Methods Inf Med. 2001;40:346.
3. Mantione KJ, Kream RM, Kuzelova H, Ptacek R, Raboch J, Samuel JM, et al. Comparing bioinformatic gene expression profiling methods: microarray and RNA-Seq. Med Sci Monit Basic Res. 2014;20:138–41.
4. Bowie J, Luthy R, Eisenberg D. A method to identify protein sequences that fold into a known three-dimensional structure. Science. 1991;253:164–70.
5. Jones MB, Schildhauer MP, Reichman OJ, Bowers S. The new bioinformatics: integrating ecological data from the gene to the biosphere. Annu Rev Ecol Evol Syst. 2006;37:519–44.
6. Wang X, Liotta L. Clinical bioinformatics: a new emerging science. J Clin Bioinform. 2011;1:1–3.
7. Belmont JW, Shaw CA. Clinical bioinformatics: emergence of a new laboratory discipline. Expert Rev Mol Diagn. 2016;16:1139.
8. Mills L. Common file formats. Curr Protoc Bioinformatics. 2003;45:A.1B.1–18.
9. Ye J, McGinnis S, Madden TL. BLAST: improvements for better sequence analysis. Nucleic Acids Res. 2006;34:W6–9.
10. Cock PJ, Fields CJ, Goto N, Heuer ML, Rice PM. The Sanger FASTQ file format for sequences with quality scores, and the Solexa/Illumina FASTQ variants. Nucleic Acids Res. 2010;38:1767–71.
11. Ewing B, Green P. Base-calling of automated sequencer traces using Phred. II. Error probabilities. Genome Res. 1998;8:186–94.
12. Ewing B, Hillier L, Wendl MC, Green P. Base-calling of automated sequencer traces UsingPhred. I. accuracy assessment. Genome Res. 1998;8:175–85.
13. Baker M. *De novo* genome assembly: what every biologist should know. Nat Methods. 2012;9:333.
14. Burrows M, Wheeler DJ. A block-sorting lossless data compression algorithm. Palo Alto: Digital Equipment Corporation; 1994.
15. Eaves HL, Gao Y. MOM: maximum oligonucleotide mapping. Bioinformatics. 2009;25:969–70.
16. Campagna D, Albiero A, Bilardi A, Caniato E, Forcato C, Manavski S, et al. PASS: a program to align short sequences. Bioinformatics. 2009;25:967–8.
17. Li H, Durbin R. Fast and accurate short read alignment with Burrows–Wheeler transform. Bioinformatics. 2009;25:1754–60.
18. Li H. Aligning sequence reads, clone sequences and assembly contigs with BWA-MEM. arXiv. 2013.
19. Pritchard CC, Salipante SJ, Koehler K, Smith C, Scroggins S, Wood B, et al. Validation and implementation of targeted capture and sequencing for the detection of actionable mutation, copy number variation, and gene rearrangement in clinical cancer specimens. J Mol Diagn. 2014;16:56–67.
20. Frampton GM, Fichtenholtz A, Otto GA, Wang K, Downing SR, He J, et al. Development and validation of a clinical cancer genomic profiling test based on massively parallel DNA sequencing. Nat Biotechnol. 2013;31:1023–31.
21. Cheng DT, Mitchell TN, Zehir A, Shah RH, Benayed R, Syed A, et al. Memorial Sloan Kettering-Integrated Mutation Profiling of Actionable Cancer Targets (MSK-IMPACT): a hybridization capture-based next-generation sequencing clinical assay for solid tumor molecular oncology. J Mol Diagn. 2015;17:251–64.
22. Mu JC, Jiang H, Kiani A, Mohiyuddin M, Asadi N, Wong WH. Fast and accurate read alignment for resequencing. Bioinformatics. 2012;28:2366–73.
23. Li H, Handsaker B, Wysoker A, Fennell T, Ruan J, Homer N, et al. The sequence alignment/map format and SAMtools. Bioinformatics. 2009;25:2078–9.

24. Robinson JT, Thorvaldsdóttir H, Winckler W, Guttman M, Lander ES, Getz G, et al. Integrative genomics viewer. Nat Biotechnol. 2011;29:24–6.
25. McKenna A, Hanna M, Banks E, Sivachenko A, Cibulskis K, Kernytsky A, et al. The Genome Analysis Toolkit: a MapReduce framework for analyzing next-generation DNA sequencing data. Genome Res. 2010;20:1297–303.
26. Mose LE, Wilkerson MD, Hayes ND, Perou CM, Parker JS. ABRA: improved coding indel detection via assembly-based realignment. Bioinformatics. 2014;30:2813–5.
27. Liu X, Han S, Wang Z, Gelernter J, Yang B-Z. Variant callers for next-generation sequencing data: a comparison study. PLoS One. 2013;8:e75619.
28. Consortium 1000. An integrated map of genetic variation from 1,092 human genomes. Nature. 2012;491:56–65.
29. Danecek P, Auton A, Abecasis G, Albers CA, Banks E, DePristo MA, et al. The variant call format and VCFtools. Bioinformatics. 2011;27:2156–8.
30. Wang K, Li M, Hakonarson H. ANNOVAR: functional annotation of genetic variants from high-throughput sequencing data. Nucleic Acids Res. 2010;38:e164.
31. Landrum MJ, Lee JM, Benson M, Brown G, Chao C, Chitipiralla S, et al. ClinVar: public archive of interpretations of clinically relevant variants. Nucleic Acids Res. 2016;44:D862–8.
32. Chakravarty D, Gao J, Phillips S, Kundra R, Zhang H, Wang J, et al. OncoKB: a precision oncology knowledge base. JCO Precis Oncol. 2017;2017:1–16.
33. Ramos AH, Lichtenstein L, Gupta M, Lawrence MS, Pugh TJ, Saksena G, et al. Oncotator: cancer variant annotation tool. Hum Mutat. 2015;36:E2423–9.
34. Roy S, LaFramboise WA, Nikiforov YE, Nikiforova MN, Routbort MJ, Pfeifer J, et al. Next-generation sequencing informatics. Arch Pathol Lab Med. 2016;140:958–75.
35. Davies KD, Farooqi MS, Gruidl M, Hill CE, Woolworth-Hirschhorn J, Jones H, et al. Multi-institutional FASTQ file exchange as a means of proficiency testing for next-generation sequencing bioinformatics and variant interpretation. J Mol Diagn. 2016;18:572–9.
36. Gargis AS, Kalman L, Lubin IM. Assuring the quality of next-generation sequencing in clinical microbiology and public health laboratories. J Clin Microbiol. 2016;54:2857–65.
37. Jennings LJ, Arcila ME, Corless C, Kamel-Reid S, Lubin IM, Pfeifer J, et al. Guidelines for validation of next-generation sequencing–based oncology panels. A Joint Consensus Recommendation of the Association for Molecular Pathology and College of American Pathologists. J Mol Diagn. 2017;19:341–65.
38. Roy S, Coldren C, Karunamurthy A, Kip NS, Klee EW, Lincoln SE, et al. Standards and guidelines for validating next-generation sequencing bioinformatics pipelines a joint recommendation of the Association for Molecular Pathology and the College of American Pathologists. J Mol Diagn. 2018;20:4.
39. Duncavage EJ, Abel HJ, Pfeifer JD. In silico proficiency testing for clinical next-generation sequencing. J Mol Diagn. 2017;19:35–42.
40. Duncavage EJ, Abel HJ, Merker JD, Bodner JB, Zhao Q, Voelkerding KV, et al. A model study of in silico proficiency testing for clinical next-generation sequencing. Arch Pathol Lab Med. 2016;140:1085–91.
41. Zhao M, Wang Q, Wang Q, Jia P, Zhao Z. Computational tools for copy number variation (CNV) detection using next-generation sequencing data: features and perspectives. BMC Bioinformatics. 2013;14:1–16.
42. Shen R, Seshan VE. FACETS: allele-specific copy number and clonal heterogeneity analysis tool for high-throughput DNA sequencing. Nucleic Acids Res. 2016;44:e131.
43. Guan P, Sung W-K. Structural variation detection using next-generation sequencing data: a comparative technical review. Methods. 2016;102:36–49.
44. Middha S, Zhang L, Nafa K, Jayakumaran G, Wong D, Kim HR, et al. Reliable pan-cancer microsatellite instability assessment by using targeted next-generation sequencing data. JCO Precis Oncol. 2017:1–17.

Chapter 5
Interpreting Genomic Reports

Alejandro Luiña Contreras

Technical Terms and Abbreviations

ACMGG	American College of Medical Genetics and Genomics
AMP	Association for Molecular Pathology
Genomic test	A laboratory test that interrogates numerous genes or regions of genes at the same time
HGNC	HUGO International Ltd. Gene Nomenclature Committee
HUGO	Human Genome Organisation
Next generation sequencing (NGS)	A diagnostic tool to determine the genetic sequence of numerous genes or regions of genes at the same time
VUS	Variant of unknown significance

Key Online Resources

- Human genome variation society [1]: hgvs.org
- HUGO Gene Nomenclature Committee [2]: Genenames.org
- HUGO [3]: www.hugo-international.org
- ClinVar [4]: https://www.ncbi.nlm.nih.gov/clinvar/
- Clinical trials.gov [5]: https://clinicaltrials.gov/
- Mutalizer website [6]: https://mutalyzer.nl/
- Sequence variant nomenclature [7]: http://varnomen.hgvs.org
- Guide to Interpreting Genomic Reports [8]: A Genomics Toolkit. A guide to genomic test results for non-genetics providers. www.ashg.org]

A. L. Contreras (✉)
Joint Pathology Center, Molecular Diagnostics Laboratory, Silver Spring, MD, USA
e-mail: Alejandro.luinacontreras.civ@mail.mil

L. J. Tafe, M. E. Arcila (eds.), *Genomic Medicine*,
https://doi.org/10.1007/978-3-030-22922-1_5

Key Points

- Genomic tests cover gene panels, the exome, or the whole genome.
- Genomic reports are different than other molecular genetic test reports and require understanding of the reportable elements.
- Familiarity with The Human Genome Variation Society standards (HGVS) for human nomenclature is recommended.

Introduction

Interpretation of genomic tests is fundamentally different than other molecular tests typically ordered to analyze individual genetic alterations. Genomic tests cover several or many genes (gene panels), the exome, or the whole genome and have the potential to identify multiple variants at the same time. The person ordering the test should be familiar with the assay and specify the reason for ordering the tests. The most common reasons to order a genomic report are to evaluate germline (inherited) conditions and somatic (acquired) mutations in neoplasia. These tests need complicated analysis pipelines (the dry bench) to analyze the data generated, and these pipelines change depending on the indication for testing. Also, several different software applications are needed to detect, annotate, and categorize each variant. After evaluation of this information, a decision is made to determine if the variant detected has clinical significance or not, a step that also requires database inquiries. The description of each step during the detection and evaluation of each variant and the decision process before reporting are beyond the scope of this chapter, and the reader is referred to the Next Generation Sequencing and Bioinformatics chapters for these.

Finally, the American College of Medical Genetics and Genomics (ACMGG) and the Association for Molecular Pathology (AMP) have developed joint consensus guidelines and recommendations for reporting and interpretation of sequence variants [9, 10] and incidental findings [11, 12]. The reader is encouraged to review these and to periodically check for updates, since the molecular genetics field is evolving rapidly.

Reporting Sequence Variants

Elements of the Molecular Pathology Report

The molecular pathology report contains multiple headers, each with different, but relevant information (Table 5.1). As recommended by The College of American Pathologists (CAP) [13], a molecular report should have seven elements, which include the identifiers, results, interpretation, comments, procedure, demographic information, and billing information (Table 5.1). It is important to note that each laboratory might include the elements of the report in different sections and might not follow this exact order.

Table 5.1 Elements of a Genomic Report [13]

Header	Body	Disclaimers, recommendations, and references
Identifiers: patient's name (first, middle, and last names); hospital ID or medical record number; date of birth; date of specimen collection; ordering healthcare provider; specimen source and indication for testing	Results using tiered system; interpretation; comment clinical trials (for somatic tests) Targeted therapies (if any)	Procedure Technical limitations Billing information (CPT code and ICD9 or ICD10 code)

Identifiers Section This section includes the name of the laboratory, its address, phone and fax, email, and website. It should also include the patient's name, an identifier like medical record or specimen number, date of birth, specimen collection time and date, date of accession in the laboratory (and an accession number), and the source of the specimen and how it was received (FFPE, fresh, etc.). Demographic information includes the name of the patient, accession number, referring clinician, location, indications for testing, and relevant clinical history.

Results The results section should include the name of the test and clearly states the result in a concise manner. It should also state the results expected in a normal individual. When abnormal results are identified, the results should be reported using the standardized genome nomenclature as set by the Human Genome Organisation (HUGO) International Ltd. Gene Nomenclature Committee (HGNC).

Interpretation This section includes the analytical interpretation, the clinical interpretation, the analytical sensitivity, and the clinical sensitivity. The analytical interpretation entails interpreting the raw data and producing a result, i.e., transforming the data to usable information. The clinical interpretation refers to the act of integrating what the analytical data means to the specific patient or to the general population. The analytical sensitivity is the ability of the test to detect the molecular event or mutation, and the clinical sensitivity is how well the assay predicts the associated disease.

Comment The comment should be used to explain, in a concise manner, aspects of the assay that might be relevant to the patient. These might include additional recommendations, limitations of the specimen (like decalcified tissue), percent tumor content, pertinent interfering substances, limitations of the test performed, or any other additional information that the person interpreting the results deems appropriate.

Procedure This is a very important part of the report, and it is often overlooked. This section includes the type of procedure that was performed (next generation sequencing, PCR, etc.), the target (using HUGO nomenclature) or analyte, how it was developed (laboratory developed test or FDA approved), and disclaimers.

Billing information: Each test should include a CPT code and ICD-9 or ICD-0 for the test.

Elements Unique to Genomic Reports

Genomic reports have unique elements, due to their complexity. They have a more universal reporting and have additional sections that might not be included in a conventional molecular pathology report. They are also stricter in the nomenclature and the definitions on how to report variants, the most important being the addition of the variant classification guidance. A sample report is provided in Fig. 5.1.

Variant Categorization

Categorization of sequence variants involves determining their clinical significance. It is dependent on whether the test was ordered to analyze germline mutations, somatic mutations, or copy number variants [9, 10, 14]. For germline mutations, the main purpose is to determine if a given variant within a gene is pathogenic for that disorder [9] or not or if there is insufficient information to determine this. Of note, the guidelines for germline mutations only apply to Mendelian (inherited) disorders and do not apply to somatic variants, pharmacogenomics, or complex or multigenic disorders. In somatic mutations, interpretation of the variant is based on the effect in clinical care [10], and characterization may depend if the variant has diagnostic, prognostic, or therapeutic implications.

Germline mutations are classified as "pathogenic," "likely pathogenic," "uncertain significance," "likely benign," and "benign" according to two sets of criteria as provided by the ACMGG. Each set of criteria is defined by combining a set of rules to classify each variant [9]. The two sets of criteria include (1) the classification of pathogenic and likely pathogenic variants and (2) the categorization as benign or likely benign. Each criterion has an assigned score, and these are added to provide a classification (Table 5.2).

Somatic mutations are categorized depending on clinical importance (therapeutic, diagnostic, or prognostic), and each of these is graded depending on the amount of information available (levels A to D) [10]. Depending on the available information, these are separated into tiers: Tier I for variants with level A or B evidence, Tier II for level C or D, Tier III for variants of unknown clinical significance, and tier IV for being or likely benign variants (Table 5.3).

Gene and Sequence Variant Nomenclature

Understanding the nomenclature used in molecular reports is essential to effectively communicate the findings on the analysis of a genome. A standard gene and gene variant nomenclature should be used in all reports as established by the Human Genome Organisation (HUGO) and the Human Genome Variation Society (HGVS). The HUGO sets the standards for human nomenclature. The HUGO Gene Nomenclature Committee (HGNC) approves a unique name for every known human

Your institution's Name and logo
Patient's name:

Patient's ID:

Phone Number
Age:

Gender:

Birth Date:

Somatic Mutation Next Generation Sequencing Report: Solid Tumor 15 Gene Panel

Provided Diagnosis: Lung adenocarcinoma

Sample location: Lymph node

Results Summary:

Variants of Strong Clinical Significance (Tier I): *EGFR* c.2573T>G (p.L858R)

Clinical significance: Drug response

Variants of Potential Clinical Significance (Tier II): None

Variants of Unknown Significance (Tier III): None

Benign or Likely Benign Variants (Tier IV): None

Interpretation: Approximately 35% of patients with lung adenocarcinoma have a mutation in the *EGFR* gene. Mutations in EGFR result in activation of the RAS/MAPK signaling pathway and patients with this mutation may respond to tyrosine kinase inhibitors and/or EGFR targeted therapies.

Clinical trials: Possible clinical trials that may benefit this patient can be found at Clinicai Trials.gov.

Procedure: Solid Tumor Mutation Panel by Next Generation Sequencing
Performance characteristics: This tests was developed to detect sequence variants in multiple cancer-related genes thai may have diagnostic, therapeutic and/or prognostic utility. Targeted next generation sequencing is performed to detect hotspot variants in 15 cancer-related genes including: *AKT1, GNA 11, NRAS, BRAF, GNAQ, PDGFRA, EGFR, KIT, PIK3CA, ERBB2, KRAS, RET, FOXL2, MET,* and *TP53. A* full list of all targeted regions within the above genes is available upon request or through our website.

Methodology: Genomic DNA is isolated from paraffin embedded tissue and enriched by microdissection, when needed. The targets are enriched and sequenced using (your vendor of choice) and analyzed using (software of choice) and the version.

Technical limitations: This test will not detect variants in areas outside the targeted genomic regions or below the limit of detection determined by our laboratory. This assay does not detect copy number alterations, translocations, microsatellite instability. it has been shown to detect >99% of single base substitutions and >90% of insertions/deletions (up to 15 bp) at an allele frequency of >5%. A negative result does not exclude a variant that falls below the detection levels of this assay. Additional testing might be indicated to determine the presence of copy number variations or rearrangements. This assay will not detect minimal residual disease. This assay cannot not distinguish between germline variants or germline variants. If a germline variant is suspected, genetic counseling and additional testing might be indicated. Variants might not be identified in pseudogenes, homologous regions and/or low map ability regions.

Limit of detection: Approximately 5% variant allele for SNV and approximately 10% for indels
Analytical sensitivity: Analytical sensitivity for all variant classes is available upon request or through our website.
Clinical disclaimer: This results should be interpreted using all available clinical and laboratory data and should not be used in isolation to diagnose a malignancy.
Billing: CPT code

References: Nat Rev clin. Oncol. 2011 Aug 23;8(11):661-8

Fig. 5.1 Example of a clinical report containing key report elements

Table 5.2 Interpreting Genomic Reports for Germline mutations [9]

Result category	Meaning	Clinical implication
Pathogenic or likely pathogenic variants[a]	Disease causing or related to the specific genotype	Genetic counseling and discussion of implications to other family members and recurrence risks is indicated
Variants of uncertain significance	A sequence that differs from the general population, but its meaning is not well understood[b]	Use for clinical decision making is not recommended; consider referral to genetic counseling; periodic review of the literature and online gene archives to see if additional information has been gathered; a mutation in this category might be reclassified as more information on its significance is accumulated. Some laboratories might reevaluate the significance at a later date, if requested
Secondary mutations	This includes variants that were found incidentally and not necessarily are related to the disease for which the test was ordered	Consider referral to genetic counseling; this results category may vary by laboratory and some laboratories might exclude from the report Current guidelines recommend reporting incidental findings for 56 diseases [11, 12] This category may vary by laboratory [18, 19]; Some laboratories might evaluate the data at a later date, if requested
Negative results and benign variants[c]	A negative result does not equate with complete absence of genetic abnormality	If the clinical suspicion for a specific disease is high, consider evaluation by other means or expanding the test panel to include other genes that might be involved in the disease process and might not be covered by the test ordered If suspicion for a specific disease is low or was a general multi-gene panel, you can perform periodic review of the literature and/or online gene archives to see if additional information has been gathered. Some laboratories might evaluate the data at a later date, if requested

[a]If there is strong evidence for disease causation, the variant will be designated as pathogenic. If there is not enough evidence, it might be classified as likely pathogenic

[b]A mutation might be classified as a variant of unknown significance if the effect on the function of the gene is unknown or if there is insufficient information to confirm that the specific change is causing the disease or risk of developing the disease. Patients from non-Caucasian ethnic groups might have an increased probability of VUS detection if their genetic composition has not been well characterized

[c]Negative results might be reported as "normal" or "not detected" depending on the laboratory. Benign variants might not be reported

genome [15], and these are available from the HGNC website [3]. In general, clinical reports follow these naming criteria. However, there are some alternate gene names that are used in the literature, and this naming is retained in clinical reports due to the clinical familiarity of the terminology. Notable examples are HER2 and MLL2 which are the non-approved names for the *ERBB2* and *KMT2A* genes, respectively.

The sequence variant nomenclature in reports should follow the recommendations of the HGVS [7]. All variants should be described at the DNA level, and a

Table 5.3 Interpreting Genomic Reports for Somatic mutations [10]

Result category	Meaning	Clinical implications
Variant of strong clinical significance (Tier I)	Disease causing, prognostically significant, or FDA-approved therapies exist for the specific variant for a specific tumor[a]	These are well documented variants that indicate a disease-causing variant, prognostically significant variants, or variants with approved therapies
Variants of potential clinical significance (Tier II)	Disease causing, prognostically significant, or FDA-approved therapies for tumor types other than the tumor being tested[a] or in early stages of evaluation[a]	Therapies and diagnostic or prognostic significance might be available for other tumor types, at early stages of investigation, only in very small studies or in preclinical trials
Variants of unknown clinical significance (Tier III)	No published data, the variant is not well represented in published databases or is a variant of unknown significance[b]	There is insufficient information to make an informed clinical decision
Benign variants or likely benign variant (Tier IV)	Includes variants that are observed in the general population	If the suspicion for a disease-causing mutation is high, consider reevaluation by other means or expanding the test panel to include other genes or areas of the gene that might not be covered by the test ordered If suspicion is low, additional test is not needed
Possible germline variant	A test designed to detect somatic mutations may detect a germline variant of clinical importance	This is an incidental finding that might necessitate additional testing to confirm the finding, genetic counseling, other risks to the patient, or discussion of possible implications to other family members

[a]In multi-gene panels, a variant might be classified as Tier 1 or Tier 2 if there is insufficient information provided to the laboratory (e.g., indicating a metastasis from colon as tumor of unknown primary)
[b]A mutation might be classified as a variant of unknown significance if the effect on the function of the gene is unknown or if there is insufficient information to confirm that the specific change is causing the disease or risk of developing the disease

Table 5.4 Prefix definitions for reference sequences

Prefix	Definition	Example[a]
m.	Mitochondrial DNA	m.123A
g.	Genomic	g.123B
c.	Coding DNA	c.123C
n.	Non-coding DNA	n.123C
p.	Protein	p.Lys892Asn
r.	RNA	r.1234A

[a]The number denotes the location from the first nucleotide of the reference sequence

prefix should be used to indicate the reference sequence that was used (Table 5.4). Variants are described according to several classes such as substitution, deletion, insertion, inversion, and duplication. Important class definitions and examples of variant descriptions are included in Table 5.5. To describe a specific variant, reports must also include the reference sequence used to describe what is observed. Next

Table 5.5 Variant class definitions

Variant class	Symbol	Definition	Format	Example
Substitution	>	One nucleotide is substituted for another	"prefix""position(s)_duplicated""dup"	m.123A>G
Duplication	dup	Insertion of one or more nucleotides directly 3'from the original copy	"prefix""position(s)_duplicated""dup"	g.123_345dup
Inversion	inv	More than one nucleotides are the reverse complement	"prefix""positions_inverted""inv"	c.123_345inv
Deletion-insertion	delins	One or more nucleotides are replaced by one or more nucleotides. Cannot be a substitution, inversion, or conversion	"prefix""position(s)_deleted""delins""inserted_sequence"	g.123_129delinsAGT
Repeated sequence	none	Repeated sequences of one or more nucleotides	"prefix" "position_first_nucleotide_first_repeat_unit""repeat_sequence" ["copy_number"],	c.123GTA[144]
Deletion	del	One or more nucleotides are deleted	"prefix""position(s)_deleted""del"	m.123_127del
Insertion	ins	One or more nucleotides are inserted The insertion cannot be a copy of the sequence immediately 5'	"prefix""positions_flanking""ins""inserted_sequence"	g.134_135insGATA
Conversion	con	A range of nucleotides that are replaced from somewhere else in the genome	"prefix""positions_converted""con""positions_replacing_sequence"	c.123_444con934_1450

generation sequencing reports will include the genomic DNA sequence denoted as "g" before the variant, a "c" for the coding DNA reference sequence, and a RefSeqGene or transcript [16].

Despite the existing guidelines, depending on the technology utilized, the degree of curation, and manual review of the data, there can be variability on how mutations are reported. A notable example where variability may be seen is in the description of insertions and duplications in *EGFR* and *ERBB2*. *ERBB2 (NM_004448) exon 20 p.Y772_A775dup (c.2313_2324dupATACGTGATGGC)*, for example, may be reported as p.A775_G776insYVMA (c. 2324_2325insATACGTGATGGC) to reflect how it is most commonly reported in the literature. There are several resources online which may be helpful in decoding these alternate nomenclature uses. A helpful resource is the Mutalizer website [6] to help with syntax checks and position conversions.

Mutation, Polymorphism, and Variants

Clinical reports commonly describe the detected genetic changes as mutations, variants, or polymorphisms. Mutations represent a change in the DNA sequence compared to the reference germline sequence and are often interpreted as a "disease-causing" change. A polymorphism is also a change in DNA sequence that is used both to indicate "a non-disease-causing change" or a change found at a frequency of 1% or more in the general population. Current guidelines, however, recommend the use of the neutral term "variant" or others such as "sequence variant," "alteration," or "allelic variant" [9]. The main reason for this is to avoid confusion and the erroneous assumption that all mutations represent a pathogenic change and all polymorphisms are benign.

Interpretation

Interpretation of genomic reports starts with reviewing the indication for testing. As noted above, the reports for inherited conditions and somatic mutations will differ in the intended meaning of the variant detected (Tables 5.2 and 5.3).

Germline Variants

In the evaluation for inherited disorders, variants classified as pathogenic or likely pathogenic are those that have direct causation or likely cause on the patient's symptoms or phenotype. The difference between these two categories is that for pathogenic variants, there is sufficient information on causation. In likely pathogenic variants, there is data, but it is incomplete. These categories should be treated the same, including discussion of appropriate therapies, recurrence risks, genetic counseling, and implications to other family members.

Variants of uncertain significance (VUS) are variants without enough information to understand their meaning. The use of these variants for clinical decision making is not recommended, and periodic review of the literature is recommended to determine if their significance changes as additional evidence evolves. Some laboratories will reevaluate data at a later date if requested and patients may incur an additional fee for this. Also, a laboratory may choose to not report these variants.

A laboratory may report a variant that is not associated with a specific disease or, alternatively, may report the result as "no significant variant detected." It is important to note that if a report indicates this, it does not necessarily mean that a variant is not present. It could be that a variant of uncertain significance or a benign variant is present. It also is possible that a variant that could have clinical impact is present but was not reported because it was outside the scope for the reason of testing. For these reasons, the ACMG issued a guidance in 2013 [11], which was updated in 2016 [12], for the reporting of 56 genes with known or expected pathogenic variants independent of the reason for testing. Patients may opt out of receiving these results prior to testing [17].

Somatic Variants

Somatic variants follow a similar tiered system that includes disease causation, but also add variants with prognostic and/or therapeutic implications. Variants of strong clinical significance and potential clinical significance include all the variants that are known to be associated with and/or probably cause the disease. These could also have a direct therapy approved by the Food and Drug Administration (FDA) for a specific tumor or for another tumor type. Also, they may confer additional information on the behavior of the tumor or serve in the risk assessment of the patient. When interpreting these, special attention should be given to the tumor type, as databases will categorize a variant as strong or of probable clinical significance depending on the context provided. For example, a *KRAS* mutation in a known metastatic colonic carcinoma may be classified as Tier I if the database is queried using the term metastatic colonic carcinoma, or it might be categorized as Tier II if the tumor is queried as a metastasis of unknown primary.

A mutation might be classified as a VUS if the effect on the function of the gene is unknown or if there is insufficient information to confirm that the specific change is causing the disease or risk of developing the disease. It is important to know that patients from a non-Caucasian ethnic group might have increased probability of VUS detection, if their genetic composition has not been well characterized. This is true for somatic as well as germline mutations.

Benign or likely benign variants indicate that a variant present has been observed in the general population. When only a benign or likely benign variant is identified and the suspicion for a disease-causing mutation is high, the clinician should discuss the findings with the laboratory in order to determine if there is the need for additional testing. The laboratory might recommend testing by another method or expanding the panel to include other genes or areas in the gene that might not be covered by that particular assay. If the suspicion was low, no further testing would be required.

One potential benefit (or pitfall) of testing for somatic mutations, without the use of a patient specific normal sample, is the potential for detection of germline variants. The ability of next generation sequencing techniques to quantify VAF allows for possible separation of these during testing for somatic mutations. As a general rule, if a patient is homozygous for a variant, the VAF should approach 100%, and heterozygous should have around 50%. Somatic mutations are generally lower than 50%, but at times might appear higher if selective amplification or deletions in one allele are present. To mitigate this, a laboratory may choose to do concurrent testing on both normal and neoplastic tissue. Conversely, if only neoplastic tissue is tested, an explanatory note indicating that a germline variant cannot be excluded is included in the report when VAFs are high.

References

1. Human Genome Variation Society [Internet]. Hgvs.org. 2019 [cited 1 April 2019]. Available from: https://www.hgvs.org/
2. Home. HUGO Gene Nomenclature Committee [Internet]. Genenames.org. 2019 [cited 1 April 2019]. Available from: https://www.genenames.org/
3. Human Genome Organisation (HUGO) International Ltd. – Home [Internet]. Hugo-international.org. 2019 [cited 1 April 2019]. Available from: http://www.hugo-international.org/
4. ClinVar [Internet]. Ncbi.nlm.nih.gov. 2019 [cited 1 April 2019]. Available from: https://www.ncbi.nlm.nih.gov/clinvar/
5. Clinicaltrials.gov. Home – ClinicalTrials.gov. 2019 [online] Available at: https://clinicaltrials.gov/. Accessed 1 April 2019.
6. Mutalyzer website [Internet]. Mutalyzer website. 2018 [cited 2 April 2019]. Available from: https://mutalyzer.nl/
7. Varnomen.hgvs.org. Sequence variant nomenclature. 2019 [online] Available at: http://varnomen.hgvs.org/. Accessed 1 April 2019.
8. Guide to Interpreting Genomic Reports: A Genomics Toolkit. A guide to genomic test results for non-genetics providers [Internet]. American Society for Human Genetics. 2018 [cited 5 December 2018]. Available from: https://www.ashg.org.
9. Richards S, Aziz N, Bale S, Bick D, Das S, Gastier-Foster J, et al. Standards and guidelines for the interpretation of sequence variants: a joint consensus recommendation of the American College of Medical Genetics and Genomics and the Association for Molecular Pathology. Genet Med. 2015;17(5):405–23. PMID: 25741868.
10. Li M, Datto M, Duncavage E, Kulkarni S, Lindeman N, Roy S, et al. Standards and guidelines for the interpretation and reporting of sequence variants in cancer. J Mol Diagn. 2017;19(1):4–23. PMID: 27993330.
11. Green R, Berg J, Grody W, Kalia S, Korf B, Martin C, et al. ACMG recommendations for reporting of incidental findings in clinical exome and genome sequencing. Genet Med. 2013;15(7):565–74. PMID: 23788249.

12. Kalia S, Adelman K, Bale S, Chung W, Eng C, Evans J, et al. Recommendations for reporting of secondary findings in clinical exome and genome sequencing, 2016 update (ACMG SF v2.0): a policy statement of the American College of Medical Genetics and Genomics. Genet Med. 2016;19(2):249–55. PMID: 27854360.
13. Gulley M, Braziel R, Halling K, Hsi E, Kant J, Nikiforova M, et al. Clinical laboratory reports in molecular pathology. Arch Pathol Lab Med. 2007;131(6):852–63. PMID: 17550311.
14. Kearney H, Thorland E, Brown K, Quintero-Rivera F, South S. American College of Medical Genetics standards and guidelines for interpretation and reporting of postnatal constitutional copy number variants. Genet Med. 2011;13(7):680–5. PMID: 21681106.
15. Wain H, Bruford E, Lovering R, Lush M, Wright M, Povey S. Guidelines for human gene nomenclature. Genomics. 2002;79(4):464–70. PMID: 11944974.
16. O'Leary N, Wright M, Brister J, Ciufo S, Haddad D, McVeigh R, et al. Reference sequence (RefSeq) database at NCBI: current status, taxonomic expansion, and functional annotation. Nucleic Acids Res. 2015;44(D1):D733–45.
17. ACMG policy statement: updated recommendations regarding analysis and reporting of secondary findings in clinical genome-scale sequencing. Genetics Med. 2014;17(1):68–69. PMID: 25356965.
18. Smith L, Douglas J, Braxton A, Kramer K. Reporting incidental findings in clinical whole exome sequencing: incorporation of the 2013 ACMG recommendations into current practices of genetic counseling. J Genet Couns. 2014;24(4):654–62. PMID: 25403901.
19. Ackerman S, Koenig B. Understanding variations in secondary findings reporting practices across U.S. genome sequencing laboratories. AJOB Empir Bioeth. 2017;9(1):48–57. PMID: 29131714.

Part II
Applications in Solid Tumors

Chapter 6
Lung Carcinoma

Maria E. Arcila, Jason C. Chang, and Laura J. Tafe

Key Points

- Recurrent alterations in EGFR, KRAS, ALK, ROS1, RET, NTRK, MET, BRAF, ERBB2, NRAS, and MAP2K1 account for the majority of driver alterations in NSCLC. These driver alterations are mutually exclusive.
- Many of these alterations represent therapeutic targets with approved targeted therapies or targeted agents undergoing clinical trials. High-throughput molecular profiling by next-generation sequencing has been increasingly used to detect these driver alterations.
- Current guidelines strongly recommend for all lung adenocarcinoma patients to be tested for genetic alterations in EGFR, ALK and ROS1, regardless of the clinical characteristics.

Key Online Resources

- https://www.amp.org/clinical-practice/practice-guidelines/updated-molecular-testing-guideline-for-the-selection-of-lung-cancer-patients-for-treatment-with-targeted-tyrosine-kinase-inhibitors/
- http://atlasgeneticsoncology.org/Tumors/LungTumOverviewID5030.html
- http://www.cbioportal.org/
- https://www.mycancergenome.org/content/disease/lung-cancer

M. E. Arcila (✉) · J. C. Chang
Department of Pathology, Memorial Sloan Kettering Cancer Center, New York, NY, USA
e-mail: arcilam@mskcc.org; changj2@mskcc.org

L. J. Tafe
Department of Pathology and Laboratory Medicine, Dartmouth-Hitchcock Medical Center, Lebanon, NH, USA

Geisel School of Medicine at Dartmouth, Hanover, NH, USA
e-mail: Laura.J.Tafe@hitchcock.org

L. J. Tafe, M. E. Arcila (eds.), *Genomic Medicine*,
https://doi.org/10.1007/978-3-030-22922-1_6

Introduction

Lung cancer is the leading cause of cancer-related death in the United States and worldwide. Historically, it has been categorized by its morphologic features into two main subgroups: non-small cell lung carcinoma (NSCLC, 85% of all lung cancers) and small cell lung carcinoma (SCLC, 15% of all lung cancers), and, for many years, treatment decisions have relied on this morphologic distinction, in conjunction with the pathologic staging. In recent years, however, accumulating evidence supports that lung cancer constitutes a highly heterogeneous disease at the molecular level, and its classification has undergone important revisions to reflect our enhanced understanding of its molecular biology. Several driver genetic alterations, including point mutations, small insertions and deletions, copy number alterations, and gene rearrangements, have been described in NSCLC, which allow the subclassification of this large category into distinct molecular subsets. The identification of key driver genetic alterations has also led to the development of newer drugs to specifically target these changes. Targeted therapies may be used alone, in combination with other types of targeted therapies or with conventional lung cancer treatments, such as chemotherapy and radiation therapy for patients with advanced disease.

The first molecular marker to be defined as a driver and predictor of treatment outcome in lung cancer was EGFR, which came about in the early 2000s with the introduction of the small molecule EGFR tyrosine kinase inhibitors (TKI), erlotinib and gefitinib. The high expression of EGFR by IHC in a large proportion on NSCLCs provided the initial rationale for the use of these agents. Although most patients in this unselected group had no response to treatment, dramatic improvements were evident in a minority of individuals. Responders were more likely females of Asian descent, non-smokers, and with adenocarcinoma histomorphology. These observations, soon lead to the discovery of activating EGFR tyrosine kinase mutations and their pivotal role in predicting response to TKIs [1–3]. This discovery not only revolutionized our understanding of the role of EGFR in lung carcinogenesis but paved the path for further research in subsequent years.

Since the discovery of activating EGFR mutations, several other driver mutations have emerged, including somatic mutations in KRAS, BRAF, HER2, ALK, MEK1, MET1, NRAS, PIK3CA, ROS1, RET, and NTRK (Fig. 6.1a). Importantly, all of these molecularly defined subsets represent "druggable" targets with agents that are either already approved for use, in various phases of clinical trials, or under development. As a result, the diagnosis and therapeutic landscape of lung carcinoma has dramatically changed and, with it, the way that we as pathologists assess and handle specimens for diagnosis.

The following text represents a basic overview of established and emerging clinically relevant driver alterations in lung carcinoma, concentrating primarily on NSCLC as their clinical role is better defined at this time.

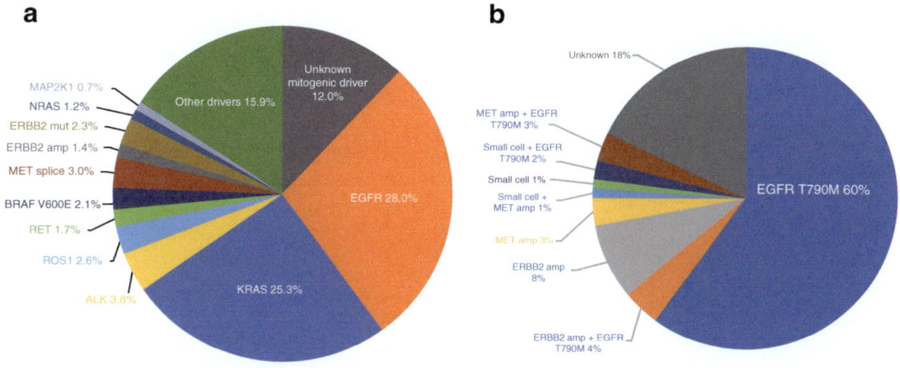

Fig. 6.1 (**a**) Frequency of various driver alterations in lung adenocarcinomas based on institutional experience at MSKCC [109]. (**b**) Frequency of various acquired resistance mechanisms in patients treated with first-generation EGFR-TKIs based on institutional experience at MSKCC [101]

Alterations with Already Approved Targeted Therapies

EGFR Mutations

The epidermal growth factor receptor 1 (EGFR/ERBB1) is a receptor tyrosine kinase of the ERBB family which includes HER2 (ERBB2), HER3 (ERBB3), and HER4 (ERBB4). Ligand binding to the extracellular domain of EGFR results in the formation of catalytically active homo- and heterodimers which, in turn, activate several downstream pathways involved in cellular proliferation, differentiation, migration, and apoptosis [4–6]. Mutations in EGFR are found in approximately 20% of lung adenocarcinomas but are rarely found in squamous cell carcinomas. Such alterations lead to the constitutive activation of the protein and unregulated downstream signaling [7].

Two types of mutations are recognized as most prevalent and clinically significant: in-frame deletions nested around amino acid residues 747–750 (exon 19) and the point mutation L858R (exon 21) [1–3, 8, 9]. Together, these encompass 80–90% of all EGFR mutations, and their association with response to currently approved tyrosine kinase inhibitors (TKIs) is well characterized. Insertions in exon 19 [10] and point mutations involving codons G719 (exon 18) and L861 (exon 21) are also associated with sensitivity, but their incidence is far less common. Although subsequent studies have identified over 50 additional rare mutations, not all have been associated with responsiveness to targeted therapy. Some mutations have been associated with primary resistance, while others remain uncharacterized due to their low prevalence (Table 6.1). Mutations commonly associated with primary resistance

Table 6.1 Common genetic alterations in non-small cell carcinoma

	Gene	Alteration	Frequency in NSCLC	Description	Most common mutations reported
Defined (approved agents)	EGFR	Mutation	10–35%	Receptor tyrosine kinase of the ERBB family. Most common mutations are sensitive to TKIs. Variable response for others depending on the mutation	Sensitizing mutations: Exon 19 indels, L858R, L861Q, G919X Exon 20 insertions (not all), T790M
	ALK	Rearrangements and mutations	3–7%	Receptor tyrosine kinase Fusions associated with sensitivity to TKIs. Mutations confer resistance to TKIs	Fusions: EML4-ALK Mutations: 1151Tins, L1152R, C1156Y, F1174L, L1196M, L1198F, G1202R
	ROS1	Rearrangement	1%	Receptor tyrosine kinase (RTK) of the insulin receptor family. Associated with sensitivity to tyrosine kinase inhibitors that have "off-target" activity against ROS1	*ROS1* rearranged with several partners *(FIG, SLC34A2, CD74, SDC, EZR, LRIG3, TPM3)*
	BRAF	Mutation	1–3%	Serine-threonine protein kinase – central mediator in the MAP kinase signaling pathway. V600E confers sensitivity to BRAF inhibitors. Recent FDA approval for dabrafenib and trametinib combination therapy in V600E mutant NSCLC	V600E, L597V, G469A/L, G466V
	NTRK1/2/3	Rearrangement	1%	Fusions associated with increased sensitivity to pan-TRK or multi-kinase inhibitors with TRK activity. Recent FDA approval for larotrectinib	*NTRK1* with several partners (*MPRIP, CD74, SQSTM1, TPR, IRF2BP2, TPM3*) *NTRK3* rearranged with *ETV6* and *SQSTM1*

Evolving	MET	Amplification, mutation	2–4%	Receptor tyrosine kinase (RTK) belonging to the MET/RON family of RTK. Associated with increased sensitivity to MET inhibitors	Exon 14 skipping mutations
	HER2	Mutation, amplification	2–4%	Receptor tyrosine kinase of the ERBB family. Variable response to TKI, depending on the mutation	3–12 bp insertions in exon 20 – YVMA insertion most common
	RET	Rearrangement	1%	Associated with increased sensitivity to multi-kinase inhibitors with RET activity (limited information)	*CCDC6-RET*, *KIF5B-RET*, and *TRIM33-RET*
	FGFR3	Mutation, rearrangement	0.5–2%	Receptor tyrosine kinase of the FGF family. Fusions associated with increased sensitivity to FGFR selective agents or TOEc1/2 inhibitors	*FGFR3-TACC3*
	KRAS	Mutation	15–25%	Small GTPase, activates several downstream effectors, including the PI3K-AKT-mTOR pathway. No direct anti-NRAS therapies available – preclinical models suggest that MEK inhibitors may be effective	G12V (A, C, D, E, F, I, R, S) G13C (R, E, D, V) Q61L (R, H)
	MAP2K1/MEK1	Mutation	1%	Serine-threonine protein kinase – of the MAP kinase signaling pathway. May respond to MEK inhibitors – not well defined	Q56P, K57N, D67N
	PIK3CA	Mutation	1–3%	Lipid kinase	E542K, E545K (Q), H1047R (I)

include some insertions in exon 20 and the point mutations S768I, L747S, D761Y, and T854A. As a group, insertions in exon 20 are the third most common mutations in EGFR, accounting for up to 10% of all mutations [11]. They are highly variable in position and size but generally occur within a hotspot region bound by codons 767 and 774 [12]. This molecular heterogeneity predicts variable interaction and potential implications for response to EGFR inhibitors [11].

ALK Fusions

The anaplastic lymphoma kinase (ALK) is a receptor tyrosine kinase of the insulin receptor superfamily. It is also known as CD246 (cluster of differentiation 246) and has significant homology with the leukocyte tyrosine kinase (LTK) receptor. ALK fusions are identified in approximately 3–7% of lung cancers [13] and are more commonly found in never or light smokers, younger age population, and those with adenocarcinoma histology, particularly of the signet ring cell subtype. The fusion partner is most commonly the EML4 gene (echinoderm microtubule–associated protein-like 4) [14–19], although fusions with other partners (KIF5B, TGF) have also been described [20, 21]. Fusions confer sensitivity to the ALK inhibitor crizotinib [22] and are associated with resistance of EGFR TKIs [23]. Unlike the sensitizing EGFR mutations, ALK rearrangements do not seem predictive of a more favorable prognosis [23].

ROS1 Fusions

ROS1 is an orphan receptor tyrosine kinase, evolutionarily related to ALK. Despite having one of the largest extracellular domains of all RTKs, no human ROS1 ligand has been identified and the protein function in humans remains largely unknown [24, 25]. In lung cancer, fusions may be present in up to 2% of tumors and involve several partner genes, including SLC34A2, CD74, TPM3, SDC4, EZR, LRIG3, and GOPC [21, 26, 27], among others. The expressed fusion genes display oncogenic properties as evidenced by transformation in vitro and tumorigenicity in in vivo models [26, 28]. Similar to ALK fusions, ROS 1 fusions are described as more prevalent in younger patients, never smokers, and those with adenocarcinoma histomorphology, which may reflect the evolutionary relatedness of these 2 RTKs. Of particular interest, ROS1 and ALK share approximately 49% amino acid sequence homology within the kinase domain [25], and several ALK inhibitors have shown ROS1 inhibitory activity in in vitro models [28–30]. ROS1 fusions define the third actionable subtype of lung cancers with crizotinib already approved by the FDA as targeted therapy for their treatment.

BRAF Mutations

The BRAF protein is a serine/threonine kinase that is activated by KRAS and transduces signals to downstream pathways which direct cellular growth and proliferation. Mutations in the BRAF gene lead to constitutive activation of the protein and are implicated in the pathogenesis of several human cancers [31]. Mutations occur in 2–3% of patients with lung adenocarcinoma [32–35] and are strongly associated with a positive smoking history. In lung adenocarcinoma, the most common mutation is the V600E, accounting for approximately 50% of all mutations. Other mutations found at lower frequencies include G466V, G469A, Y472C, D594G, and L597V in exons 11 and 15 [34, 36]. At this time, evidence of response to BRAF inhibitors is only [37] available for BRAF V600E mutated tumors. Case reports document response to vemurafenib [37]) or dabrafenib [38], but these agents are not yet approved for this specific use. More recently, combination therapy dabrafenib and trametinib has been approved for use by the FDA in this setting [39, 40].

NTRK Fusions

The neurotropic tyrosine kinase receptors, NTRK1, NTRK2, and NTRK3, are receptor tyrosine kinases which play a critical role in neuronal survival and differentiation. Fusions involving NTRK are reported in a wide variety of solid tumors and have been shown to function as oncogenic drivers by the expression of constitutively active fusion proteins that harbor a functional kinase domain. NTRK fusions are rare in NSCLC with its frequency estimated at 1% or less. Rearrangements of NTRK1 are the most common and involve several fusion partners, including MPRIP, CD74, SQSTM1, TPR, IRF2BP2, and TPM3. NTRK3 fusions with ETV6 and SQSTM1 are also reported [41–44]. Inhibition of NRK signaling has shown dramatic responses across multiple tumor types providing the supportive evidence for the recent accelerated approval by the FDA to larotrectinib for adult and pediatric patients with advanced solid tumors, including lung cancer.

KRAS Mutations

KRAS is a GTPase protein encoded by the KRAS proto-oncogene, also known as V-Ki-ras2 Kirsten rat sarcoma viral oncogene homolog. The normal protein plays a critical role in the activation of several signal transduction pathways downstream of EGFR. Mutations lead the constitutive activation of KRAS signaling pathways and are implicated in the pathogenesis of several cancers, particularly colon, lung, and pancreatic malignancies. In lung adenocarcinomas, KRAS mutations may be found in up to 30% of tumors, but significantly lower frequencies, <10%, are reported in Asian patients [45, 46]. The vast majority of mutations are identified in codons 12 and 13, and less frequently in codon 61. As a group, KRAS mutations are more common in former or current smokers [47]. However, when stratified into specific subtypes, some mutations are far more common in never smokers. Transition mutations (substitution of purine to purine or pyrimidine to pyrimidine) such as those seen in G12D and G12S are more common in never smokers, while transversions (substitution from purine to pyrimidine and vice versa) as seen in mutations G12C, G12V, and G13C are more common in former or current smokers [45, 47–49].

Despite considerable attempts, the quest for effective therapeutic inhibition of KRAS has not been productive; currently, there are no direct anti-KRAS therapies available. A major obstacle to the development of specific KRAS inhibitors is that the mutated KRAS proteins lose their normal enzymatic function, making them far more difficult to inhibit compared to those with gain of function. Downstream targeting therefore represents a more promising approach. Mutations are a strong negative predictor of response to EGFR TKIs [45, 47], but unlike colon carcinoma, they have not yet been shown to be negative predictors of benefit to anti-EGFR antibodies.

HER2 Mutations

The human epidermal growth factor receptor 2 (HER2/ERBB2) is a receptor tyrosine kinase of the ERBB family. In contrast to other members of this family, HER2 does not have a direct ligand but constitutes the preferred dimerization partner for EGFR and other ERBB receptors. Duc to this association, *HER2* plays a pivotal role in EGFR signal transduction with corresponding significant roles in cancer development and progression when its function is deregulated. Activating mutations in the TK domain of the gene have been described in 2–4% of lung adenocarcinomas, with highest prevalence among never smokers [50, 51]. In-frame insertions in exon 20 represent the vast majority of mutations, but point mutations along the tyrosine kinase domain have also been identified [52]. Insertions range from 3 to 12 bp in length and are confined to a hotspot region between codons 775 and 881. The A775_G776insYVMA mutation is the most common, representing over 80% of the cases. Other insertions and point mutations include G776>VC, V777_G778insCG, P780_Y781insGSP, L755S, D769H, V777L, and V777M but are less common. Patients with HER2 mutations may benefit from HER2 targeted therapy. The sensitivity of HER2 mutant tumor cells to HER2 inhibitors has been demonstrated under clinical trials with partial responses [53–57]. Treatments such as trastuzumab, afatinib, and other compounds offer promising therapeutic options, but further studies are needed [57, 58]. To date, no FDA-approved agents are available.

MET Alterations

MET is a receptor tyrosine kinase, also known at the hepatocyte growth factor receptor, which plays a key role in embryonic development and wound healing. Deregulation, through mutation or amplification, is associated with cancer development by the activation of key oncogenic pathways, including RAS, PI3K, STAT3, and beta-catenin, and through promotion of angiogenesis, invasion, migration, and metastasis. In lung cancer, both mutation and amplification are reported. Activating somatic mutations that affect the splice site regions of exon 14 are seen in approximately 4% of lung adenocarcinomas. These mutations lead to exon 14 skipping and deletion of the juxtamembrane domain of the MET receptor with resulting enhanced signaling through the MET receptor pathway [59–68]. Mutations confer sensitivity to targeted MET inhibitors.

MET activation through gene amplification is also reported in lung carcinoma. In previously untreated patients, amplification is found in only a small proportion of tumors, 2–4% [64, 69–74], and is associated with primary resistance to EGFR inhibitors and poor prognosis [70, 74–76]. More commonly, however, MET amplification is associated with the development of acquired resistance in patients who are EGFR mutation positive and have received EGFR inhibitors [69, 71, 72, 77–79]. In this setting, it is reported in 5–20% of tumors; in over 50% of cases it is concurrently seen with the secondary T790M mutation [77].

RET Fusions

RET (rearranged during transfection) is a receptor tyrosine kinase that plays a pivotal role in neural crest development [80]. Normal RET signaling involves the formation of a complex between GFL (glial cell line-derived neurotropic factor (GDFN) family of ligands) and the co-receptor GRFa1 (glial-cell line-derived neurotropic factor family receptor a1). In turn, this GFL/GFRa1 complex brings together two molecules of RET to form an activated kinase complex which will transduce the signal to several downstream signaling pathways [81, 82]. Fusions involving RET and several partner genes (CCDC6, KIF5B, NCOA4, TRIM33, CUX1, KIAA1468) have been described in lung adenocarcinomas at a frequency of approximately 1%. While the functional consequences of these RET fusions in lung carcinogenesis are not yet fully understood, both in vivo and in vitro studies confirm their activating [83, 84] and transforming [26, 83] oncogenic potential.

Inhibition of RET is possible through multi-targeted inhibitors with anti-RET activity but RET-specific inhibitors are not yet available. Several clinical trials are currently underway but, to date, there are no FDA-approved agents for treatment.

PIK3CA Mutations

The PIK3CA gene encodes the p110α catalytic subunit of the mitogenic signaling protein phosphoinositide 3-kinase (PI3K), which is linked numerous cellular functions including cell growth, proliferation, differentiation, and cell survival. PIK3 is activated by receptor tyrosine kinases such as EGFR and transduces signals through activation of AKT in the PI3K/AKT/mTOR pathway. PIK3CA mutations are found in up to 2% of lung adenocarcinomas [85] but are more common in squamous cell carcinomas [86]; they have also been detected in a very small percentage of lung cancers with acquired resistance [78]. Mutations occur in two hotspot regions in exons 9 and 20, coding for the helical and kinase domains of the protein, respectively. E545K and H1047R variants encompass approximately 80% of the mutations reported in lung adenocarcinomas; H1047L, E542K, and E545Q [36, 85] are less frequently reported.

In contrast to the mutual exclusivity of other driver oncogene mutations seen in lung adenocarcinoma, PIK3CA mutations are often found concurrently with other alterations. At least 70% of PIK3 CA mutations are identified in conjunction with mutations in EGFR, KRAS, and ALK [46, 85, 86]. The clinical impact of this finding on the efficacy of targeted therapies such as erlotinib and crizotinib is not well defined at this time. Multiple PI3K inhibitors are currently under investigation in clinical trials [87–90].

MAP2K1/MEK1 Mutations

The mitogen-activated protein kinase kinase 1 (MAP2K1), also known as MEK1, is a dual specificity kinase of the MAP2K/STE7 kinase family with pivotal role in the signal integration of the MAPK/ERK cascade. Mutations in the activation segment of the gene have been shown to constitutively activate the protein, enhancing cell proliferation and differentiation and promoting transformation [91–94]. Mutations in MAP2K1 are found in approximately 1% of all NSCLC and are more common in adenocarcinoma with higher prevalence among smokers. The most common mutations are K57N and Q56P [94, 95]. The selective MAP2K1 inhibitor trametinib is currently available and FDA approved for patients with BRAF-mutant melanoma only. There are no approved agents or trials of MEK-selective inhibitors for MEK-mutant patients with non-small cell lung cancer, at this time.

FGFR3 Alterations

The fibroblast growth factor receptor 3 (*FGFR3*) is a receptor tyrosine kinase family belonging to the immunoglobulin superfamily and is involved in downstream signaling in the MAPK, JAK/STAT, and PI3K/AKT signaling pathways. Oncogenic activation through both mutations and fusions has been reported in 1–2% of NSCLC, primarily squamous cell carcinomas. Mutations R248C, S249C, G370C, and K650E have been most commonly reported [96, 97]. FGFR3-TACC3 fusions have been reported in both squamous and adenocarcinomas. The same fusions have been reported in bladder cancer with documented partial response to FGFR1-4 inhibitors. Response to this type of targeted therapy is not yet documented in patients with lung cancer. Importantly, the same fusion has also been reported as acquired events post-EGFR TKI suggesting it may also represent a recurrent resistance mechanism in EGFR-positive tumors [98].

Acquired Resistance Mechanisms to TKIs

Despite high initial response rates to targeted therapy, all patients inevitably develop progression of disease through acquired resistance to TKIs by various mechanisms [99]. The resistance mechanisms to EGFR-TKIs (Fig. 6.1b) and ALK-TKIs are best studied and are discussed below.

The most frequent mechanism of acquired resistance to first- and second-generation EGFR-TKIs is the EGFR T790M point mutation within exon 20 [100, 101], accounting for 60% of acquired resistance to EGFR-TKIs. This secondary mutation occurs on the same *EGFR* allele harboring the original sensitizing mutation and is thought to increase tyrosine kinase affinity for ATP, thus reducing the interaction between EGFR with reversible EGFR-TKIs [102]. The detection of the *EGFR* T790M mutation has significant clinical impact because third-generation EGFR TKIs such as osimertinib are irreversible EGFR inhibitors that are active in the presence of T790M mutation. Other less common acquired resistance mechanisms to first- and second-generation EGFR TKIs include *MET* amplification, *ERBB2* (HER2) amplification, and small cell transformation [101]. Recently, osimertinib has been approved as standard first-line treatment for *EGFR*-mutant NSCLC [103]. In patients who develop acquired resistance to osimertinib, mechanisms including *EGFR* C797S mutation, *MET* amplification, and fusions involving other RTKs have been reported [104, 105].

Similarly, a broad spectrum of acquired resistance mechanisms has been identified in *ALK*-positive NSCLC treated with ALK-TKIs. Various *ALK* resistance mutations have been observed in approximately 20% of patients progressing on first-generation ALK-TKIs and 50% of patients progressing on second-generation ALK-TKIs [106]. Less commonly, *ALK* amplification can be seen in patients without *ALK* resistance mutations.

Molecular Testing Guidelines for Therapy Selection

In 2013, an evidence-based guideline for molecular testing of patients with lung cancer was published as a concerted effort from the College of American Pathologists (CAP), the International Association for the Study of Lung Cancer (IASLC), and the Association for Molecular Pathology (AMP), to set standards for the molecular analysis of lung cancers which would guide treatment decisions with targeted inhibitors [107]. This guideline was subsequently updated in 2018, based on emerging evidence for other markers [108]. A detailed description of the current guidelines is beyond the scope of this chapter, and the readers are therefore referred to the complete guideline for further information. Highlights of the guidelines are summarized in the bulleted section below.

- Current guidelines strongly recommend for all lung cancer patients to be tested for genetic alterations in EGFR, ALK, and ROS1, regardless of the clinical characteristics.
- For ALK fusions, immunohistochemistry was incorporated in the new guidelines as a suitable alternative to fluorescence in situ hybridization testing. The use of IHC for EGFR mutations using mutation-specific antibodies was not endorsed.
- Multiplex genetic sequencing panels that can simultaneously test for alterations in these prioritized genes and other clinically relevant genes are preferred over multiple single-gene tests. If testing is performed by NGS, assessment of BRAF, ERBB2, MET, RET, and KRAS is also recommended.
- For patients undergoing targeted therapy for tumors harboring EGFR-sensitizing mutations and acquired resistance is suspected, testing for the EGFR T790M mutation is required. Testing may be done by biopsy or cell-free DNA (cfDNA).
- Based on the evidence available at the time of preparation of the guidelines, it is emphasized that cfDNA is not recommended for initial diagnosis if tissue or cytology material can be obtained.

Conclusions

Lung cancer is a common disease encountered daily in pathology practice. With the discovery of activating mutations as drivers of lung carcinogens, we can now redefine this disease using morphologic and molecular attributes that have direct clinicopathologic impact. In this setting, pathologists are becoming key providers of personalized medicine information. A well-rounded understanding of the molecular biology and the technical aspects of testing is required to effectively deliver critical answers to questions of diagnosis, prognosis, and predictive parameters of the tumor.

References

1. Lynch TJ, Bell DW, Sordella R, Gurubhagavatula S, Okimoto RA, Brannigan BW, et al. Activating mutations in the epidermal growth factor receptor underlying responsiveness of non-small-cell lung cancer to gefitinib. N Engl J Med. 2004;350(21):2129–39. https://doi.org/10.1056/NEJMoa040938.
2. Paez JG, Janne PA, Lee JC, Tracy S, Greulich H, Gabriel S, et al. EGFR mutations in lung cancer: correlation with clinical response to gefitinib therapy. Science. 2004;304(5676):1497–500. https://doi.org/10.1126/science.1099314.

3. Pao W, Miller V, Zakowski M, Doherty J, Politi K, Sarkaria I, et al. EGF receptor gene mutations are common in lung cancers from "never smokers" and are associated with sensitivity of tumors to gefitinib and erlotinib. Proc Natl Acad Sci U S A. 2004;101(36):13306–11. https://doi.org/10.1073/pnas.0405220101.
4. Daly JM, Jannot CB, Beerli RR, Graus-Porta D, Maurer FG, Hynes NE. Neu differentiation factor induces ErbB2 down-regulation and apoptosis of ErbB2-overexpressing breast tumor cells. Cancer Res. 1997;57(17):3804–11.
5. Graus-Porta D, Beerli RR, Hynes NE. Single-chain antibody-mediated intracellular retention of ErbB-2 impairs Neu differentiation factor and epidermal growth factor signaling. Mol Cell Biol. 1995;15(3):1182–91.
6. Riese DJ 2nd, Stern DF. Specificity within the EGF family/ErbB receptor family signaling network. Bioessays. 1998;20(1):41–8. https://doi.org/10.1002/(SICI)1521-1878(199801)20:1<41::AID-BIES7>3.0.CO;2-V.
7. Sordella R, Bell DW, Haber DA, Settleman J. Gefitinib-sensitizing EGFR mutations in lung cancer activate anti-apoptotic pathways. Science. 2004;305(5687):1163–7. https://doi.org/10.1126/science.1101637.
8. D'Angelo SP, Park B, Azzoli CG, Kris MG, Rusch V, Ladanyi M, et al. Reflex testing of resected stage I through III lung adenocarcinomas for EGFR and KRAS mutation: report on initial experience and clinical utility at a single center. J Thorac Cardiovasc Surg. 2011;141(2):476–80. https://doi.org/10.1016/j.jtcvs.2010.08.026.
9. Cappuzzo F, Hirsch FR, Rossi E, Bartolini S, Ceresoli GL, Bemis L, et al. Epidermal growth factor receptor gene and protein and gefitinib sensitivity in non-small-cell lung cancer. J Natl Cancer Inst. 2005;97(9):643–55. https://doi.org/10.1093/jnci/dji112.
10. He M, Capelletti M, Nafa K, Yun CH, Arcila ME, Miller VA, et al. EGFR exon 19 insertions: a new family of sensitizing EGFR mutations in lung adenocarcinoma. Clin Cancer Res. 2012;18(6):1790–7. https://doi.org/10.1158/1078-0432.CCR-11-2361.
11. Arcila ME, Nafa K, Chaft JE, Rekhtman N, Lau C, Reva BA, et al. EGFR exon 20 insertion mutations in lung adenocarcinomas: prevalence, molecular heterogeneity, and clinicopathologic characteristics. Mol Cancer Ther. 2013;12(2):220–9. https://doi.org/10.1158/1535-7163.MCT-12-0620.
12. Yasuda H, Kobayashi S, Costa DB. EGFR exon 20 insertion mutations in non-small-cell lung cancer: preclinical data and clinical implications. Lancet Oncol. 2012;13(1):e23–31. https://doi.org/10.1016/S1470-2045(11)70129-2.
13. Pillai RN, Ramalingam SS. The biology and clinical features of non-small cell lung cancers with EML4-ALK translocation. Curr Oncol Rep. 2012;14(2):105–10. https://doi.org/10.1007/s11912-012-0213-4.
14. Choi YL, Takeuchi K, Soda M, Inamura K, Togashi Y, Hatano S, et al. Identification of novel isoforms of the EML4-ALK transforming gene in non-small cell lung cancer. Cancer Res. 2008;68(13):4971–6. https://doi.org/10.1158/0008-5472.CAN-07-6158.
15. Horn L, Pao W. EML4-ALK: honing in on a new target in non-small-cell lung cancer. J Clin Oncol. 2009;27(26):4232–5. https://doi.org/10.1200/JCO.2009.23.6661.
16. Koivunen JP, Mermel C, Zejnullahu K, Murphy C, Lifshits E, Holmes AJ, et al. EML4-ALK fusion gene and efficacy of an ALK kinase inhibitor in lung cancer. Clin Cancer Res. 2008;14(13):4275–83. https://doi.org/10.1158/1078-0432.CCR-08-0168.
17. Soda M, Choi YL, Enomoto M, Takada S, Yamashita Y, Ishikawa S, et al. Identification of the transforming EML4-ALK fusion gene in non-small-cell lung cancer. Nature. 2007;448(7153):561–6. https://doi.org/10.1038/nature05945.
18. Takeuchi K, Choi YL, Soda M, Inamura K, Togashi Y, Hatano S, et al. Multiplex reverse transcription-PCR screening for EML4-ALK fusion transcripts. Clin Cancer Res. 2008;14(20):6618–24. https://doi.org/10.1158/1078-0432.CCR-08-1018.
19. Wong DW, Leung EL, So KK, Tam IY, Sihoe AD, Cheng LC, et al. The EML4-ALK fusion gene is involved in various histologic types of lung cancers from nonsmokers with wild-type EGFR and KRAS. Cancer. 2009;115(8):1723–33. https://doi.org/10.1002/cncr.24181.

20. Takeuchi K, Choi YL, Togashi Y, Soda M, Hatano S, Inamura K, et al. KIF5B-ALK, a novel fusion oncokinase identified by an immunohistochemistry-based diagnostic system for ALK-positive lung cancer. Clin Cancer Res. 2009;15(9):3143–9. https://doi.org/10.1158/1078-0432.CCR-08-3248.
21. Rikova K, Guo A, Zeng Q, Possemato A, Yu J, Haack H, et al. Global survey of phosphotyrosine signaling identifies oncogenic kinases in lung cancer. Cell. 2007;131(6):1190–203. https://doi.org/10.1016/j.cell.2007.11.025.
22. Camidge DR, Bang YJ, Kwak EL, Iafrate AJ, Varella-Garcia M, Fox SB, et al. Activity and safety of crizotinib in patients with ALK-positive non-small-cell lung cancer: updated results from a phase 1 study. Lancet Oncol. 2012;13(10):1011–9. https://doi.org/10.1016/S1470-2045(12)70344-3.
23. Shaw AT, Yeap BY, Solomon BJ, Riely GJ, Gainor J, Engelman JA, et al. Effect of crizotinib on overall survival in patients with advanced non-small-cell lung cancer harbouring ALK gene rearrangement: a retrospective analysis. Lancet Oncol. 2011;12(11):1004–12. https://doi.org/10.1016/S1470-2045(11)70232-7.
24. Robinson DR, Wu YM, Lin SF. The protein tyrosine kinase family of the human genome. Oncogene. 2000;19(49):5548–57. https://doi.org/10.1038/sj.onc.1203957.
25. Ou SH, Tan J, Yen Y, Soo RA. ROS1 as a 'druggable' receptor tyrosine kinase: lessons learned from inhibiting the ALK pathway. Expert Rev Anticancer Ther. 2012;12(4):447–56. https://doi.org/10.1586/era.12.17.
26. Takeuchi K, Soda M, Togashi Y, Suzuki R, Sakata S, Hatano S, et al. RET, ROS1 and ALK fusions in lung cancer. Nat Med. 2012;18(3):378–81. https://doi.org/10.1038/nm.2658.
27. Suehara Y, Arcila M, Wang L, Hasanovic A, Ang D, Ito T, et al. Identification of KIF5B-RET and GOPC-ROS1 fusions in lung adenocarcinomas through a comprehensive mRNA-based screen for tyrosine kinase fusions. Clin Cancer Res. 2012;18:6599. https://doi.org/10.1158/1078-0432.CCR-12-0838.
28. Gu TL, Deng X, Huang F, Tucker M, Crosby K, Rimkunas V, et al. Survey of tyrosine kinase signaling reveals ROS kinase fusions in human cholangiocarcinoma. PLoS One. 2011;6(1):e15640. https://doi.org/10.1371/journal.pone.0015640.
29. McDermott U, Iafrate AJ, Gray NS, Shioda T, Classon M, Maheswaran S, et al. Genomic alterations of anaplastic lymphoma kinase may sensitize tumors to anaplastic lymphoma kinase inhibitors. Cancer Res. 2008;68(9):3389–95. https://doi.org/10.1158/0008-5472.CAN-07-6186.
30. Bergethon K, Shaw AT, Ou SH, Katayama R, Lovly CM, McDonald NT, et al. ROS1 rearrangements define a unique molecular class of lung cancers. J Clin Oncol. 2012;30(8):863–70. https://doi.org/10.1200/JCO.2011.35.6345.
31. Davies H, Bignell GR, Cox C, Stephens P, Edkins S, Clegg S, et al. Mutations of the BRAF gene in human cancer. Nature. 2002;417(6892):949–54. https://doi.org/10.1038/nature00766.
32. Brose MS, Volpe P, Feldman M, Kumar M, Rishi I, Gerrero R, et al. BRAF and RAS mutations in human lung cancer and melanoma. Cancer Res. 2002;62(23):6997–7000.
33. Naoki K, Chen TH, Richards WG, Sugarbaker DJ, Meyerson M. Missense mutations of the BRAF gene in human lung adenocarcinoma. Cancer Res. 2002;62(23):7001–3.
34. Paik PK, Arcila ME, Fara M, Sima CS, Miller VA, Kris MG, et al. Clinical characteristics of patients with lung adenocarcinomas harboring BRAF mutations. J Clin Oncol. 2011;29(15):2046–51. https://doi.org/10.1200/JCO.2010.33.1280.
35. Pratilas CA, Hanrahan AJ, Halilovic E, Persaud Y, Soh J, Chitale D, et al. Genetic predictors of MEK dependence in non-small cell lung cancer. Cancer Res. 2008;68(22):9375–83. https://doi.org/10.1158/0008-5472.CAN-08-2223.
36. Forbes SA, Bhamra G, Bamford S, Dawson E, Kok C, Clements J, et al. The catalogue of somatic mutations in cancer (COSMIC). Curr Protoc Hum Genet 2008;Chapter 10:Unit 10.11. https://doi.org/10.1002/0471142905.hg1011s57.

37. Gautschi O, Pauli C, Strobel K, Hirschmann A, Printzen G, Aebi S, et al. A patient with BRAF V600E lung adenocarcinoma responding to vemurafenib. J Thorac Oncol. 2012;7(10):e23–4. https://doi.org/10.1097/JTO.0b013e3182629903.
38. Rudin CM, Hong K, Streit M. Molecular characterization of acquired resistance to the BRAF inhibitor dabrafenib in a patient with BRAF-mutant non-small-cell lung cancer. J Thorac Oncol. 2013;8(5):e41–2. https://doi.org/10.1097/JTO.0b013e31828bb1b3.
39. Planchard D, Smit EF, Groen HJM, Mazieres J, Besse B, Helland A, et al. Dabrafenib plus trametinib in patients with previously untreated BRAF(V600E)-mutant metastatic non-small-cell lung cancer: an open-label, phase 2 trial. Lancet Oncol. 2017;18(10):1307–16. https://doi.org/10.1016/S1470-2045(17)30679-4.
40. www.FDA.GOV. FDA grants regular approval to dabrafenib and trametinib combination for metastatic NSCLC with BRAF V600E mutation. 2018.
41. Vaishnavi A, Capelletti M, Le AT, Kako S, Butaney M, Ercan D, et al. Oncogenic and drug-sensitive NTRK1 rearrangements in lung cancer. Nat Med. 2013;19(11):1469–72. https://doi.org/10.1038/nm.3352.
42. Farago AF, Taylor MS, Doebele RC, Zhu VW, Kummar S, Spira AI, et al. Clinicopathologic features of non-small-cell lung cancer harboring an NTRK gene fusion. JCO Precis Oncol. 2018;2018. https://doi.org/10.1200/PO.18.00037.
43. Farago AF, Azzoli CG. Beyond ALK and ROS1: RET, NTRK, EGFR and BRAF gene rearrangements in non-small cell lung cancer. Transl Lung Cancer Res. 2017;6(5):550–9. https://doi.org/10.21037/tlcr.2017.08.02.
44. Farago AF, Le LP, Zheng Z, Muzikansky A, Drilon A, Patel M, et al. Durable clinical response to entrectinib in NTRK1-rearranged non-small cell lung cancer. J Thorac Oncol. 2015;10(12):1670–4. https://doi.org/10.1097/01.JTO.0000473485.38553.f0.
45. Riely GJ, Marks J, Pao W. KRAS mutations in non-small cell lung cancer. Proc Am Thorac Soc. 2009;6(2):201–5. https://doi.org/10.1513/pats.200809-107LC.
46. Sun Y, Ren Y, Fang Z, Li C, Fang R, Gao B, et al. Lung adenocarcinoma from East Asian never-smokers is a disease largely defined by targetable oncogenic mutant kinases. J Clin Oncol. 2010;28(30):4616–20. https://doi.org/10.1200/JCO.2010.29.6038.
47. Riely GJ, Kris MG, Rosenbaum D, Marks J, Li A, Chitale DA, et al. Frequency and distinctive spectrum of KRAS mutations in never smokers with lung adenocarcinoma. Clin Cancer Res. 2008;14(18):5731–4. https://doi.org/10.1158/1078-0432.CCR-08-0646.
48. Arcila M, Lau C, Nafa K, Ladanyi M. Detection of KRAS and BRAF mutations in colorectal carcinoma roles for high-sensitivity locked nucleic acid-PCR sequencing and broad-spectrum mass spectrometry genotyping. J Mol Diagn. 2011;13(1):64–73. https://doi.org/10.1016/j.jmoldx.2010.11.005.
49. Le Calvez F, Mukeria A, Hunt JD, Kelm O, Hung RJ, Taniere P, et al. TP53 and KRAS mutation load and types in lung cancers in relation to tobacco smoke: distinct patterns in never, former, and current smokers. Cancer Res. 2005;65(12):5076–83. https://doi.org/10.1158/0008-5472.CAN-05-0551.
50. Shigematsu H, Takahashi T, Nomura M, Majmudar K, Suzuki M, Lee H, et al. Somatic mutations of the HER2 kinase domain in lung adenocarcinomas. Cancer Res. 2005;65(5):1642–6.
51. Stephens P, Hunter C, Bignell G, Edkins S, Davies H, Teague J, et al. Lung cancer: intragenic ERBB2 kinase mutations in tumours. Nature. 2004;431(7008):525–6.
52. Arcila ME, Chaft JE, Nafa K, Roy-Chowdhuri S, Lau C, Zaidinski M, et al. Prevalence, clinicopathologic associations, and molecular spectrum of ERBB2 (HER2) tyrosine kinase mutations in lung adenocarcinomas. Clin Cancer Res. 2012;18(18):4910–8. https://doi.org/10.1158/1078-0432.CCR-12-0912.
53. Ross HJ, Blumenschein GR Jr, Aisner J, Damjanov N, Dowlati A, Garst J, et al. Randomized phase II multicenter trial of two schedules of lapatinib as first- or second-line monotherapy in patients with advanced or metastatic non-small cell lung cancer. Clin Cancer Res. 2010;16(6):1938–49.

54. Yap TA, Vidal L, Adam J, Stephens P, Spicer J, Shaw H, et al. Phase I trial of the irreversible EGFR and HER2 kinase inhibitor BIBW 2992 in patients with advanced solid tumors. J Clin Oncol. 2010;28(25):3965–72.
55. Engelman JA, Zejnullahu K, Gale CM, Lifshits E, Gonzales AJ, Shimamura T, et al. PF00299804, an irreversible pan-ERBB inhibitor, is effective in lung cancer models with EGFR and ERBB2 mutations that are resistant to gefitinib. Cancer Res. 2007;67(24):11924–32.
56. Li BT, Shen R, Buonocore D, Olah ZT, Ni A, Ginsberg MS, et al. Ado-trastuzumab emtansine for patients with HER2-mutant lung cancers: results from a phase II basket trial. J Clin Oncol. 2018;36(24):2532–7. https://doi.org/10.1200/JCO.2018.77.9777.
57. Kris MG, Camidge DR, Giaccone G, Hida T, Li BT, O'Connell J, et al. Targeting HER2 aberrations as actionable drivers in lung cancers: phase II trial of the pan-HER tyrosine kinase inhibitor dacomitinib in patients with HER2-mutant or amplified tumors. Ann Oncol. 2015;26(7):1421–7. https://doi.org/10.1093/annonc/mdv186.
58. Azzoli CG, Krug LM, Miller VA, Kris MG, Mass R. Trastuzumab in the treatment of non-small cell lung cancer. Semin Oncol. 2002;29(1 Suppl 4):59–65.
59. Awad MM, Oxnard GR, Jackman DM, Savukoski DO, Hall D, Shivdasani P, et al. MET exon 14 mutations in non-small-cell lung cancer are associated with advanced age and stage-dependent MET genomic amplification and c-met overexpression. J Clin Oncol. 2016;34(7):721–30. https://doi.org/10.1200/JCO.2015.63.4600.
60. Frampton GM, Ali SM, Rosenzweig M, Chmielecki J, Lu X, Bauer TM, et al. Activation of MET via diverse exon 14 splicing alterations occurs in multiple tumor types and confers clinical sensitivity to MET inhibitors. Cancer Discov. 2015;5(8):850–9. https://doi.org/10.1158/2159-8290.CD-15-0285.
61. Jenkins RW, Oxnard GR, Elkin S, Sullivan EK, Carter JL, Barbie DA. Response to crizotinib in a patient with lung adenocarcinoma harboring a MET splice site mutation. Clin Lung Cancer. 2015;16(5):e101–4. https://doi.org/10.1016/j.cllc.2015.01.009.
62. Kollmannsberger CK, Sharma S, Shapiro G, Chi KN, Christensen J, Tassell VR. Phase I study of receptor tyrosine kinase (RTK) inhibitor, MGCD265, in patients (pts) with advanced solid tumors. ASCO Annual Meeting 2015. J Clin Oncol. 2015;33(15_suppl):2589.
63. Liu X, Jia Y, Stoopler MB, Shen Y, Cheng H, Chen J, et al. Next-generation sequencing of pulmonary sarcomatoid carcinoma reveals high frequency of actionable MET gene mutations. J Clin Oncol. 2016;34(8):794–802. https://doi.org/10.1200/JCO.2015.62.0674.
64. Onozato R, Kosaka T, Kuwano H, Sekido Y, Yatabe Y, Mitsudomi T. Activation of MET by gene amplification or by splice mutations deleting the juxtamembrane domain in primary resected lung cancers. J Thorac Oncol. 2009;4(1):5–11. https://doi.org/10.1097/JTO.0b013e3181913e0e.
65. Paik PK, Drilon A, Fan PD, Yu H, Rekhtman N, Ginsberg MS, et al. Response to MET inhibitors in patients with stage IV lung adenocarcinomas harboring MET mutations causing exon 14 skipping. Cancer Discov. 2015;5(8):842–9. https://doi.org/10.1158/2159-8290.CD-14-1467.
66. Seo JS, Ju YS, Lee WC, Shin JY, Lee JK, Bleazard T, et al. The transcriptional landscape and mutational profile of lung adenocarcinoma. Genome Res. 2012;22(11):2109–19. https://doi.org/10.1101/gr.145144.112.
67. Cancer Genome Atlas Research N. Comprehensive molecular profiling of lung adenocarcinoma. Nature. 2014;511(7511):543–50. https://doi.org/10.1038/nature13385.
68. Kong-Beltran M, Seshagiri S, Zha J, Zhu W, Bhawe K, Mendoza N, et al. Somatic mutations lead to an oncogenic deletion of met in lung cancer. Cancer Res. 2006;66(1):283–9. https://doi.org/10.1158/0008-5472.CAN-05-2749.
69. Bean J, Brennan C, Shih JY, Riely G, Viale A, Wang L, et al. MET amplification occurs with or without T790M mutations in EGFR mutant lung tumors with acquired resistance to gefitinib or erlotinib. Proc Natl Acad Sci U S A. 2007;104(52):20932–7. https://doi.org/10.1073/pnas.0710370104.
70. Cappuzzo F, Marchetti A, Skokan M, Rossi E, Gajapathy S, Felicioni L, et al. Increased MET gene copy number negatively affects survival of surgically resected non-small-cell lung cancer patients. J Clin Oncol. 2009;27(10):1667–74. https://doi.org/10.1200/JCO.2008.19.1635.

71. Chen HJ, Mok TS, Chen ZH, Guo AL, Zhang XC, Su J, et al. Clinicopathologic and molecular features of epidermal growth factor receptor T790M mutation and c-MET amplification in tyrosine kinase inhibitor-resistant Chinese non-small cell lung cancer. Pathol Oncol Res. 2009;15(4):651–8. https://doi.org/10.1007/s12253-009-9167-8.
72. Engelman JA, Zejnullahu K, Mitsudomi T, Song Y, Hyland C, Park JO, et al. MET amplification leads to gefitinib resistance in lung cancer by activating ERBB3 signaling. Science. 2007;316(5827):1039–43. https://doi.org/10.1126/science.1141478.
73. Kubo T, Yamamoto H, Lockwood WW, Valencia I, Soh J, Peyton M, et al. MET gene amplification or EGFR mutation activate MET in lung cancers untreated with EGFR tyrosine kinase inhibitors. Int J Cancer. 2009;124(8):1778–84. https://doi.org/10.1002/ijc.24150.
74. Okuda K, Sasaki H, Yukiue H, Yano M, Fujii Y. Met gene copy number predicts the prognosis for completely resected non-small cell lung cancer. Cancer Sci. 2008;99(11):2280–5. https://doi.org/10.1111/j.1349-7006.2008.00916.x.
75. Cappuzzo F, Janne PA, Skokan M, Finocchiaro G, Rossi E, Ligorio C, et al. MET increased gene copy number and primary resistance to gefitinib therapy in non-small-cell lung cancer patients. Ann Oncol. 2009;20(2):298–304. https://doi.org/10.1093/annonc/mdn635.
76. Go H, Jeon YK, Park HJ, Sung SW, Seo JW, Chung DH. High MET gene copy number leads to shorter survival in patients with non-small cell lung cancer. J Thorac Oncol. 2010;5(3):305–13. https://doi.org/10.1097/JTO.0b013e3181ce3d1d.
77. Arcila ME, Oxnard GR, Nafa K, Riely GJ, Solomon SB, Zakowski MF, et al. Rebiopsy of lung cancer patients with acquired resistance to EGFR inhibitors and enhanced detection of the T790M mutation using a locked nucleic acid-based assay. Clin Cancer Res. 2011;17(5):1169–80. https://doi.org/10.1158/1078-0432.CCR-10-2277.
78. Sequist LV, Waltman BA, Dias-Santagata D, Digumarthy S, Turke AB, Fidias P, et al. Genotypic and histological evolution of lung cancers acquiring resistance to EGFR inhibitors. Sci Transl Med. 2011;3(75):75ra26. https://doi.org/10.1126/scitranslmed.3002003.
79. Turke AB, Zejnullahu K, Wu YL, Song Y, Dias-Santagata D, Lifshits E, et al. Preexistence and clonal selection of MET amplification in EGFR mutant NSCLC. Cancer Cell. 2010;17(1):77–88. https://doi.org/10.1016/j.ccr.2009.11.022.
80. Takahashi M, Ritz J, Cooper GM. Activation of a novel human transforming gene, ret, by DNA rearrangement. Cell. 1985;42(2):581–8.
81. Phay JE, Shah MH. Targeting RET receptor tyrosine kinase activation in cancer. Clin Cancer Res. 2010;16(24):5936–41. https://doi.org/10.1158/1078-0432.CCR-09-0786.
82. Arighi E, Borrello MG, Sariola H. RET tyrosine kinase signaling in development and cancer. Cytokine Growth Factor Rev. 2005;16(4–5):441–67. https://doi.org/10.1016/j.cytogfr.2005.05.010.
83. Kohno T, Ichikawa H, Totoki Y, Yasuda K, Hiramoto M, Nammo T, et al. KIF5B-RET fusions in lung adenocarcinoma. Nat Med. 2012;18(3):375–7. https://doi.org/10.1038/nm.2644.
84. Lipson D, Capelletti M, Yelensky R, Otto G, Parker A, Jarosz M, et al. Identification of new ALK and RET gene fusions from colorectal and lung cancer biopsies. Nat Med. 2012;18(3):382–4. https://doi.org/10.1038/nm.2673.
85. Chaft JE, Arcila ME, Paik PK, Lau C, Riely GJ, Pietanza MC, et al. Coexistence of PIK3CA and other oncogene mutations in lung adenocarcinoma-rationale for comprehensive mutation profiling. Mol Cancer Ther. 2012;11(2):485–91. https://doi.org/10.1158/1535-7163.MCT-11-0692.
86. Kawano O, Sasaki H, Endo K, Suzuki E, Haneda H, Yukiue H, et al. PIK3CA mutation status in Japanese lung cancer patients. Lung Cancer. 2006;54(2):209–15. https://doi.org/10.1016/j.lungcan.2006.07.006.
87. Bendell JC, Rodon J, Burris HA, de Jonge M, Verweij J, Birle D, et al. Phase I, dose-escalation study of BKM120, an oral pan-Class I PI3K inhibitor, in patients with advanced solid tumors. J Clin Oncol. 2012;30(3):282–90. https://doi.org/10.1200/JCO.2011.36.1360.
88. Hyman DM, Snyder AE, Carvajal RD, Gerecitano JF, Voss MH, Ho AL, et al. Parallel phase Ib studies of two schedules of buparlisib (BKM120) plus carboplatin and paclitaxel (q21 days or q28 days) for patients with advanced solid tumors. Cancer Chemother Pharmacol. 2015;75(4):747–55. https://doi.org/10.1007/s00280-015-2693-z.

89. Mayer IA, Abramson VG, Isakoff SJ, Forero A, Balko JM, Kuba MG, et al. Stand up to cancer phase Ib study of pan-phosphoinositide-3-kinase inhibitor buparlisib with letrozole in estrogen receptor-positive/human epidermal growth factor receptor 2-negative metastatic breast cancer. J Clin Oncol. 2014;32(12):1202–9. https://doi.org/10.1200/JCO.2013.54.0518.
90. Vansteenkiste JF, Canon JL, De Braud F, Grossi F, De Pas T, Gray JE, et al. Safety and efficacy of buparlisib (BKM120) in patients with PI3K pathway-activated non-small cell lung cancer: results from the phase II BASALT-1 study. J Thorac Oncol. 2015;10(9):1319–27. https://doi.org/10.1097/JTO.0000000000000607.
91. Cowley S, Paterson H, Kemp P, Marshall CJ. Activation of MAP kinase kinase is necessary and sufficient for PC12 differentiation and for transformation of NIH 3T3 cells. Cell. 1994;77(6):841–52.
92. Mansour SJ, Candia JM, Gloor KK, Ahn NG. Constitutively active mitogen-activated protein kinase kinase 1 (MAPKK1) and MAPKK2 mediate similar transcriptional and morphological responses. Cell Growth Differ. 1996;7(2):243–50.
93. Mansour SJ, Matten WT, Hermann AS, Candia JM, Rong S, Fukasawa K, et al. Transformation of mammalian cells by constitutively active MAP kinase kinase. Science. 1994;265(5174):966–70.
94. Arcila ME, Drilon A, Sylvester BE, Lovly CM, Borsu L, Reva B, et al. MAP2K1 (MEK1) mutations define a distinct subset of lung adenocarcinoma associated with smoking. Clin Cancer Res. 2015;21(8):1935–43. https://doi.org/10.1158/1078-0432.CCR-14-2124.
95. Marks JL, Gong Y, Chitale D, Golas B, McLellan MD, Kasai Y, et al. Novel MEK1 mutation identified by mutational analysis of epidermal growth factor receptor signaling pathway genes in lung adenocarcinoma. Cancer Res. 2008;68(14):5524–8. https://doi.org/10.1158/0008-5472.CAN-08-0099.
96. Helsten T, Elkin S, Arthur E, Tomson BN, Carter J, Kurzrock R. The FGFR landscape in cancer: analysis of 4,853 tumors by next-generation sequencing. Clin Cancer Res. 2016;22(1):259–67. https://doi.org/10.1158/1078-0432.CCR-14-3212.
97. Majewski IJ, Mittempergher L, Davidson NM, Bosma A, Willems SM, Horlings HM, et al. Identification of recurrent FGFR3 fusion genes in lung cancer through kinome-centred RNA sequencing. J Pathol. 2013;230(3):270–6. https://doi.org/10.1002/path.4209.
98. Ou SI, Horn L, Cruz M, Vafai D, Lovly CM, Spradlin A, et al. Emergence of FGFR3-TACC3 fusions as a potential by-pass resistance mechanism to EGFR tyrosine kinase inhibitors in EGFR mutated NSCLC patients. Lung Cancer. 2017;111:61–4. https://doi.org/10.1016/j.lungcan.2017.07.006.
99. Riely GJ, Yu HA. EGFR: the paradigm of an oncogene-driven lung cancer. Clin Cancer Res. 2015;21(10):2221–6. https://doi.org/10.1158/1078-0432.CCR-14-3154.
100. Kobayashi S, Boggon TJ, Dayaram T, Janne PA, Kocher O, Meyerson M, et al. EGFR mutation and resistance of non-small-cell lung cancer to gefitinib. N Engl J Med. 2005;352(8):786–92. https://doi.org/10.1056/NEJMoa044238.
101. Yu HA, Arcila ME, Rekhtman N, Sima CS, Zakowski MF, Pao W, et al. Analysis of tumor specimens at the time of acquired resistance to EGFR-TKI therapy in 155 patients with EGFR-mutant lung cancers. Clin Cancer Res. 2013;19(8):2240–7. https://doi.org/10.1158/1078-0432.CCR-12-2246.
102. Yun CH, Mengwasser KE, Toms AV, Woo MS, Greulich H, Wong KK, et al. The T790M mutation in EGFR kinase causes drug resistance by increasing the affinity for ATP. Proc Natl Acad Sci U S A. 2008;105(6):2070–5. https://doi.org/10.1073/pnas.0709662105.
103. Soria JC, Ramalingam SS. Osimertinib in EGFR mutation-positive advanced NSCLC. N Engl J Med. 2018;378(13):1262–3. https://doi.org/10.1056/NEJMc1801669.
104. Offin M, Rizvi H, Tenet M, Ni A, Sanchez-Vega F, Li BT, et al. Tumor mutation burden and efficacy of EGFR-tyrosine kinase inhibitors in patients with EGFR-mutant lung cancers. Clin Cancer Res. 2018;25:1063. https://doi.org/10.1158/1078-0432.CCR-18-1102.
105. Piotrowska Z, Isozaki H, Lennerz JK, Gainor JF, Lennes IT, Zhu VW, et al. Landscape of acquired resistance to osimertinib in EGFR-mutant NSCLC and clinical validation of com-

bined EGFR and RET inhibition with osimertinib and BLU-667 for acquired RET fusion. Cancer Discov. 2018;8(12):1529–39. https://doi.org/10.1158/2159-8290.CD-18-1022.

106. Gainor JF, Dardaei L, Yoda S, Friboulet L, Leshchiner I, Katayama R, et al. Molecular mechanisms of resistance to first- and second-generation ALK inhibitors in ALK-rearranged lung cancer. Cancer Discov. 2016;6(10):1118–33. https://doi.org/10.1158/2159-8290.CD-16-0596.
107. Lindeman NI, Cagle PT, Beasley MB, Chitale DA, Dacic S, Giaccone G, et al. Molecular testing guideline for selection of lung cancer patients for EGFR and ALK tyrosine kinase inhibitors: guideline from the College of American Pathologists, International Association for the Study of Lung Cancer, and Association for Molecular Pathology. J Mol Diagn. 2013;15(4):415–53. https://doi.org/10.1016/j.jmoldx.2013.03.001.
108. Lindeman NI, Cagle PT, Aisner DL, Arcila ME, Beasley MB, Bernicker EH, et al. Updated molecular testing guideline for the selection of lung cancer patients for treatment with targeted tyrosine kinase inhibitors: guideline from the College of American Pathologists, the International Association for the Study of Lung Cancer, and the Association for Molecular Pathology. J Mol Diagn. 2018;20(2):129–59. https://doi.org/10.1016/j.jmoldx.2017.11.004.
109. Jordan EJ, Kim HR, Arcila ME, Barron DA, Chakravarty D, Gao J, et al. Prospective comprehensive molecular characterization of lung adenocarcinomas for efficient patient matching to approved and emerging therapies. Cancer Discov. 2017;7:596. https://doi.org/10.1158/2159-8290.CD-16-1337.

Chapter 7
GI Including GIST

Efsevia Vakiani

Key Points

- Microsatellite instability testing is recommended for all patients with colorectal adenocarcinoma and advanced gastric adenocarcinoma.
- Patients with colorectal adenocarcinoma being considered for anti-EGFR therapy should be tested for hotspot mutations in all exons of the *KRAS* and *NRAS* genes.
- Patients with gastrointestinal stromal tumors being considered for treatment with tyrosine kinase inhibitors should undergo mutational testing for mutations in the *KIT* and *PDGFRA* genes.

Key Online Resources

- NCCN guidelines for the management of colorectal cancer: https://www.nccn.org/professionals/physician_gls/pdf/colon.pdf
- NCCN guidelines for the management of gastric cancer: https://www.nccn.org/professionals/physician_gls/pdf/gastric.pdf
- NCCN guidelines for the management of gastrointestinal stromal tumors: https://www.nccn.org/professionals/physician_gls/pdf/sarcoma.pdf
- ASCP/CAP/AMP/ASCO Colorectal Biomarker Guidelines: https://www.amp.org/clinical-practice/practice-guidelines/colorectal-biomarker-guideline

E. Vakiani (✉)
Department of Pathology, Memorial Sloan-Kettering Cancer Center, New York, NY, USA
e-mail: vakianie@mskcc.org

L. J. Tafe, M. E. Arcila (eds.), *Genomic Medicine*,
https://doi.org/10.1007/978-3-030-22922-1_7

Introduction

The era of precision oncology has placed the spotlight on molecular biomarkers that can stratify patients and predict response to therapy. In gastrointestinal (GI) carcinomas, several molecular biomarkers, such as KRAS mutations in colorectal cancer (CRC) and *HER2* gene amplification in gastroesophageal (GE) carcinomas, are a critical part of patient management, while other biomarkers are gaining increasing attention as new targeted therapies are being developed and/or novel resistance mechanisms are identified. This chapter discusses both established and emerging molecular biomarkers in the most common adenocarcinomas of the GI tract, namely, CRC and GE adenocarcinomas. It also outlines key genetic alterations important in the management of gastrointestinal stromal tumors (GISTs), which are the most common mesenchymal tumor of the GI tract. Finally, it summarizes common hereditary GI cancer syndromes and the genetic aberrations that underlie them. Detecting these alterations in the patient's germline DNA has important implications for the management of both patients and their family members.

Microsatellite Instability in Colorectal and Gastric Adenocarcinomas

Microsatellites are short sequences of genomic DNA that contain tandem repeats 1–6 base pairs in length. They are especially prone to mistakes during replication, and, when tumors have defects in DNA mismatch repair (MMR) proteins, microsatellites show variability in their size, a phenomenon referred to as microsatellite instability (MSI). Determination of MSI status is important both in CRC and gastric adenocarcinomas both for identifying families with germline deleterious mutations and for treatment purposes.

In CRC MSI is seen in approximately 15% of cases, the majority arising sporadically. These sporadic cases have a predilection for the right colon of elderly female patients and commonly show hypermethylation of the *MLH1* gene promoter and/or a BRAF V600E mutation. Recently, the presence of somatic biallelic mutations in the MMR genes, *MLH1*, *MSH2*, *MSH6*, and *PMS2*, has also been documented [1]. In contrast to sporadic cases, approximately 3% of microsatellite unstable (MSI-H) tumors are seen in patients with Lynch syndrome who harbor germline deleterious mutations in MMR genes and *EPCAM*. In gastric cancer MSI is detected in approximately 20% of adenocarcinomas, though it is probably lower in Caucasian populations [2]. These tumors are commonly of intestinal type, located in the distal stomach of elderly female patients and similar to CRC are sporadic in the vast majority of cases [2, 3].

Determination of MSI status with the goal of identifying families with Lynch syndrome has been an important component of the clinical management of patients with CRC for two decades. More recently, MSI has emerged as at least one positive predictor of response to immunotherapy in many types of solid tumors, further expanding the patient population that may benefit from MSI testing [4]. The current

2018 NCCN guidelines for CRC recommend universal testing in all patients with a personal history of CRC, while for gastric cancer they state that MMR or MSI testing should be considered on locally advanced, recurrent, or metastatic carcinomas, in patients who are candidates for treatment with PD-1 inhibitors [5, 6].

Microsatellite instability can be assessed in several ways. The approach most often used is immunohistochemistry (IHC) using antibodies against MLH1, MSH2, MSH6, and PMS2. In the molecular pathology laboratory, the traditional method of testing has been polymerase chain reaction (PCR) using fluorescently labeled primers against select microsatellites. Guidelines on the number and type of microsatellites that constitute the most sensitive panel have changed over the years, and currently it is recommended by the National Cancer Institute/International Collaborative Group/HNPCC that five mononucleotide repeats be used [7]. Both tumor and normal DNA from the same patient are required with this method and assessment of MSI is done by comparing the results from the normal and tumor specimen (Fig. 7.1). Microsatellite stable (MSS) tumors are expected to show the same size between tumor and normal DNA in all microsatellite sequences, while MSI-H tumors are characterized by altered size in ≥40% of loci.

More recently, investigators have begun looking into using next generation sequencing (NGS) data, which normally includes information on multiple genes, to assess for the presence of MSI [8]. Such methods allow for MSI status to be reported as part of broader profiling and can also yield germline information in patients that have been

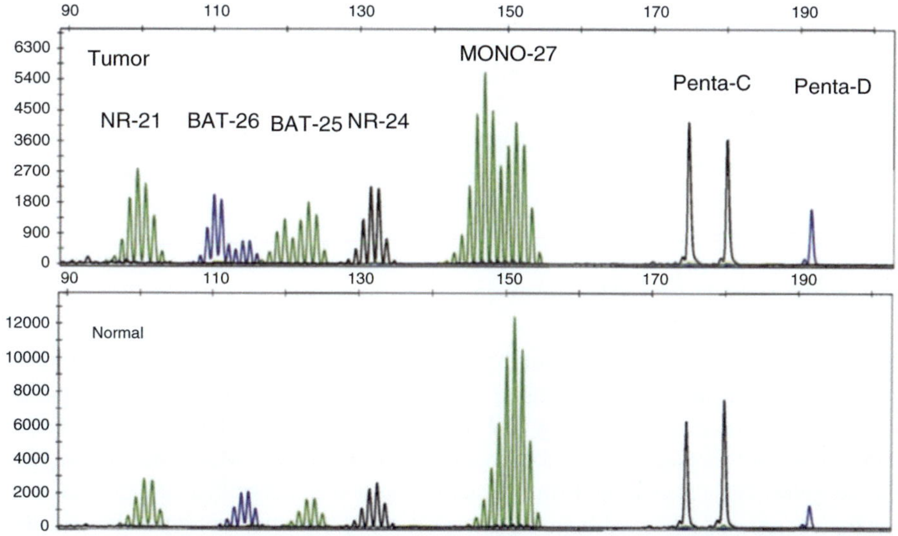

Fig. 7.1 Microsatellite analysis using five mononucleotides repeat markers (NR-21, NR-24, BAT-25, BAT-26, MONO-27). The appearance of new alleles in the tumor sample in two or more loci allows for the tumor to be classified as microsatellite unstable (MSI-H). Polymorphic pentanucleotide markers are used to confirm that the tumor and normal samples are from the same patient

consented for germline testing. They do have a longer turnaround time compared to IHC and PCR and can only be performed in laboratories with NGS platforms.

MLH1 *Promoter Hypermethylation in CRC*

As most MSI-H tumors are sporadic, the diagnosis of Lynch syndrome is ultimately based on identifying germline pathogenic events by sequencing germline DNA. As this process can be costly and time consuming, it is recommended that, after a tumor is categorized as MSI-H, additional tests be performed that can discriminate between sporadic and familial MSI-H cases. *MLH1* promoter hypermethylation is common among sporadic MSI-H tumors and its presence argues against Lynch syndrome. It is important, however, to keep in mind that exceptions do occur and rare cases of patients with Lynch syndrome showing *MLH1* promoter hypermethylation have been reported [9]. This has led some authors to recommend that cases showing *MLH1* promoter hypermethylation be considered for follow-up testing for a germline *MLH1* mutation and/or epimutation, if they present under the age of 60 years and/or the tumor does not harbor a *BRAF* mutation [10].

The first step in determining *MLH1* gene promoter methylation involves treatment of DNA with bisulfite which converts cytosine residues without methylation to uracil but does not affect 5-methylcytosine residues. The altered DNA can then be examined by various methods such as PCR, pyrosequencing, and high-resolution melting analysis. A popular method is methylation-specific PCR which uses methylated and unmethylated specific primer pairs, and determination of methylation status is based on which specific primers result in amplification. More recently, there is increasing interest in the use of microarray-based methods which can be used to generate genome-wide methylation, although they can be costly and time consuming [11].

RAS Mutations in CRC

Members of the RAS family are small guanine nucleotide-binding proteins that alternate between an inactive GDP-bound and an active GTP-bound state and regulate many cellular processes including proliferation and apoptosis. They are encoded by three genes *KRAS*, *NRAS*, and *HRAS* with four coding exons. Mutations in key parts of the genes can result in constitutive activation and uncontrolled cell growth, and such mutations are observed frequently in a variety of human tumor types. In CRC the majority of patients (~30–40%) harbor mutations in KRAS codons 12 and 13 located in exon 2. Another 10% of CRC patients have mutations in exons 3 (codon 61) and 4 (codons 117 and 146) of *KRAS* as well as mutations in *NRAS* exons 2–4 (Table 7.1).

The RAS proteins act as a key signal transducer for a number of cellular receptors including the epidermal growth factor receptor (EGFR) (Fig. 7.2). The latter is a transmembrane receptor tyrosine kinase which is a member of the ErbB family of

Table 7.1 Clinically significant genetic alterations in CRC

	Gene	Alteration(s)	Frequency	Common mutations	Clinical relevance
Established biomarkers	*KRAS*	Single-base substitution Amplification (less common)	30–40%	Exon 2: G12D/V/C/A/S/R G13D/C Exon 3: Q61H/K/R/L Exon 4: K117N, A146P/T/V	Confer resistance to EGFR inhibitors
	NRAS	Single-base substitution Amplification (less common)	4–9%	Exon 2: G12D/C/A/S G13D/R/C Exon 3: Q61R/L/K/H	Confer resistance to EGFR inhibitors
	BRAF	Single-base substitution Fusions (less common) Amplification (less common)	8–15%	V600E	Supports sporadic origin of an MSI-H tumor Renders tumor eligible for treatment with BRAF inhibitors (in combination with other drugs, including an EGFR inhibitor)
	MLH1 *MSH2* *MSH6* *PMS2* *EPCAM*	Single-base substitution Small indels Large deletions or duplications	15%	Alterations distributed throughout the genes	Result in MSI-H phenotype Confer sensitivity to immunotherapy Germline mutations seen in patients with Lynch syndrome
	MLH1 promoter	Hypermethylation	10%	NA	Supports sporadic origin of a microsatellite unstable tumor
Emerging biomarkers	*PIK3CA*	Single-base substitution	15–20%	R88Q, G106V, C420R, E542K, E545K/G, Q546R, M1043I, H1047R/L	Possible benefit from aspirin May confer resistance to EGFR inhibitors
	ERBB2	Amplification Single-base substitution	4–8%	A293T, S310F, R678Q, L755S, D769N/Y, V777L, V824I	Confer resistance to EGFR inhibitors Confer sensitivity to targeted therapy with ERBB2 inhibitors
	EGFR	Single-base substitution Amplification Fusions (rare)	4%	G465E/R, D761N, V843I, L861Q	Amplifications associated with response to EGFR inhibitors Some mutations confer resistance to EGFR inhibitors
	FGFR1–4	Amplification Rearrangement	2–3%	NA	Confer sensitivity to FGFR inhibitors Associated with resistance to EGFR inhibitors
	MAP2K1/ MEK1	Single-base substitution	2%	Q56P, K57N/T/E, E102_I103del	Associated with resistance to EGFR and BRAF inhibitors
	MET	Amplification	1–2%	NA	Confer sensitivity to MET inhibitors Associated with resistance to EGFR inhibitors
	RET	Rearrangement	<0.5%	NCO4-RET	Confer sensitivity to targeted therapy with RET inhibitors
	NTRK1–3	Rearrangement	<0.5%	NTRK1-LMNA	Confer sensitivity to NTRK inhibitors

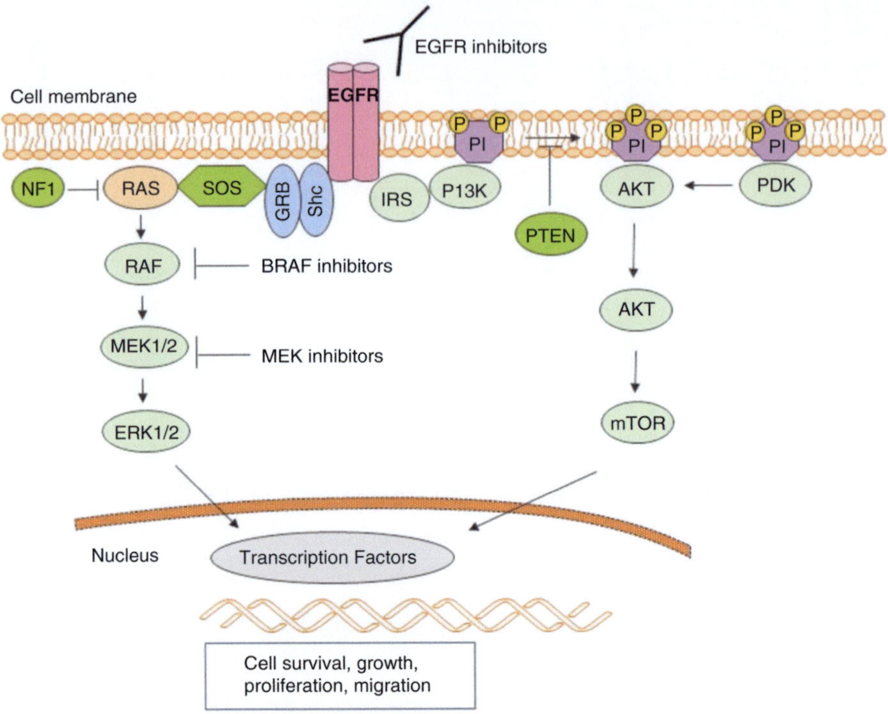

Fig. 7.2 Schematic representation of the EGFR signaling pathway. Binding of growth factors to the extracellular domain of EGFR activates the receptor, which in turn activates cytoplasmic proteins that are part of signaling pathways including the RAS/RAF/MEK1/2 and PI3K/AKT pathways. The 2 EGFR inhibitors used in the treatment of colon cancer are antibodies that bind to the extracellular domain of EGFR preventing ligand binding and activation

receptors. Upon binding of its specific ligands, it forms an active dimer and signals through several pathways. Inhibition of the EGFR protein by the humanized antibodies cetuximab and panitumumab blocks signaling and is approved for the treatment of stage IV CRC. According to current NCCN criteria and the American Society of Clinical Oncology, these drugs should not be given to patients with any known *KRAS* or *NRAS* mutation as tumors harboring such mutations are not responsive to EGFR inhibition [12]. Although initial testing had focused on the most common KRAS mutations, namely, those in codons 12 and 13 of exon 2, it is important that current testing in patients who are candidates for an EGFR inhibitor encompasses KRAS and NRAS hotspot mutations in all exons [5, 13].

BRAF Alterations in CRC

BRAF is a serine/threonine protein, which similar to RAS proteins is an integral mediator of EGFR signaling (Fig. 7.2). The *BRAF* gene is mutated in 8–15% of

CRC cases and the most prevalent mutation is a valine to glutamate change at residue 600 (V600E). This amino acid change leads to a constitutively active protein activation leading to unregulated cell proliferation, and testing for this mutation is important in several contexts.

Identification of *BRAF* mutations in CRC is helpful in two clinical contexts. First, similar to *MLH1* gene promoter hypermethylation, the presence of a V600E mutation can be useful in categorizing an MSI-H tumor as sporadic or familial [14]. The mutation is especially prevalent among sporadic MSI-H tumors, where approximately 50% of cases are positive. In contrast, it is typically not encountered in patients with Lynch syndrome. As with *MLH1* gene promoter hypermethylation exceptions have been reported, highlighting again the importance of interpreting test results in the context of all available clinical data including family history [15].

Identifying a BRAF V600E mutation is also used for treatment purposes, although some of these data are more controversial. Although there isn't universal agreement that BRAF mutations mediate resistance to EGFR inhibitors, the current NCCN guidelines state that BRAF V600E mutation makes response to cetuximab or panitumumab highly unlikely unless given with a BRAF inhibitor and recommend *BRAF* genotyping of tumor tissue in patients with stage IV disease [5, 16]. In contrast to melanoma, the BRAF inhibitor vemurafenib has very limited activity in V600E mutant CRC as monotherapy [17]. Combining vemurafenib and cetuximab with or without conventional chemotherapy shows better results, although the response rates do not exceed 35% [18]. More recently, the combination of a BRAF inhibitor encorafenib and cetuximab and the MEK inhibitor binimetinib showed promising results, and a phase III trial is currently under way to evaluate the efficacy of this regimen for the treatment of BRAF V600E mutant CRC.

A small number of CRC harbor mutations outside V600 and many of these are considered to be oncogenic. Their clinical implications are not fully understood because of their rarity, and it is not clear if they mediate resistance to EGFR inhibitors. They differ from V600E mutant proteins by signaling as dimers as well as in the degree in which they activate ERK signaling. Most importantly, they are not sensitive to BRAF V600E inhibitors such as vemurafenib, and novel targeted therapies are being developed for these tumors [19]. BRAF fusions and amplifications may also be seen in a small number of CRC cases (<0.5%); they are deemed to be oncogenic though clinical response of such tumors to various inhibitors is not well studied.

HER2 Alterations in Upper Gastrointestinal Adenocarcinomas and CRC

The human epidermal growth factor receptor 2 (HER2, HER2/neu, ERBB2) is a transmembrane tyrosine kinase receptor protein with the same basic molecular structure as EGFR. HER2 is overexpressed in a number of different cancer types, including breast, stomach, esophagus, and colon, and in the vast majority of cases, this is a result of *HER2* gene amplification. In gastroesophageal adenocarcinomas,

HER2 is overexpressed in approximately 15–20% of cases, and among gastric tumors overexpression is significantly more common in intestinal-type adenocarcinomas compared to diffuse type [20]. These HER2-positive tumors show clinical response to HER2 inhibition with anti-HER2 antibodies like trastuzumab, and for this reason HER2 testing has become standard of practice in the treatment of patients with GE adenocarcinomas [21].

In clinical practice advanced carcinomas are routinely assessed for HER2 status by performing IHC and scoring the stained slides using the Hofmann-modified criteria [22]. Cases scored as 2+ are considered equivocal and further analyzed by fluorescence in situ hybridization (FISH). More recently, investigators have also been looking into using NGS data to derive copy number alterations and determine HER2 status, as this would be more efficient compared to a single-gene assay [23]. This approach is more dependent on tumor content, and false-negative results may be obtained in cases with tumor content, especially in the context of low level amplification in the *HER2* gene. It is also important to keep in mind that compared to breast adenocarcinomas, GE tumors show increased heterogeneity in HER2 expression, and this can also lead to a negative result by NGS, even if there is a clone showing amplification.

In CRC *HER2* amplification is observed in 3% of cases, while another 4–5% of cases harbor somatic mutations including the hotspot kinase domain mutations V777L and V824I which activate HER2 signaling [24]. Currently testing for *HER2* amplification is not part of standard of care for CRC patients, but there is emerging data that it might be a useful predictive biomarker, and testing is often performed for enrollment in clinical trials. Both *HER2*-amplified and *HER2* mutant cases have been reported to show de novo and acquired resistance to EGFR inhibitors [25, 26] as they cause persistent ERK signaling even in the presence of cetuximab. Furthermore, *HER2*-amplified (*KRAS* exon 2 wild-type) metastatic CRC tumors appear to respond to treatment with a combination of trastuzumab and lapatinib [27]. Whether the presence of a HER2 hotspot mutation can serve as a positive predictor of response to treatment remains to be determined. Preliminary results of a trial using the pan-HER2 tyrosine kinase inhibitor, neratinib, to treat HER2 and HER3 mutant tumors did not show a response in CRC or GE adenocarcinomas, and investigators are currently attempting dual inhibition using a second HER2 inhibitor in addition to neratinib [28].

PIK3CA Mutations in CRC

The *PIK3CA* gene encodes the catalytic subunit of phosphatidylinositol 3-kinase (PI3K) which is also a downstream effector of EGFR signaling (Fig. 7.2). Mutations in *PIK3CA* occur in 15–20% of CRC with the majority of these mutations being in the helical (exon 9) or catalytic (exon 20) domain and resulting in the functional activation of PI3K (Table 7.1). Testing for these mutations is currently not part of standard clinical practice. Initial studies provided conflicting results regarding response of PIK3CA mutant tumors to EGFR inhibitor therapy with some investigators reporting resistance to panitumumab or cetuximab among tumors harboring *PIK3CA* mutations [29], while others failed to find a correlation [30]. Two recent retrospective studies reported an interesting association between *PIK3CA* mutations and better outcomes in patients taking aspirin following diagnosis of CRC [31, 32]. They suggested that in CRC patients PIK3CA mutations may serve as a predictive molecular biomarker for adjuvant aspirin therapy, but prospective studies are warranted before this can be incorporated into clinical practice.

Other Emerging Biomarkers in CRC and Upper Gastrointestinal Adenocarcinomas

MET Amplification

The mesenchymal-epithelial transition (MET) protein is a receptor tyrosine kinase that is activated by binding its ligand, HGF, and signals via multiple pathways including the RAS and PI3K pathways, regulating cell proliferation and migration. *MET* gene amplification which is found in approximately 5% of GE adenocarcinomas and 1–2% of CRC leads to constitutive receptor activation independent of ligand. Inhibitors of MET are under development with some showing efficacy in MET-amplified GE tumors [33]. MET amplification was also shown to mediate resistance to HER2 inhibitors in GE adenocarcinomas with *HER2* amplification, and these tumors may respond to dual inhibition of MET and HER2 [34]. Similarly to what was observed in GE adenocarcinomas, MET amplification has been implicated in both primary and acquired resistance to EGFR inhibition in CRC.

EGFR Alterations

Contrary to non-small cell lung cancer, EGFR mutations are infrequent in CRC and GE adenocarcinomas, but have been reported in the context of secondary resistance following treatment of CRC tumors with anti-EGFR antibodies. The majority of mutations found in this setting are in the extracellular domain of the protein that is involved in the binding of the EGFR inhibitor (S464L, G465R, I491M, and S492R), though rare mutations in the kinase domain of EGFR have also been reported [25, 35].

Amplifications in *EGFR* are found in approximately 6% and 2% of GE adenocarcinomas and CRCs, respectively. In CRC *EGFR* amplification is associated with response to EGFR inhibitors, but it is not used clinically to select patients as tumors without amplification also show response. In GE adenocarcinomas, *EGFR* amplification has been associated with resistance to trastuzumab [36]. Tumors with co-amplification in HER2 and EGFR were found to respond clinically to treatment with afatinib which is an inhibitor of both HER2 and EGFR [34].

MAP2K1 Mutations

Mitogen-activated protein kinase 1 (MAP2K1), also called MEK1, is a dual-specific serine/threonine and tyrosine kinase that lies downstream of RAS and is activated when phosphorylated by RAF kinase (Fig. 7.2). Mutations in MEK1 that cause constitutive activation occur in approximately 1% of CRC and have been reported to mediate resistance to EGFR and BRAF inhibitors [37, 38].

FGFR Alterations

Fibroblast growth factor receptors (FGFRs) are a family of tyrosine kinase receptors encoded by four different genes (FGFR1–4). These receptors share the same canonical protein structure and affect signaling pathways involved in cell proliferation, differentiation, and angiogenesis. FGFR aberrations are found in approximately 7% of carcinomas with amplification being the most common abnormality [39]. FGFR1 amplifications are seen in up to 2% of cases both in CRC and GE adenocarcinomas, while FGFR2 amplifications are seen in approximately 4% of GE adenocarcinomas and are rare in CRC. Fusions are seen in less than 0.6% of cases and most of them involve FGFR1 and FGFR2. FGFR inhibitors are currently under development in the hope that they can prove effective for the treatment of tumors with FGFR amplifications and/or fusions. Detection of FGFR alterations might also be useful in patients being treated with EGFR inhibitors, as amplifications in FGFR genes have been implicated in resistance to EGFR inhibitors [25].

NTRK Rearrangements

The TRK proteins (TRKA/NTRK1, TRKB/NTRK2, TRKC/NTRK3) are a family of transmembrane receptor kinases whose intracellular kinase domain is activated following binding of neurotrophins on the extracellular part of the receptor. Dysregulation of the TRK signaling pathway is a driver event in multiple tumor types, and fusions involving all three genes are the most common mechanisms of oncogenic activation [40]. Typically, 3′ sequences of *NTRK1*, *NTRK2*, or *NTRK3* that include the kinase domain are juxtaposed to 5′ sequences of a different gene, and the product of the fusion is a chimeric oncoprotein characterized by ligand-independent constitutive activation of the TRK kinase. Tumors harboring these fusions show response to first-generation TRK inhibitors; one of them larotrectinib was recently approved for the treatment of solid tumors with NTRK fusions regardless of histology, and other TRK inhibitors are also under development. NTRK fusions are not frequent in adenocarcinomas of the GI tract but several cases have been reported in CRC.

RET, ALK, and ROS1 Rearrangements

RET is another receptor tyrosine protein which can undergo rearrangement resulting in ligand independence, constitutive activation, aberrant proliferation, and tumor growth. RET kinase fusions are rare in CRC occurring in fewer than 0.5% of cases [41], but their identification may become clinically important as RET inhibitors are currently under development. Recurrent gene fusions involving anaplastic lymphoma kinase (*ALK)* and *ROS*1 have been described primarily in lung non-small cell carcinomas, but can be found in up to 2.4% of CRC [42]. ROS1 fusions but not ALK fusions were also identified in 1% of gastric adenocarcinomas [43]. Targeted therapies such as crizotinib, ceritinib, and alectinib are FDA approved for the treatment of lung tumors harboring these fusions, and this raises the possibility that they may also be effective in other tumor types, although clinical experience outside the lung is limited.

Mutational Testing in Gastrointestinal Stromal Tumors

KIT and PDGFRA Mutant GISTs

Gastrointestinal stromal tumors (GISTs) are the most common mesenchymal neoplasm of the gastrointestinal tract. They can arise from any site, although their most frequent location is the small intestine followed by stomach. The vast majority of tumors (~75%) harbor mutations in the KIT gene, while another 10% have mutations in the *PDGFRA* gene. The *KIT* and *PDGFRA* genes are on chromosome 4q12 and both encode for type III tyrosine kinase receptors (Fig. 7.3). They are composed of an extracellular domain consistent of IG-like motifs, a transmembrane section, a juxtamembrane (JM) domain, and an intracellular tyrosine kinase domain that has two regions (TK1, TK2) separated by a kinase insert domain. Oncogenic alterations in KIT and PDGFRA are gain of function events and result in constitutive ligand-independent activation of the receptor. Imatinib is a protein-tyrosine kinase inhibitor that inhibits both KIT and PDGFRA, but tumor response depends on the underlying mutation.

The majority of *KIT* mutations occur in the JM domain of the protein which is encoded by exon 11 (Table 7.2). They are typically deletions and single-nucleotide substitutions that involve codons 550–560. Prognostic significance of various exon 11 mutations varies, but they all tend to respond to treatment with imatinib. In approximately 10% of cases, mutations are found in *KIT* exon 9 which encodes part of the extracellular domain. The most common aberration is A502_Y505dup, a duplication that replicates the conformational change that the KIT receptor undergoes upon ligand binding. Tumors with *KIT* exon 9 mutations

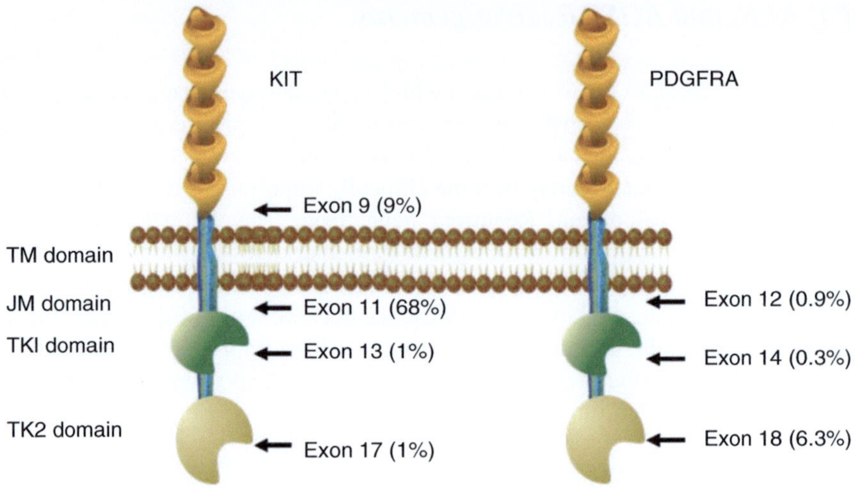

Fig. 7.3 Schematic representation of the KIT and PDGFRA proteins. Arrows indicate the regions that harbor most of the mutations encountered in gastrointestinal stromal tumors. Approximate mutational frequencies are shown in parentheses. Abbreviations: TM, transmembrane; JM, juxtamembrane; TK1, tyrosine kinase 1; TK2, tyrosine kinase 2

are usually in the small bowel and require a higher dose of imatinib for clinical response. Primary mutations in *KIT* exons 13, 14, and 17 occur infrequently in GISTs, and some of these tumors have shown response to imatinib treatment [44]. Nonetheless, mutations in these three exons are more frequent in the setting of secondary imatinib resistance. The most common mutations in exons 13 and 14 are V654A and T670I, and they both affect the ATP binding site, which is also the binding site for imatinib. Tumors with V654A and T670I mutations respond to sunitinib which is another tyrosine kinase receptor inhibitor less specific than imatinib. Similarly to exon 13 and 14 mutations, exon 17 mutations arise more frequently in the context of secondary imatinib resistance. These mutations stabilize the active confirmation of the activation loop and are also resistant to sunitinib.

PDGFRA mutations are seen in the majority of KIT-negative tumors, are most common in tumors arising in the stomach, and are associated with indolent behavior. Most mutations are in exon 18 which encodes the TK2 domain (Table 7.2). Less commonly *PDGFRA* mutations occur in exon 12 (JM domain) and exon 14 (TK1 domain). Many PDGFRA mutant tumors respond to imatinib, but the most common mutation D842V, which occurs in exon 18 is associated with resistance to imatinib. Notably a novel, potent PDGFRA inhibitor, crenolanib, has been reported that can inhibit D842V mutation in vitro, and a phase III clinical trial designed to test the efficacy of crenolanib in advanced GIST is ongoing [45].

Table 7.2 Clinically significant genetic alterations in GISTs

Gene	Exon	Type(s) of genetic alteration	Frequency	Most common event(s)	Treatment implications
KIT	Exon 9	Codon duplication Single-nucleotide substitution (less common)	10%	A502_Y503dup	Respond better to high-dose imatinib Respond better to sunitinib compared to exon 11 alterations
	Exon 11	In-frame deletion Single-nucleotide substitution	65%	W557_K558del V559A/D/G, V560D, W557R, L576P	Respond to imatinib
	Exon 13	Single-nucleotide substitution	2%	K642E, V654A	Associated with secondary resistance to imatinib Respond to sunitinib
	Exon 14	Single-nucleotide substitution	<1%	T670I	Associated with secondary resistance to imatinib
	Exon 17	Single-nucleotide substitution	1%	D820G, N822V, Y823D	Associated with secondary resistance to imatinib
PDGFRA	Exon 12	Single-nucleotide substitution	1%	V561D	Respond to imatinib
	Exon 14	Single-nucleotide substitution	<1%	V658A, N659Y/K	Respond to imatinib
	Exon 18	Single-nucleotide substitution Deletion	6%	D842V I843_D846del	D842V resistant to imatinib I843_D846del respond to imatinib
BRAF	Exon 15	Single-nucleotide substitution	4%	V600E	Resistant to imatinib May respond to BRAF inhibitors
NF1	NA	Single-nucleotide substitution Frameshift indels	6%	Loss of function events	Poor response rates to imatinib Ongoing trials with MEK inhibitors
SDH A/B/C/D	NA	Single-nucleotide substitution Deletion SDHC promoter methylation	5%	Loss of function events	Poor response to imatinib

KIT/PDGFRA-Negative GISTs

Approximately 15% of GISTs do not show mutations in KIT or PDGFRA. About half of those "wild-type" GISTs show functional loss of the SDH complex (SDH deficient). This complex is encoded by four separate genes, *SDHA*, *SDHB*, *SDHC*, and *SDHD*, is located in the inner mitochondrial membrane, and plays an important role in the electron transport chain and the citric acid cycle. SDH-deficient GISTs occur in the stomach, typically in children and young adults. At least half of SDH-deficient GISTs harbor mutations in one of the four subunit genes, with the most common being *SDHA*. These mutations include frameshift deletions, missense, and nonsense mutations and occasionally splice site mutations. Tumors with underlying *SDH* mutations often show simultaneous allelic loss at the respective gene locus, consistent with biallelic loss that is classically seen in tumor suppressor genes. SDH-deficient tumors do not respond to imatinib but may show response to sunitinib.

Alterations in the neurofibromin-1 (*NF1*) gene are thought to occur in approximately 6% of GISTs. *NF1* is a very large tumor suppressor gene, and mutations that disrupt its normal function result in constitutive RAS activation. As such loss of function, mutations are identified throughout the gene and are seen both in patients with neurofibromatosis type I and sporadically. Most NF1-associated GISTs arise in the small intestine, including the duodenum, and show a low response rate to imatinib treatment; a clinical trial using a MEK inhibitor, selumetinib, is currently underway for patients with NF1 mutant GISTs.

In about 5% of cases, the driver mutation is BRAF V600E. These GISTs show a predilection for the small intestine, arise in middle-aged females, and exhibit a high mitotic rate. Accumulating data suggest that BRAF mutant GISTs are resistant to imatinib, but may respond to BRAF inhibitors [46].

Molecular Testing for Familial Syndromes

Hereditary forms of GI cancers and GISTs comprise only a very small subset of cases; nonetheless, their recognition is critical for the clinical management of both patients and their families. The most common genes associated with these syndromes are shown in Table 7.3, and many of these genes are also associated with carcinomas outside the GI tract. Most current panels offered to patients that meet clinical criteria for a hereditary cancer syndrome are NGS-based and can detect single-nucleotide substitutions and small insertions and deletions in the targeted genes. It is important to keep in mind that some events identified in hereditary cases consist of large deletions and duplications, which can be more challenging in their detection, and laboratories may vary in their testing methods.

Approximately 5% of all CRCs occur in the setting of highly penetrant autosomal dominant susceptibility syndromes, the most common being Lynch syndrome. Patients who fulfill the revised Bethesda criteria are identified clinically for testing [7]. Nonetheless, because reliance on these criteria does not identify all patients, there is a recommendation for MSI testing in all CRC as a first step toward identifying Lynch syndrome patients that may not fulfill clinical criteria.

Table 7.3 Familial syndromes and genes associated with GI cancers or GISTs

Syndrome	Gene(s)	Gene(s) description	Germline genetic alteration(s)	Associated features
Familial GISTs	*KIT* (4q12)	Type III RTK	Mutations[a] in exons 11, 8, 13, 17	Multiple GISTs, pigmented cutaneous lesions, dysphagia
	PDGFRA (4q12)	Type III RTK	Mutations in exons 12, 18	Multiple GISTs, "large hands"
Neurofibromatosis	*NF1* (17q11)	Negative regulator of RAS pathway	Mutations	Multiple GISTs, café au lait spots, neurofibromas, Lisch nodules, optic nerve gliomas, skeletal defects
Carney triad (not hereditary)	*SDHA* (5p15) *SDHB* (1p36) *SDHC* (1q23) *SDHD* (11q23)	Regulators of electron transport chain and citric acid cycle	SDHC promoter hypermethylation	Multiple GISTs, pulmonary chondromas, paragangliomas
Carney-Stratakis			Mutations (most common in SDHB)	Multiple GISTs, paragangliomas
Lynch Syndrome	*MLH1* (3p22) *MSH2* (2p21-p16) *MSH6* (2p16.3) *PMS2* (7p22.1)	Mismatch repair proteins	Mutations Large deletions or rearrangements	Increased risk of multiple cancers (e.g., CRC, endometrial, small bowel, prostate, ovarian, urinary tract)
	EPCAM (2p21)	Glycoprotein mediating cell adhesion	Deletion of 3′ end resulting in inactivation of MSH2	
Constitutional mismatch repair deficiency (CMMRD)	*MLH1, MSH2, MSH6, PMS2*	Mismatch repair proteins	Biallelic mutations	Adenomas, early onset CRC and other GI cancers, skin lesions, hematologic malignancies, brain tumors
Familial adenomatous polyposis (FAP)	*APC* (5q21)	Negative regulator of Wnt/β-catenin pathway	Mutations Large deletions	>100 colonic adenomas, early onset CRC, gastric fundic gland polyps
Attenuated familial adenomatous polyposis	*APC*	Negative regulator of Wnt/β-catenin pathway	Mutations near 5′ and 3′ end of APC Exon 9 mutations leading to alternative splicing	10–100 colonic adenomas
MUTYH-associated polyposis	*MUTYH* (1p34)	Base excision repair glycosylase	Mutations	10–100 colonic adenomas, increased risk of multiple cancers (e.g., CRC, ovarian)
Peutz-Jeghers	*STK11* (19p13)	Negative regulator of mTOR pathway	Mutations Large deletions	Hamartomatous polyps, pigmented cutaneous macules, increased risk for multiples cancers (e.g., breast, CRC, gastric, pancreas)

(continued)

Table 7.3 (continued)

Syndrome	Gene(s)	Gene(s) description	Germline genetic alteration(s)	Associated features
Juvenile polyposis syndrome	*SMAD4* (18q21)	Mediator of TGF-β signaling	Mutations Large deletions	Hamartomatous polyps, increased risk of gastric CA and CRC
	BMPR1A (10q23)	Type I RTK		
Cowden	*PTEN* (10q23)	Negative regulator of PI3K/AKT pathway	Mutations Large deletions	Hamartomatous and ganglioneuromatous polyps, macrocephaly, mucocutaneous lesions, increased risk of multiple cancers (e.g., breast, colon, kidney)
Hereditary diffuse gastric cancer	*CDH1* (16q22)	Glycoprotein involved in cell adhesion	Loss of function mutations Large rearrangements Promoter methylation	Increased risk of gastric (diffuse type), breast, prostate, colon cancer
Gastric adenocarcinoma and proximal polyposis of the stomach	*APC*	Negative regulator of Wnt/β-catenin pathway	Mutations in promoter 1B	Fundic gland polyposis (>100), increased risk of gastric CA
Hereditary mixed polyposis syndrome	*GREM1* (15q13)	Secreted protein that inhibits BMP (bone morphogenetic protein)	Large duplications including enhancer elements	Multiple types of colorectal polyps; Increased risk of CRC
NA	*CHEK2* (22q21)	Cell cycle checkpoint regulator	Mutations throughout the gene	Increased risk of multiple cancers (e.g., colon, gastric, breast, prostate, thyroid)
NA	*ATM* (11q22)	Cell cycle checkpoint regulator	Mutations throughout the gene	Increased risk for multiple cancers including colon, pancreas, breast
NA	*AXIN2* (17q24)	Negative regulator of Wnt/β-catenin pathway		Increased risk of colon cancer
NA	*POLE* (12q24)	DNA polymerase	Mutations in exonuclease domain	Multiple adenomas and increased risk of CRC
NA	*POLD1* (19q13)	DNA polymerase	Mutations in exonuclease domain	Multiple adenomas and increased risk of CRC
NA	*NTHL1* (16p13)	Base excision repair glycosylase	Mutations	Multiple adenomas and increased risk of CRC

Abbreviations: *CA* carcinoma, *CRC* colorectal cancer, *RTK* receptor tyrosine kinase, *GIST* gastrointestinal stromal tumor, *GI* gastrointestinal

[a]Mutations include single-nucleotide substitutions and small insertions and deletions (indels)

The second most common syndrome occurring in fewer than 1% of patients affected with CRC is familial adenomatous polyposis (FAP). In classic FAP, patients have >100 adenomas throughout the colon and rectum and, if they do not undergo prophylactic colectomy, develop CRC by age 40. The underlying genetic aberrations are mutations in the *APC* gene which is a negative regulator of Wnt/β-catenin signaling pathway. Inactivation of *APC* results in nuclear translocation of β-catenin and increased transcription of multiple genes that affect cell proliferation. Patients with classic FAP usually have mutations between codons 157 and 1595, while *APC* mutations between codons 1250 and 1464 result in a more severe phenotype with >2000 adenomas. In attenuated FAP, patients have fewer adenomas (approx. 20–100) and tend to develop CRC at a later age. These patients usually have *APC* mutations near the 5′ or 3′ end of the gene and alternatively spliced regions in exon 9 of *APC*. Patients with an attenuated FAP phenotype may also show mutations in *MUTYH*, a gene that encodes a base excision repair glycosylase involved in repair of 8-oxoG:A mismatches.

Hamartomatous polyposis syndromes such as Peutz-Jeghers (PJS), juvenile polyposis syndrome (JPS), and Cowden's syndrome (PTEN hamartoma tumor syndrome) are implicated in <0.5% of CRC cases. They are characterized by hamartomatous GI polyps and increased risk of intestinal or gastric CA as well as other tumors outside the GI tract.

The most well-characterized gastric cancer syndrome to date is hereditary diffuse gastric cancer (HDGC) syndrome. Patients are at increased risk for developing diffuse-type gastric cancer and have germline mutations in the *CDH1* gene, which encodes for E-cadherin, a type I transmembrane glycoprotein that regulates cell-cell adhesion. Another gene involved in intracellular cell adhesion (*CTNNA1*) has also been implicated in HDGC [47]. Recent exome and targeted sequencing identified other candidate genes such as *BRCA2*, *STK11*, *SDHB*, *PRSS1*, *ATM*, *MSR1*, and *PALB2*, but these remain to be validated by future studies [48].

A less frequent syndrome associated with gastric cancer is GAPPS (gastric adenocarcinoma and proximal polyposis of the stomach), a syndrome characterized by >100 polyps in the gastric fundus and body and increased risk of gastric adenocarcinoma at early age. These patients harbor a germline mutation in the *APC* 1B promoter.

Similar to GI adenocarcinomas, less than 5% of GIST cases are thought to occur due to hereditary tumor syndromes. Germline mutations in either *KIT* or *PDGFRA* have been identified in several families with familial GISTs; *KIT* exon 11 mutations appear to be the most common ones paralleling the high frequency of these mutations in sporadic GISTs. GISTs seen in patients with neurofibromatosis type 1 are associated with germline loss of function events in *NF1*, while GISTs in patients with Carney-Stratakis syndrome are associated with germline loss of function mutations in the SDH complex genes, most commonly in *SDHB*. In contrast to Carney-Stratakis, patients with Carney's triad have a non-inherited, rare condition characterized by GISTs, paragangliomas, and pulmonary chondromas, and in these patients GISTs show methylation of SDHC promoter.

References

1. Sourrouille I, Coulet F, Lefevre JH, Colas C, Eyries M, Svrcek M, et al. Somatic mosaicism and double somatic hits can lead to MSI colorectal tumors. Familial Cancer. 2013;12(1):27–33.
2. Cancer Genome Atlas Research N. Comprehensive molecular characterization of gastric adenocarcinoma. Nature. 2014;513(7517):202–9.
3. Yamamoto H, Perez-Piteira J, Yoshida T, Terada M, Itoh F, Imai K, et al. Gastric cancers of the microsatellite mutator phenotype display characteristic genetic and clinical features. Gastroenterology. 1999;116(6):1348–57.
4. Le DT, Uram JN, Wang H, Bartlett BR, Kemberling H, Eyring AD, et al. PD-1 blockade in tumors with mismatch-repair deficiency. N Engl J Med. 2015;372(26):2509–20.
5. NCCN. Clinical Practice Guidelines in Oncology: Colon Cancer 2018. Version 4.2018. Available from: https://www.nccn.org/professionals/physician_gls/pdf/colon.pdf.
6. NCCN. Clinical Practice Guidelines in Oncology: Gastric Cancer 2018. Version 2.2018. Available from: https://www.nccn.org/professionals/physician_gls/pdf/gastric.pdf.
7. Umar A, Boland CR, Terdiman JP, Syngal S, de la Chapelle A, Ruschoff J, et al. Revised Bethesda Guidelines for hereditary nonpolyposis colorectal cancer (Lynch syndrome) and microsatellite instability. J Natl Cancer Inst. 2004;96(4):261–8.
8. Hechtman JF, Middha S, Stadler ZK, Zehir A, Berger MF, Vakiani E, et al. Universal screening for microsatellite instability in colorectal cancer in the clinical genomics era: new recommendations, methods, and considerations. Familial Cancer. 2017;16(4):525–9.
9. Niessen RC, Hofstra RM, Westers H, Ligtenberg MJ, Kooi K, Jager PO, et al. Germline hypermethylation of MLH1 and EPCAM deletions are a frequent cause of Lynch syndrome. Genes Chromosomes Cancer. 2009;48(8):737–44.
10. Hitchins MP, Lynch HT. Dawning of the epigenetic era in hereditary cancer. Clin Genet. 2014;85(5):413–6.
11. Chatterjee A, Rodger EJ, Morison IM, Eccles MR, Stockwell PA. Tools and strategies for analysis of genome-wide and gene-specific DNA methylation patterns. Methods Mol Biol. 2017;1537:249–77.
12. Allegra CJ, Rumble RB, Hamilton SR, Mangu PB, Roach N, Hantel A, et al. Extended RAS gene mutation testing in metastatic colorectal carcinoma to predict response to anti-epidermal growth factor receptor monoclonal antibody therapy: American Society of Clinical Oncology Provisional Clinical Opinion Update 2015. J Clin Oncol. 2016;34(2):179–85.
13. Sepulveda AR, Hamilton SR, Allegra CJ, Grody W, Cushman-Vokoun AM, Funkhouser WK, et al. Molecular biomarkers for the evaluation of colorectal cancer: guideline from the American Society for Clinical Pathology, College of American Pathologists, Association for Molecular Pathology, and American Society of Clinical Oncology. J Mol Diagn. 2017;19(2):187–225.
14. Domingo E, Laiho P, Ollikainen M, Pinto M, Wang L, French AJ, et al. BRAF screening as a low-cost effective strategy for simplifying HNPCC genetic testing. J Med Genet. 2004;41(9):664–8.
15. Walsh MD, Buchanan DD, Walters R, Roberts A, Arnold S, McKeone D, et al. Analysis of families with Lynch syndrome complicated by advanced serrated neoplasia: the importance of pathology review and pedigree analysis. Familial Cancer. 2009;8(4):313–23.
16. Rowland A, Dias MM, Wiese MD, Kichenadasse G, McKinnon RA, Karapetis CS, et al. Meta-analysis of BRAF mutation as a predictive biomarker of benefit from anti-EGFR monoclonal antibody therapy for RAS wild-type metastatic colorectal cancer. Br J Cancer. 2015;112(12):1888–94.
17. Kopetz S, Desai J, Chan E, Hecht JR, O'Dwyer PJ, Maru D, et al. Phase II Pilot Study of vemurafenib in patients with metastatic BRAF-mutated colorectal cancer. J Clin Oncol. 2015;33(34):4032–8.
18. Hong DS, Morris VK, El Osta B, Sorokin AV, Janku F, Fu S, et al. Phase 1B study of vemurafenib in combination with irinotecan and cetuximab in patients with metastatic colorectal cancer with BRAF V600E mutation. Cancer Discov. 2016;6:1352.

19. Dankner M, Rose AAN, Rajkumar S, Siegel PM, Watson IR. Classifying BRAF alterations in cancer: new rational therapeutic strategies for actionable mutations. Oncogene. 2018;37(24):3183–99.
20. Tafe LJ, Janjigian YY, Zaidinski M, Hedvat CV, Hameed MR, Tang LH, et al. Human epidermal growth factor receptor 2 testing in gastroesophageal cancer: correlation between immunohistochemistry and fluorescence in situ hybridization. Arch Pathol Lab Med. 2011;135(11):1460–5.
21. Bang YJ, Van Cutsem E, Feyereislova A, Chung HC, Shen L, Sawaki A, et al. Trastuzumab in combination with chemotherapy versus chemotherapy alone for treatment of HER2-positive advanced gastric or gastro-oesophageal junction cancer (ToGA): a phase 3, open-label, randomised controlled trial. Lancet. 2010;376(9742):687–97.
22. Hofmann M, Stoss O, Shi D, Buttner R, van de Vijver M, Kim W, et al. Assessment of a HER2 scoring system for gastric cancer: results from a validation study. Histopathology. 2008;52(7):797–805.
23. Ross DS, Zehir A, Cheng DT, Benayed R, Nafa K, Hechtman JF, et al. Next-generation assessment of human epidermal growth factor receptor 2 (ERBB2) amplification status: clinical validation in the context of a hybrid capture-based, comprehensive solid tumor genomic profiling assay. J Mol Diagn. 2017;19(2):244–54.
24. Kavuri SM, Jain N, Galimi F, Cottino F, Leto SM, Migliardi G, et al. HER2 activating mutations are targets for colorectal cancer treatment. Cancer Discov. 2015;5(8):832–41.
25. Bertotti A, Papp E, Jones S, Adleff V, Anagnostou V, Lupo B, et al. The genomic landscape of response to EGFR blockade in colorectal cancer. Nature. 2015;526(7572):263–7.
26. Yonesaka K, Zejnullahu K, Okamoto I, Satoh T, Cappuzzo F, Souglakos J, et al. Activation of ERBB2 signaling causes resistance to the EGFR-directed therapeutic antibody cetuximab. Sci Transl Med. 2011;3(99):99ra86.
27. Sartore-Bianchi A, Trusolino L, Martino C, Bencardino K, Lonardi S, Bergamo F, et al. Dual-targeted therapy with trastuzumab and lapatinib in treatment-refractory, KRAS codon 12/13 wild-type, HER2-positive metastatic colorectal cancer (HERACLES): a proof-of-concept, multicentre, open-label, phase 2 trial. Lancet Oncol. 2016;17(6):738–46.
28. Hyman DM, Piha-Paul SA, Won H, Rodon J, Saura C, Shapiro GI, et al. HER kinase inhibition in patients with HER2- and HER3-mutant cancers. Nature. 2018;554(7691):189–94.
29. Sartore-Bianchi A, Martini M, Molinari F, Veronese S, Nichelatti M, Artale S, et al. PIK3CA mutations in colorectal cancer are associated with clinical resistance to EGFR-targeted monoclonal antibodies. Cancer Res. 2009;69(5):1851–7.
30. Prenen H, De Schutter J, Jacobs B, De Roock W, Biesmans B, Claes B, et al. PIK3CA mutations are not a major determinant of resistance to the epidermal growth factor receptor inhibitor cetuximab in metastatic colorectal cancer. Clin Cancer Res. 2009;15(9):3184–8.
31. Domingo E, Church DN, Sieber O, Ramamoorthy R, Yanagisawa Y, Johnstone E, et al. Evaluation of PIK3CA mutation as a predictor of benefit from nonsteroidal anti-inflammatory drug therapy in colorectal cancer. J Clin Oncol. 2013;31(34):4297–305.
32. Liao X, Lochhead P, Nishihara R, Morikawa T, Kuchiba A, Yamauchi M, et al. Aspirin use, tumor PIK3CA mutation, and colorectal-cancer survival. N Engl J Med. 2012;367(17):1596–606.
33. Van Cutsem E, Karaszewska B, Kang YK, Chung HC, Shankaran V, Siena S, et al. A multicenter phase 2 study of AMG 337 in patients with MET-amplified gastric/gastroesophageal junction/esophageal adenocarcinoma and other solid tumors. Clin Cancer Res. 2019;25(8):2414–23.
34. Sanchez-Vega F, Hechtman JF, Castel P, Ku GY, Tuvy Y, Won H, et al. EGFR and MET amplifications determine response to HER2 inhibition in ERBB2-amplified esophagogastric cancer. Cancer Discov. 2019;9(2):199–209.
35. Barber TD, Vogelstein B, Kinzler KW, Velculescu VE. Somatic mutations of EGFR in colorectal cancers and glioblastomas. N Engl J Med. 2004;351(27):2883.
36. Pietrantonio F, Fuca G, Morano F, Gloghini A, Corso S, Aprile G, et al. Biomarkers of primary resistance to trastuzumab in HER2-positive metastatic gastric cancer patients: the AMNESIA Case-Control Study. Clin Cancer Res. 2018;24(5):1082–9.

37. Ahronian LG, Sennott EM, Van Allen EM, Wagle N, Kwak EL, Faris JE, et al. Clinical acquired resistance to RAF inhibitor combinations in BRAF-mutant colorectal cancer through MAPK pathway alterations. Cancer Discov. 2015;5(4):358–67.
38. Siravegna G, Mussolin B, Buscarino M, Corti G, Cassingena A, Crisafulli G, et al. Clonal evolution and resistance to EGFR blockade in the blood of colorectal cancer patients. Nat Med. 2015;21(7):795–801.
39. Helsten T, Elkin S, Arthur E, Tomson BN, Carter J, Kurzrock R. The FGFR landscape in cancer: analysis of 4,853 tumors by next-generation sequencing. Clin Cancer Res. 2016;22(1):259–67.
40. Vaishnavi A, Le AT, Doebele RC. TRKing down an old oncogene in a new era of targeted therapy. Cancer Discov. 2015;5(1):25–34.
41. Le Rolle AF, Klempner SJ, Garrett CR, Seery T, Sanford EM, Balasubramanian S, et al. Identification and characterization of RET fusions in advanced colorectal cancer. Oncotarget. 2015;6(30):28929–37.
42. Aisner DL, Nguyen TT, Paskulin DD, Le AT, Haney J, Schulte N, et al. ROS1 and ALK fusions in colorectal cancer, with evidence of intratumoral heterogeneity for molecular drivers. Mol Cancer Res. 2014;12(1):111–8.
43. Lee J, Lee SE, Kang SY, Do IG, Lee S, Ha SY, et al. Identification of ROS1 rearrangement in gastric adenocarcinoma. Cancer. 2013;119(9):1627–35.
44. Heinrich MC, Owzar K, Corless CL, Hollis D, Borden EC, Fletcher CD, et al. Correlation of kinase genotype and clinical outcome in the North American Intergroup Phase III Trial of imatinib mesylate for treatment of advanced gastrointestinal stromal tumor: CALGB 150105 Study by Cancer and Leukemia Group B and Southwest Oncology Group. J Clin Oncol. 2008;26(33):5360–7.
45. Heinrich MC, Griffith D, McKinley A, Patterson J, Presnell A, Ramachandran A, et al. Crenolanib inhibits the drug-resistant PDGFRA D842V mutation associated with imatinib-resistant gastrointestinal stromal tumors. Clin Cancer Res. 2012;18(16):4375–84.
46. Falchook GS, Trent JC, Heinrich MC, Beadling C, Patterson J, Bastida CC, et al. BRAF mutant gastrointestinal stromal tumor: first report of regression with BRAF inhibitor dabrafenib (GSK2118436) and whole exomic sequencing for analysis of acquired resistance. Oncotarget. 2013;4(2):310–5.
47. Majewski IJ, Kluijt I, Cats A, Scerri TS, de Jong D, Kluin RJ, et al. An alpha-E-catenin (CTNNA1) mutation in hereditary diffuse gastric cancer. J Pathol. 2013;229(4):621–9.
48. Hansford S, Kaurah P, Li-Chang H, Woo M, Senz J, Pinheiro H, et al. Hereditary diffuse gastric cancer syndrome: CDH1 mutations and beyond. JAMA Oncol. 2015;1(1):23–32.

Chapter 8
Breast

Dara S. Ross

Key Points

- Biomarkers, multigene expression assays, and mutation profiling may facilitate diagnosis, provide potential treatment options, and identify mechanisms of resistance in breast cancer.
- Genetic alterations and dysregulation of signaling pathways involving hormones (ER, PR, AR), growth factors (HER2, FGFR1), cell cycle regulation (cyclin D1, CDK4, CDK6, RB1, TP53), and PI3K/AKT/MTOR underlie the pathogenesis of breast cancer.
- Somatic alterations in metastatic breast tumors associated with acquired resistance to endocrine therapy include *ESR1* mutations involving the ligand-binding domain, *ERBB2*-activating mutations, *NF1* loss-of-function mutations, and alterations in other MAPK pathway genes (*EGFR*, *KRAS*) and ER transcriptional regulators (*MYC*, *CTCF*, *FOXA1*, *TBX3*).

Key Online Resource

- NCCN Version 3.2018: https://www.nccn.org/professionals/physician_gls/pdf/breast.pdf

D. S. Ross (✉)
Department of Pathology, Memorial Sloan Kettering Cancer Center, New York, NY, USA
e-mail: rossd@mskcc.org

L. J. Tafe, M. E. Arcila (eds.), *Genomic Medicine*,
https://doi.org/10.1007/978-3-030-22922-1_8

Introduction

Breast cancer is one of the leading causes of cancer-related death in women worldwide. In the United States, 266,120 new cases of invasive breast cancer and 40,920 deaths are estimated in women for 2018 [1]. After the histologic assessment and diagnosis of an invasive breast carcinoma, the use of biomarkers, multigene expression assays, and mutation profiling may be utilized. Estrogen receptor (ER), progesterone receptor (PR), and human epidermal growth factor receptor 2 (HER2) are predictive biomarkers in breast cancer, and the American Society of Clinical Oncology/College of American Pathologists (ASCO/CAP) guidelines recommend testing on every primary invasive breast cancer, recurrence, and metastasis (if stage IV and specimen is available) to guide decisions regarding therapy [2–4]. Multigene expression assays provide prognostic and therapy-predictive information that complements staging (T, N, M) and biomarker information. The multigene assays listed in the National Comprehensive Cancer Network (NCCN) Clinical Practice Guidelines in Oncology (NCCN Guidelines Version 3.2018) for breast cancer include Oncotype Dx (21 gene), MammaPrint (70 gene), Prosigna (PAM 50), EndoPredict (12 gene), and Breast Cancer Index [5]. With the development of improved molecular profiling assays with faster turnaround times, the identification of "driver" and "actionable" somatic genetic alterations (i.e., missense mutations, copy number alterations, insertions or deletions, and rearrangements) in key oncogenes and tumor suppressor genes now play an essential role in the diagnosis and treatment of many cancers, and this is evolving in the treatment of breast cancer as well. This chapter summarizes the most clinically significant somatic genetic alterations in breast cancer and how this information can be used to facilitate diagnosis, provide potential treatment options, and identify mechanisms of resistance.

Molecular Diagnostics in Breast Cancer

Breast cancer is a heterogenous disease histologically and at the molecular level and next-generation sequencing (NGS) has broadened our understanding of these tumors. Genetic alterations and subsequent dysregulation of signaling pathways involving hormones (ER, PR, androgen receptor (AR)), growth factors (HER2, FGFR1), cell cycle regulation (cyclin D1, CDK4, CDK6, RB1, TP53), and PI3K/AKT/MTOR underlie the pathogenesis of breast cancer. In addition, molecular profiles vary for ER-positive and ER-negative tumors and can be characterized even further among the intrinsic subtypes of breast cancer (luminal A, luminal B, HER2-enriched, and basal-like) [6]. The Cancer Genome Atlas Network (TCGA) showed that the most common recurrent molecular alterations across all breast cancers involve the genes *TP53*, *PIK3CA*, and *GATA3* [7]. Further classification among the intrinsic subtypes showed that somatic *PIK3CA* mutations were more commonly seen in luminal tumors (45% of luminal A subtype, 29% of luminal B subtype) and

Table 8.1 Diagnostic somatic alterations in invasive breast cancer

Gene	Alteration	Description	Available assays	Significance
CDH1	Truncating mutations, loss of heterozygosity, promoter methylation	Located on 16q22, encodes E-cadherin, an intercellular adhesion protein	IHC, SGA, NGS	Diagnostic for lobular carcinoma (5–15% of invasive BC) [8]
ETV6-NTRK3	Translocation	t(12;15)(p13;q25) leading to *ETV6-NTRK3* gene fusion	FISH, NGS	Diagnostic for secretory carcinoma (<0.15% of invasive BC) [8]
MYB-NFIB	Translocation	t(6;9)(q22-23;p23-24), leading to *MYB-NF1B* gene fusion	FISH, NGS	Diagnostic for adenoid cystic carcinoma (<0.1% of invasive BC) [8]

IHC immunohistochemistry, *SGA* single-gene assay, *NGS* next-generation sequencing, *FISH* fluorescence in situ hybridization, *BC* breast cancer

in 39% of HER2-enriched tumors [7]. These types of findings allow the tailoring of therapy to specific tumor types. Despite the large number of mutations that may be found in breast cancer, there are a limited amount of clinically significant somatic alterations, including those that contribute to the appropriate histologic classification (Table 8.1) and those that can be targets of therapy, including FDA-approved or ongoing clinical trials (Table 8.2). In addition to NGS, alternate methods of detection for genomic alterations may include immunohistochemistry, fluorescence in situ hybridization, chromogenic in situ hybridization, and various single-gene assays.

Resistance Mechanisms in Breast Cancer

Resistance to targeted therapy is a major clinical challenge in the treatment of breast cancer. Various resistance mechanisms for all tumor types exist, including primary (intrinsic) resistance and secondary (acquired) resistance after treatment. Biopsy upon progression of disease is becoming more common to explore mechanisms of resistance and new therapeutic options. Somatic alterations in metastatic breast tumors associated with resistance to endocrine therapy, in particular, have been identified (Table 8.3), and the clinical significance of this information in a practical setting is evolving.

Antiestrogen therapy is an effective treatment strategy for women with ER-positive breast cancer [35, 36] and includes estrogen deprivation therapy (aromatase inhibitors, gonadotropin-releasing hormone agonists) and direct inhibitors of ER (selective ER modulators and selective ER degraders) [37, 38]. Despite the benefits of these drugs, *ESR1* mutations involving the ligand-binding domain can develop, resulting in a constitutively active receptor and acquired resistance to

Table 8.2 Clinically significant and emerging somatic alterations for targeted therapy in invasive breast cancer

Gene (chromosome)	Alteration	Frequency	Description	Most common alteration(s)	Available assays	Significance
ERBB2 (17q12)	Amplification	18–25% [9–11]	Oncogene, encodes HER2, a transmembrane receptor tyrosine kinase	N/A	IHC, CISH, FISH, NGS	Response to monoclonal antibodies (trastuzumab, pertuzumab, ado-trastuzumab emtansine) and tyrosine kinase inhibitors (lapatinib) [12]
ERBB2 (17q12)	Mutation	1.6–3.7% [13, 14]	Oncogene, encodes HER2, a transmembrane receptor tyrosine kinase (most common mutations cluster around 2 domains: exon 8, affecting aa 309–310 of HER2 extracellular domain, and exons 19–20, affecting aa 755–781 of tyrosine kinase domain)	S310F/Y, L755S, D769H/Y, Y772_A775dup V777L	SGA, NGS	Response to irreversible pan-HER tyrosine kinase inhibitor (neratinib) (NCT01953926) [15]
PIK3CA (3q26)	Mutation	30–36.1% [14, 16–18]	Oncogene, catalytic subunit of PI3-kinase (most common mutations cluster around 2 domains: exon 9, affecting aa 542–546 of helical domain, and exon 20, affecting aa 1047 of kinase domain)	E542K, E545K/A/Q, H1047L/R/Y	SGA, NGS	Response to PI3-kinase targeted inhibitors (alpelisib, buparlisib, copanlisib, GDC-0077, serabelisib, taselisib), either alone or in combination with ER-antagonists (fulvestrant) [19–26]
AKT1 (14q32)	Mutation	5.1% [14]	Oncogene, serine/threonine intracellular kinase, downstream effector in the PI3K signaling pathway	E17K	SGA, NGS	Response to ATP-competitive, AKT1 inhibitors (NCT01226316, NCT03337724) [27]
PTEN (10q23)	Mutation, deletion	7.1% [14]	Tumor suppressor, lipid and protein phosphatase that converts PIP3 to PIP2	T319*, R130*/G/P/Q	SGA, NGS	Loss-of-function *PTEN* alterations may be sensitive to PI3Kβ-selective inhibitor (GSK2636771 and AZD8186) (NCT01458067, NCT03218826, NCT01884285) [28]

IHC immunohistochemistry, *SGA* single-gene assay, *NGS* next-generation sequencing, *CISH* chromogenic in situ hybridization, *FISH* fluorescence in situ hybridization, *aa* amino acids, *NCT* ClinicalTrials.gov Identifier, *PI3K* phosphoinositide 3-kinase, *PIP3* phosphatidylinositol (3,4,5)-triphosphate, *PIP2* phosphatidylinositol (4,5)-bisphosphate

Table 8.3 Clinically significant somatic alterations in invasive breast cancer associated with resistance to therapy

Gene (chromosome)	Alteration	Mechanism	Most common alteration(s)	Available assays	Significance
ESR1 (6q25)	Mutation	Constitutive ligand-independent activation of ER transcription and ERα expression	E380Q, L536H/P/R, Y537C/D/N/S, D538G	SGA, NGS	Resistance to estrogen deprivation therapies, alternate therapy with AZD9496 or fulvestrant may be warranted
FGFR1 (8p11)	Amplification	Resistance to hormonal therapies	N/A	FISH, NGS	Response to pan-FGFR inhibitors AZD4547 (NCT01791985, NCT01202591, NCT01795768), debio 1347 (NCT03344536), erdafitinib (NCT03238196)
RB1 (13q14)	Mutation (inactivating)	Tumor suppressor; wild-type RB1 downstream of CDK4/6 is required for CDK4/6 inhibitors to work properly	N/A	NGS	Resistance to CDK 4/6 inhibitors (palbociclib, ribociclib, abemaciclib) in ER-positive BC [29–32]. The combination of endocrine therapy, CDK4/6 inhibitors, and PI3 kinase inhibitors can prevent acquired resistance to treatment
AR splice variants	Splicing mutation	Lacks ligand binding domain and is constitutively active	Splice variant 7 (AR-V7)	NGS	Resistance to androgen deprivation therapy [33, 34]

SGA single-gene assay, *NGS* next-generation sequencing, *FISH* fluorescence in situ hybridization, *NCT* ClinicalTrials.gov Identifier, *BC* breast cancer

estrogen deprivation therapies [39–45]. Activating *ESR1* mutations occur in up to 35–40% of hormone-resistant ER-positive breast cancer, including studies assessing tissue samples and circulating tumor DNA [43–50]. The most common *ESR1* mutations are D538G and Y537S, which are reported as being associated with a worse overall prognosis [47]. These mutations rarely occur in untreated primary tumors but were detected in nearly 30% of ER-positive metastatic breast cancer previously treated with aromatase inhibitors [46, 47].

Additional mutations associated with resistance to endocrine therapy have been identified by sequencing of metastatic lesions. Amplification and overexpression of *FGFR1* (~10%) [51] may contribute to poor prognosis in luminal A and luminal B breast cancers leading to subsequent endocrine therapy resistance. The cyclin D1-CDK4/6-Rb pathway has been implicated in resistance to endocrine therapy as well. Targeted CDK4/6 inhibitors (palbociclib, ribociclib, abemaciclib) that act upstream of Rb are now routinely used in clinical practice for ER-positive breast cancer [29–32]; however, inactivating mutations of RB1 (which is wild type in the majority of ER-positive breast cancers [7]) will result in resistance to this targeted therapy.

The AR pathway has also emerged as a potential therapeutic target in breast cancer, with many ongoing clinical trials in triple-negative breast cancer (i.e., ClinicalTrials.gov identifier NCT02605486, NCT03090165, NCT02457910, NCT02750358) and other subtypes (i.e., NCT02007512, NCT02676986, NCT02955394, NCT02091960). In prostate cancer, resistance to androgen deprivation therapy is frequently associated with the emergence of androgen-independent splice variants of the androgen receptor, and women with breast cancer may be prone to a similar mechanism of resistance [33, 34].

With more frequent sequencing of metastases, we learn more about the mutation profile of tumors exposed to systemic therapy. A recent large study with sequencing data from breast tumors previously exposed to hormonal therapy showed an enrichment in *ERBB2*-activating mutations, *NF1* loss-of-function mutations, and alterations in other MAPK pathway genes (*EGFR*, *KRAS*) and ER transcriptional regulators (*MYC*, *CTCF*, *FOXA1*, *TBX3*) [52]. The incorporation of these findings into clinical practice is ongoing.

For the Practicing Clinician

Selection of the appropriate material for molecular testing is crucial for useful results. Although biopsy of metastatic breast lesions for molecular profiling can be very informative, this can be a challenge clinically as many patients have bone-only metastases which can be difficult to biopsy/rebiopsy. Decalcified bone specimens are unsuitable for molecular testing. Solutions to this problem include (1) performing a concurrent fine-needle aspiration so a cell block can be prepared, (2) alerting the Pathology department of the need for molecular testing by adding a note that the core biopsy should not be decalcified, and/or (3) making at least two passes and request that one core will not undergo decalcification. In addition, there is a growing interest in utilizing circulating tumor cells (CTCs) and circulating DNA (ctDNA) as potential tools for "liquid biopsy."

The primary tumor or metastatic tumor (preferred) can be sent for molecular profiling. When tissue is received in the Molecular department, the tumor percentage will be evaluated. It is important to be familiar with the technical/analytic sensitivity and diagnostic sensitivity of the molecular profiling assay being performed. The technical sensitivity of an assay will determine the minimum tumor percentage necessary in the submitted tissue in order to exclude the possibility of a false-negative result. In addition, there are technical limitations inherent in analysis of formalin-fixed paraffin-embedded tissue due to the degradation of DNA and mRNA that occurs during the fixation process which can lead to alteration in the sensitivity and specificity of an assay as well. An understanding of these limitations is always important when interpreting molecular results.

References

1. American Cancer Society. Cancer facts & figures 2018. Atlanta; 2018. Available from: https://www.cancer.org/content/dam/cancer-org/research/cancer-facts-and-statistics/annual-cancer-facts-and-figures/2018/cancer-facts-and-figures-2018.pdf.
2. Hammond ME, Hayes DF, Dowsett M, Allred DC, Hagerty KL, Badve S, et al. American Society of Clinical Oncology/College Of American Pathologists guideline recommendations for immunohistochemical testing of estrogen and progesterone receptors in breast cancer. J Clin Oncol. 2010;28(16):2784–95.
3. Wolff AC, Hammond ME, Hicks DG, Dowsett M, McShane LM, Allison KH, et al. Recommendations for human epidermal growth factor receptor 2 testing in breast cancer: American Society of Clinical Oncology/College of American Pathologists clinical practice guideline update. J Clin Oncol. 2013;31(31):3997–4013.
4. Wolff AC, Hammond MEH, Allison KH, Harvey BE, Mangu PB, Bartlett JMS, et al. Human epidermal growth factor receptor 2 testing in breast cancer: American Society of Clinical Oncology/College of American Pathologists Clinical Practice Guideline Focused Update. J Clin Oncol. 2018;36(20):2105–22.
5. NCCN Clinical Practice Guidelines in Oncology (NCCN Guidelines), Breast Cancer (Version 3.2018). Available from: https://www.nccn.org/professionals/physician_gls/pdf/breast.pdf.
6. Perou CM, Sorlie T, Eisen MB, van de Rijn M, Jeffrey SS, Rees CA, et al. Molecular portraits of human breast tumours. Nature. 2000;406(6797):747–52.
7. Cancer Genome Atlas Network. Comprehensive molecular portraits of human breast tumours. Nature. 2012;490(7418):61–70.
8. WHO classification of tumours of the breast, 4th ed. Lyon: International Agency for Research on Cancer; 2012.
9. Slamon DJ, Clark GM, Wong SG, Levin WJ, Ullrich A, McGuire WL. Human breast cancer: correlation of relapse and survival with amplification of the HER-2/neu oncogene. Science. 1987;235(4785):177–82.
10. Owens MA, Horten BC, Da Silva MM. HER2 amplification ratios by fluorescence in situ hybridization and correlation with immunohistochemistry in a cohort of 6556 breast cancer tissues. Clin Breast Cancer. 2004;5(1):63–9.
11. Yaziji H, Goldstein LC, Barry TS, Werling R, Hwang H, Ellis GK, et al. HER-2 testing in breast cancer using parallel tissue-based methods. JAMA. 2004;291(16):1972–7.
12. Giordano SH, Temin S, Kirshner JJ, Chandarlapaty S, Crews JR, Davidson NE, et al. Systemic therapy for patients with advanced human epidermal growth factor receptor 2-positive breast cancer: American Society of Clinical Oncology clinical practice guideline. J Clin Oncol. 2014;32(19):2078–99.
13. Bose R, Kavuri SM, Searleman AC, Shen W, Shen D, Koboldt DC, et al. Activating HER2 mutations in HER2 gene amplification negative breast cancer. Cancer Discov. 2013;3(2):224–37.

14. Zehir A, Benayed R, Shah RH, Syed A, Middha S, Kim HR, et al. Erratum: mutational landscape of metastatic cancer revealed from prospective clinical sequencing of 10,000 patients. Nat Med. 2017;23(8):1004.
15. Hyman DM, Piha-Paul SA, Won H, Rodon J, Saura C, Shapiro GI, et al. HER kinase inhibition in patients with HER2- and HER3-mutant cancers. Nature. 2018;554(7691):189–94.
16. Saal LH, Holm K, Maurer M, Memeo L, Su T, Wang X, et al. PIK3CA mutations correlate with hormone receptors, node metastasis, and ERBB2, and are mutually exclusive with PTEN loss in human breast carcinoma. Cancer Res. 2005;65(7):2554–9.
17. Stemke-Hale K, Gonzalez-Angulo AM, Lluch A, Neve RM, Kuo WL, Davies M, et al. An integrative genomic and proteomic analysis of PIK3CA, PTEN, and AKT mutations in breast cancer. Cancer Res. 2008;68(15):6084–91.
18. O'Brien C, Wallin JJ, Sampath D, GuhaThakurta D, Savage H, Punnoose EA, et al. Predictive biomarkers of sensitivity to the phosphatidylinositol 3′ kinase inhibitor GDC-0941 in breast cancer preclinical models. Clin Cancer Res. 2010;16(14):3670–83.
19. Bosch A, Li Z, Bergamaschi A, Ellis H, Toska E, Prat A, et al. PI3K inhibition results in enhanced estrogen receptor function and dependence in hormone receptor-positive breast cancer. Sci Transl Med. 2015;7(283):283ra51.
20. Miller TW, Balko JM, Fox EM, Ghazoui Z, Dunbier A, Anderson H, et al. ERalpha-dependent E2F transcription can mediate resistance to estrogen deprivation in human breast cancer. Cancer Discov. 2011;1(4):338–51.
21. Juric D, Rodon J, Tabernero J, Janku F, Burris HA, Schellens JHM, et al. Phosphatidylinositol 3-kinase alpha-selective inhibition with alpelisib (BYL719) in PIK3CA-altered solid tumors: results from the first-in-human study. J Clin Oncol. 2018;36(13):1291–9.
22. Juric D, de Bono JS, LoRusso PM, Nemunaitis J, Heath EI, Kwak EL, et al. A first-in-human, phase I, dose-escalation study of TAK-117, a selective PI3Kalpha isoform inhibitor, in patients with advanced solid malignancies. Clin Cancer Res. 2017;23(17):5015–23.
23. Rodon J, Brana I, Siu LL, De Jonge MJ, Homji N, Mills D, et al. Phase I dose-escalation and -expansion study of buparlisib (BKM120), an oral pan-Class I PI3K inhibitor, in patients with advanced solid tumors. Invest New Drugs. 2014;32(4):670–81.
24. Fritsch C, Huang A, Chatenay-Rivauday C, Schnell C, Reddy A, Liu M, et al. Characterization of the novel and specific PI3Kalpha inhibitor NVP-BYL719 and development of the patient stratification strategy for clinical trials. Mol Cancer Ther. 2014;13(5):1117–29.
25. Maira SM, Pecchi S, Huang A, Burger M, Knapp M, Sterker D, et al. Identification and characterization of NVP-BKM120, an orally available pan-class I PI3-kinase inhibitor. Mol Cancer Ther. 2012;11(2):317–28.
26. Patnaik A, Appleman LJ, Tolcher AW, Papadopoulos KP, Beeram M, Rasco DW, et al. First-in-human phase I study of copanlisib (BAY 80-6946), an intravenous pan-class I phosphatidylinositol 3-kinase inhibitor, in patients with advanced solid tumors and non-Hodgkin's lymphomas. Ann Oncol. 2016;27(10):1928–40.
27. Hyman DM, Smyth LM, Donoghue MTA, Westin SN, Bedard PL, Dean EJ, et al. AKT inhibition in solid tumors with AKT1 mutations. J Clin Oncol. 2017;35(20):2251–9.
28. Mateo J, Ganji G, Lemech C, Burris HA, Han SW, Swales K, et al. A first-time-in-human study of GSK2636771, a phosphoinositide 3 kinase Beta-selective inhibitor, in patients with advanced solid tumors. Clin Cancer Res. 2017;23(19):5981–92.
29. Finn RS, Crown JP, Lang I, Boer K, Bondarenko IM, Kulyk SO, et al. The cyclin-dependent kinase 4/6 inhibitor palbociclib in combination with letrozole versus letrozole alone as first-line treatment of oestrogen receptor-positive, HER2-negative, advanced breast cancer (PALOMA-1/TRIO-18): a randomised phase 2 study. Lancet Oncol. 2015;16(1):25–35.
30. Hortobagyi GN, Stemmer SM, Burris HA, Yap YS, Sonke GS, Paluch-Shimon S, et al. Ribociclib as first-line therapy for HR-positive, advanced breast cancer. N Engl J Med. 2016;375(18):1738–48.
31. Goetz MP, Toi M, Campone M, Sohn J, Paluch-Shimon S, Huober J, et al. MONARCH 3: abemaciclib as initial therapy for advanced breast cancer. J Clin Oncol. 2017;35(32):3638–46.

32. Finn RS, Martin M, Rugo HS, Jones S, Im SA, Gelmon K, et al. Palbociclib and letrozole in advanced breast cancer. N Engl J Med. 2016;375(20):1925–36.
33. Aceto N, Bardia A, Wittner BS, Donaldson MC, O'Keefe R, Engstrom A, et al. AR expression in breast cancer CTCs associates with bone metastases. Mol Cancer Res. 2018;16(4):720–7.
34. Hickey TE, Irvine CM, Dvinge H, Tarulli GA, Hanson AR, Ryan NK, et al. Expression of androgen receptor splice variants in clinical breast cancers. Oncotarget. 2015;6(42):44728–44.
35. Early Breast Cancer Trialists' Collaborative G. Effects of chemotherapy and hormonal therapy for early breast cancer on recurrence and 15-year survival: an overview of the randomised trials. Lancet. 2005;365(9472):1687–717.
36. Mouridsen H, Gershanovich M, Sun Y, Perez-Carrion R, Boni C, Monnier A, et al. Phase III study of letrozole versus tamoxifen as first-line therapy of advanced breast cancer in postmenopausal women: analysis of survival and update of efficacy from the International Letrozole Breast Cancer Group. J Clin Oncol. 2003;21(11):2101–9.
37. Ariazi EA, Ariazi JL, Cordera F, Jordan VC. Estrogen receptors as therapeutic targets in breast cancer. Curr Top Med Chem. 2006;6(3):181–202.
38. Patel HK, Bihani T. Selective estrogen receptor modulators (SERMs) and selective estrogen receptor degraders (SERDs) in cancer treatment. Pharmacol Ther. 2018;186:1–24.
39. Musgrove EA, Sutherland RL. Biological determinants of endocrine resistance in breast cancer. Nat Rev Cancer. 2009;9(9):631–43.
40. Strasser-Weippl K, Goss PE. Advances in adjuvant hormonal therapy for postmenopausal women. J Clin Oncol. 2005;23(8):1751–9.
41. Arimidex, Tamoxifen, Alone or in Combination (ATAC) Trialists' Group, Forbes JF, Cuzick J, Buzdar A, Howell A, Tobias JS, et al. Effect of anastrozole and tamoxifen as adjuvant treatment for early-stage breast cancer: 100-month analysis of the ATAC trial. Lancet Oncol. 2008;9(1):45–53.
42. Peng J, Sengupta S, Jordan VC. Potential of selective estrogen receptor modulators as treatments and preventives of breast cancer. Anticancer Agents Med Chem. 2009;9(5):481–99.
43. Toy W, Shen Y, Won H, Green B, Sakr RA, Will M, et al. ESR1 ligand-binding domain mutations in hormone-resistant breast cancer. Nat Genet. 2013;45(12):1439–45.
44. Robinson DR, Wu YM, Vats P, Su F, Lonigro RJ, Cao X, et al. Activating ESR1 mutations in hormone-resistant metastatic breast cancer. Nat Genet. 2013;45(12):1446–51.
45. Jeselsohn R, Yelensky R, Buchwalter G, Frampton G, Meric-Bernstam F, Gonzalez-Angulo AM, et al. Emergence of constitutively active estrogen receptor-alpha mutations in pretreated advanced estrogen receptor-positive breast cancer. Clin Cancer Res. 2014;20(7):1757–67.
46. Fribbens C, O'Leary B, Kilburn L, Hrebien S, Garcia-Murillas I, Beaney M, et al. Plasma ESR1 mutations and the treatment of estrogen receptor-positive advanced breast cancer. J Clin Oncol. 2016;34(25):2961–8.
47. Chandarlapaty S, Chen D, He W, Sung P, Samoila A, You D, et al. Prevalence of ESR1 mutations in cell-free DNA and outcomes in metastatic breast Cancer: a secondary analysis of the BOLERO-2 clinical trial. JAMA Oncol. 2016;2(10):1310–5.
48. Merenbakh-Lamin K, Ben-Baruch N, Yeheskel A, Dvir A, Soussan-Gutman L, Jeselsohn R, et al. D538G mutation in estrogen receptor-alpha: a novel mechanism for acquired endocrine resistance in breast cancer. Cancer Res. 2013;73(23):6856–64.
49. Spoerke JM, Gendreau S, Walter K, Qiu J, Wilson TR, Savage H, et al. Heterogeneity and clinical significance of ESR1 mutations in ER-positive metastatic breast cancer patients receiving fulvestrant. Nat Commun. 2016;7:11579.
50. Schiavon G, Hrebien S, Garcia-Murillas I, Cutts RJ, Pearson A, Tarazona N, et al. Analysis of ESR1 mutation in circulating tumor DNA demonstrates evolution during therapy for metastatic breast cancer. Sci Transl Med. 2015;7(313):313ra182.
51. Turner N, Pearson A, Sharpe R, Lambros M, Geyer F, Lopez-Garcia MA, et al. FGFR1 amplification drives endocrine therapy resistance and is a therapeutic target in breast cancer. Cancer Res. 2010;70(5):2085–94.
52. Razavi P, Chang MT, Xu G, Bandlamudi C, Ross DS, Vasan N, et al. The genomic landscape of endocrine-resistant advanced breast cancers. Cancer Cell. 2018;34(3):427–38.e6.

Chapter 9
Genitourinary Tumors

Marie-Lisa Eich and George J. Netto

Key Points

- Consider tumor-based molecular assays like Decipher, Oncotype Dx Prostate, Prolaris, or Promark for patients with low-risk or favorable intermediate-risk disease with at least 10 years life expectancy for initial workup and risk stratification.
- Consider testing for homologous gene mutations and for microsatellite instability (MSI-H) or mismatch repair deficiency (dMMR) in patients with visceral or lymph node metastasis. Mutations in DNA repair genes may be predictive of sensitivity to PARP inhibitors and platinum-based chemotherapy. Patients with MSI or dMMR are eligible for pembrolizumab in CRPC.
- Germline testing should be considered in metastatic, high-risk, very-high-risk or regional disease. Furthermore in all patients with a family history suspicious for inherited cancer syndrome.
- According to NCCN guidelines, urinary tumor markers can be considered in addition to urine cytology and cystoscopy for surveillance in patients with high-risk NMIBC.
- Novel molecular taxonomy for MIBC with two major subclasses of luminal and basal/squamous tumors promises a new approach to therapy guidance.
- Luminal-infiltrated and the basal/squamous subtypes tend to benefit most from treatment with checkpoint inhibitors.

M.-L. Eich · G. J. Netto (✉)
Department of Pathology, The University of Alabama at Birmingham, Birmingham, AL, USA
e-mail: gnetto@uabmc.edu

L. J. Tafe, M. E. Arcila (eds.), *Genomic Medicine*,
https://doi.org/10.1007/978-3-030-22922-1_9

Key Online Resources
Prostate Cancer

- National Comprehensive Cancer Network (NCCN): https://www.nccn.org/store/login/login.aspx?ReturnURL=https://www.nccn.org/professionals/physician_gls/pdf/prostate.pdf
- American Urological Association (AUA):
  - Early detection of prostate cancer: http://www.auanet.org/guidelines/prostate-cancer-castration-resistant-(2013-amended-2018)
  - Localized prostate cancer: http://www.auanet.org/guidelines/prostate-cancer-clinically-localized-(2017)
  - Castration-resistant prostate cancer: http://www.auanet.org/guidelines/prostate-cancer-castration-resistant-(2013-amended-2018)
- European Association of Urology (EAU): http://uroweb.org/guideline/prostate-cancer/

Bladder Cancer

- National Comprehensive Cancer Network (NCCN): https://www.nccn.org/store/login/login.aspx?ReturnURL=https://www.nccn.org/professionals/physician_gls/PDF/bladder.pdf
- American Urological Association (AUA):
  - Non-muscle invasive bladder cancer: http://www.auanet.org/guidelines/bladder-cancer-non-muscle-invasive-(2016)
  - Muscle-invasive bladder cancer: http://www.auanet.org/guidelines/bladder-cancer-non-metastatic-muscle-invasive-(2017)
- European Association of Urology (EAU):
  - Non-muscle invasive bladder cancer: http://uroweb.org/guideline/non-muscle-invasive-bladder-cancer/
  - Muscle-invasive bladder cancer: http://uroweb.org/guideline/bladder-cancer-muscle-invasive-and-metastatic/

Introduction

Neoplasms of the prostate and bladder are among the most common solid tumors. Recent genomic advances have contributed to our understanding of the key driver genetic alterations in these malignancies offering new opportunities for targeted therapy. Prostate cancers can be stratified into very-low-risk, low-risk, favorable intermediate-risk, and unfavorable intermediate-risk categories. Tumor-based molecular biomarker testing is currently recommended for low-risk and favorable intermediate-risk groups, and germline testing is also recommended for potentially all prostate cancer patients considering clinical characteristics.

Urothelial carcinoma can be non-muscle-invasive bladder cancer (NMIBC) or muscle-invasive disease (MIBC) both with different treatment and prognostic significance. A novel molecular genomic-based taxonomy for bladder cancer has recently been proposed, and associated potential practical implications are discussed.

This chapter lists salient predictive and prognostic biomarkers in prostate cancer and urothelial neoplasms as well as molecular approaches examining eligibility for therapeutic targets and novel immunotherapy strategies. A summary of noninvasive urine-based assays for early detection and surveillance of urothelial carcinoma is provided. Practice-based key points and references are emphasized.

Prostate

Molecular Diagnostics in Prostate Cancer

Adenocarcinoma of the prostate is the most prevalent cancer type in American men with estimated 164,690 new cases diagnosed in 2018 men [1]. Given the wide variability in clinical behavior of prostate cancer (PCa), its management strategies span the spectrum from active surveillance for patients with very-low-risk disease to definitive treatment with radical prostatectomy (RP) and radiation therapy for patients with localized higher-risk disease. In advanced metastatic setting, therapeutic options include androgen-deprivation therapy, chemotherapy, and more recently immunotherapy.

Salient molecular events in PCa development are shown in Fig. 9.1. *TMPRSS2-ERG* rearrangement occurs in approximately half of PCa making it the most common alteration in human solid tumors [2]. In progression from localized to metastatic PCa, *PTEN* loss and telomerase activation play a critical role. Amplification of the androgen receptor gene locus, *TP53* mutation or deletion, and RB deletion are common in late-stage disease [3].

PCa is now recognized as one of the most heritable cancer types driven by numerous inherited germline genetic risk variants. Most established among these are germline mutations in *BRCA 2* tumor suppressor gene and *HOXB13 (G84E)* that carries a 4.5- and 2.93-fold risk of PCa development [4, 5]. Patients with Lynch syndrome harbor a 2.13-fold risk for developing PCa [6].

Prognostic Molecular Assays in PCa

Recently, the value of prostatic-specific antigen (PSA) screening strategy in affecting overall prostate cancer survivorship has been questioned. In this regard, molecular assays may assist in avoidance of overtreatment of clinically indolent disease and identifying patient with a higher probability of developing lethal disease. Several commercially available genomic/proteomic tests are now available at the disposal of urologists and urologic oncologists to guide management. Some of these

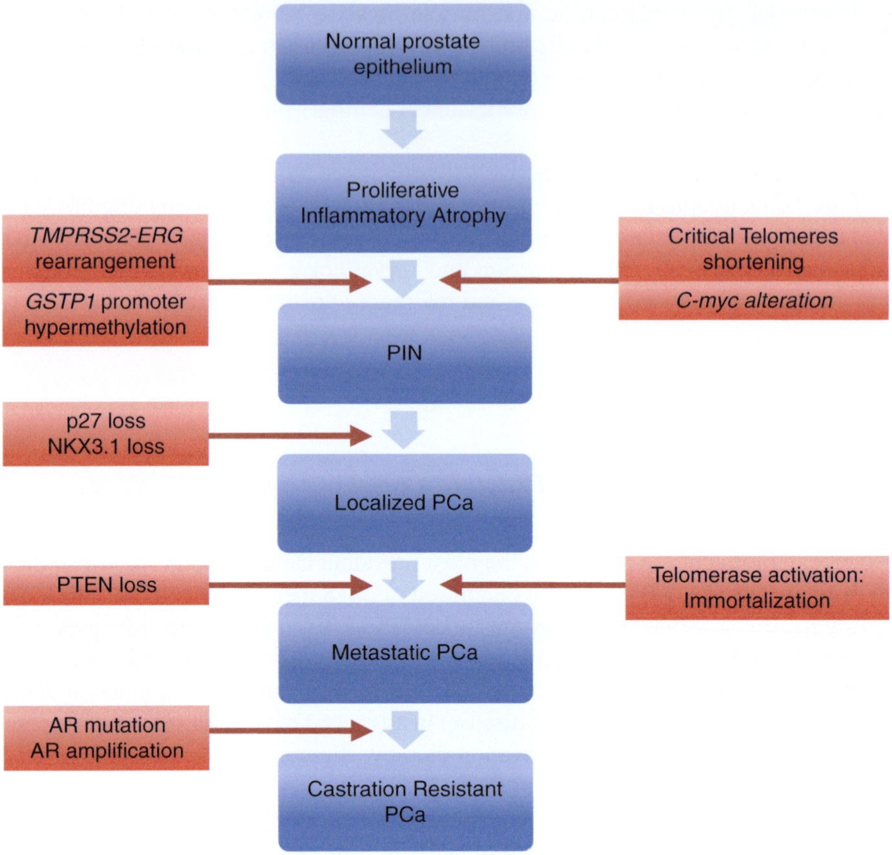

Fig. 9.1 Salient molecular events in PCa development

assays are shown in Table 9.1. Current NCCN guidelines recommend a consideration of these test only in men with low-risk or favorable intermediate-risk disease with a life expectancy of at least 10 years during initial risk stratification. Molecular assays performed on prostate needle biopsy or RP specimens carry prognostic information independent of NCCN risk groups. These include, but are not limited to, likelihood of death with conservative management, likelihood of biochemical progression or metastasis after RP, or external beam therapy [7].

Targets of Therapy and Predictive Molecular Markers

The Cancer Genome Atlas Network has recently carried out a detailed molecular analysis of 333 primary prostate cancers. Based on genetic, epigenetic, and proteomic analysis, 74% of tumor were assigned to one of seven molecular subtypes defined by a specific oncogenic driver. These include four gene fusions (*ERG, ETV1, ETV4,*

Table 9.1 Commercially available genomic/proteomic tests in prostate cancer

Assay (manufacturer)	Sample	Platform	Assessed genes	Clinical application	Molecular Diagnostic Services Program (MolDx) Recommendations
Prolaris®[8] (Myriad Genetics)	FFPE needle biopsy or prostatectomy tissue	*Cell cycle progression (CCP) score*: expression of 31 cell cycle genes; quantitative RT-PCR	FOXM1, ASPM, TK1, PRC1, CDC20, BUB1B, PBK, DTL, CDKN3, RRM2, ASF1B, CEP55, CDC2, DLGAP5, C18orf24, RAD51, KIF11, BIRC5, RAD54L, CENPM, KIAA0101, KIF20A, PTTG1, CDCA8, NUSAP1, PLK1, CDCA3, ORC6L, CENPF, TOP2A, MCM10	Calculate risk of BCR or metastasis post RP Predict, on needle biopsy, death of disease in conservatively treated Predict, on needle biopsy, presence of Gleason pattern ≥ 4 disease at RP	Use for post-biopsy for NCCN very-low-risk, low-risk, and favorable intermediate-risk prostate cancer in patients with at least 10 years life expectancy who have not received treatment for prostate cancer and are candidates for active surveillance or definitive therapy [7]
Oncotype DX® [9] (Genomic Health)	FFPE needle biopsy tissue	*Genomic predictor score (GPS):* expression of 12 genes; (androgen pathway, cellular organization, cell proliferation, and stromal response); quantitative RT-PCR	Androgen pathway: AZGP1, KLK2, SRD5A2, FAM13C Cellular organization: FLNC, GSN, TPM2, GSTM2 Proliferation: TPX2 Stromal response: BGN, COL1A1, SFRP4	Risk assessment prior to treatment intervention Predict non-organ-confined (pT3) or Gleason pattern 4 disease on RP	Use for post-biopsy for NCCN very-low-risk, low risk, and favorable intermediate-risk prostate cancer in patients with at least 10 years life expectancy who have not received treatment for prostate cancer and are candidates for active surveillance or definitive therapy [7]

(continued)

Table 9.1 (continued)

Assay (manufacturer)	Sample	Platform	Assessed genes	Clinical application	Molecular Diagnostic Services Program (MolDx) Recommendations
Decipher™ [10, 11] (GenomeDx)	FFPE needle biopsy or prostatectomy tissue	*Genomic classifier (GC):* expression of 22 genes; gene expression profiling arrays	Cell proliferation, differentiation: LASP1, IQGAP3, NFIB, S1PR4 Cell structure, adhesion, motility: THBS2, ANO7 (3' UTR, non-coding transcript), PCDH7, MYBPC1 (coding, intronic), EPPK1 Immune response: TSBP, PBX1 Cell cycle progression, mitosis: NUSAP1, ZWILCH, UBE2C (3'UTR, coding antisense), CAMK2N1, RABGAP1 Other, unknown function: PCAT-32, GLYATL1P4/ PCAT-80, TNFRSF19	Calculate risk for prostate cancer-specific mortality and metastasis post RP Guide clinical decision for radiotherapy in adjuvant or salvage setting Predict, on needle biopsy, metastasis and Gleason pattern ≥4 disease post RP and metastasis post EBRT	Use for post-RP for: 1. pT2 with positive margins 2. Any pT3 disease 3. Rising PSA (above nadir) [7]
ProMark™ [12] (Metamark Genetics Inc.)	FFPE needle biopsy sections	*Metamark's automated proteomic imaging platform* tissue sections subjected to multiplex immunofluorescent staining	DERL1, PDSS1, pS6, YBX1, HSPA9, FUS, SMAD4, CUL2	Predict presence of non-organ-confined (pT3) disease or Gleason pattern 4 on RP	Use for post-biopsy for NCCN very-low-risk and low risk prostate cancer in patients with at least 10 years life expectancy who have not received treatment for prostate cancer and are candidates for active surveillance or definitive therapy [7]

FLI1: 46%, 8%, 4%, and 1% of cases, respectively) and three genetic mutations (*SPOP, FOXA1, IDH1*: 11%, 3%, and 1%, respectively). The TCGA study identified therapeutically targetable alterations in PI3K and MAPK (RAS) pathways affecting 25% of all PCa tumors [13]. Distribution of most common genetic alterations in another dataset (MSK-IMPACT dataset) are shown by pathway across locoregional, metastatic non-castrate, and metastatic castration resistant, shown in Fig. 9.2 [14].

Several independent studies identified mutations in DNA repair genes in 12–27% of all PCa. These are more frequent in metastatic castration-resistant prostate cancer (CRPC) than in localized cancer [13, 15–17]. Germline DNA repair gene mutations occur in 11.8% of men with metastatic and in 6% of men with localized high-risk PCa [16]. Preliminary studies have suggested that either germline or somatically acquired mutations in these genes might be predictive of the therapeutic benefit of poly-ADP ribose polymerase (PARP) inhibitors, e.g., olaparib [17, 18]. Furthermore, presence of BRCA/ATM germline mutations may predict better response to next-generation hormonal therapy in CRPC patients [15]. Distribution of inherited DNA repair gene mutations in men with metastatic PCa is shown in Fig. 9.3.

Similar to other solid tumors, DNA mismatch repair deficiency (dMMR) has been suggested to predict response to immune checkpoint blockade with antibodies to programmed death receptor-1 (PD-1) [19]. CRPC patients with tumors harboring these alterations are now eligible for treatment with the immune checkpoint inhibitor pembrolizumab. dMMR status may also be predictive for the sensitivity to platinum agents [20]. Therefore, testing tumor for microsatellite instability (MSI-H) or dMMR should be considered in PCa patients with visceral and/or lymph node metastasis.

The current NCCN guidelines recommend considering germline testing for all men with metastatic, regional, or high-/very-high-risk clinically localized prostate cancer. Furthermore, if a familial cancer syndrome is suspected, germline testing can be considered also in patients with very low, low, favorable intermediate, and unfavorable intermediate risk [7].

Bladder

Molecular Diagnostics in Bladder Cancer

Urothelial carcinoma is the most common malignancy of the bladder with estimated 81,190 new cases and 17,240 cancer-related deaths in 2018 in the USA [1]. Invasive bladder cancer evolves through two distinct precursor lesions: noninvasive papillary tumors and “flat” urothelial carcinoma in situ (CIS). Due to high recurrence rates (up to 75%) [21] and likelihood for progression (up to 25%) [22], patients diagnosed with non-muscle-invasive bladder cancer (NMIBC) are regularly followed by cystoscopy and cytology. Treatment options for NMIBC include transurethral tumor resection and for high-risk patients intravesical instillation of an attenuated strain of *Mycobacterium bovis* (bacillus Calmette-Guérin “BCG”) [23–25]. Muscle-invasive disease (MIBC) is treated with radical cystectomy/cystoprostatectomy with or without chemotherapy (or less frequently radiotherapy) in the neoadjuvant or adjuvant

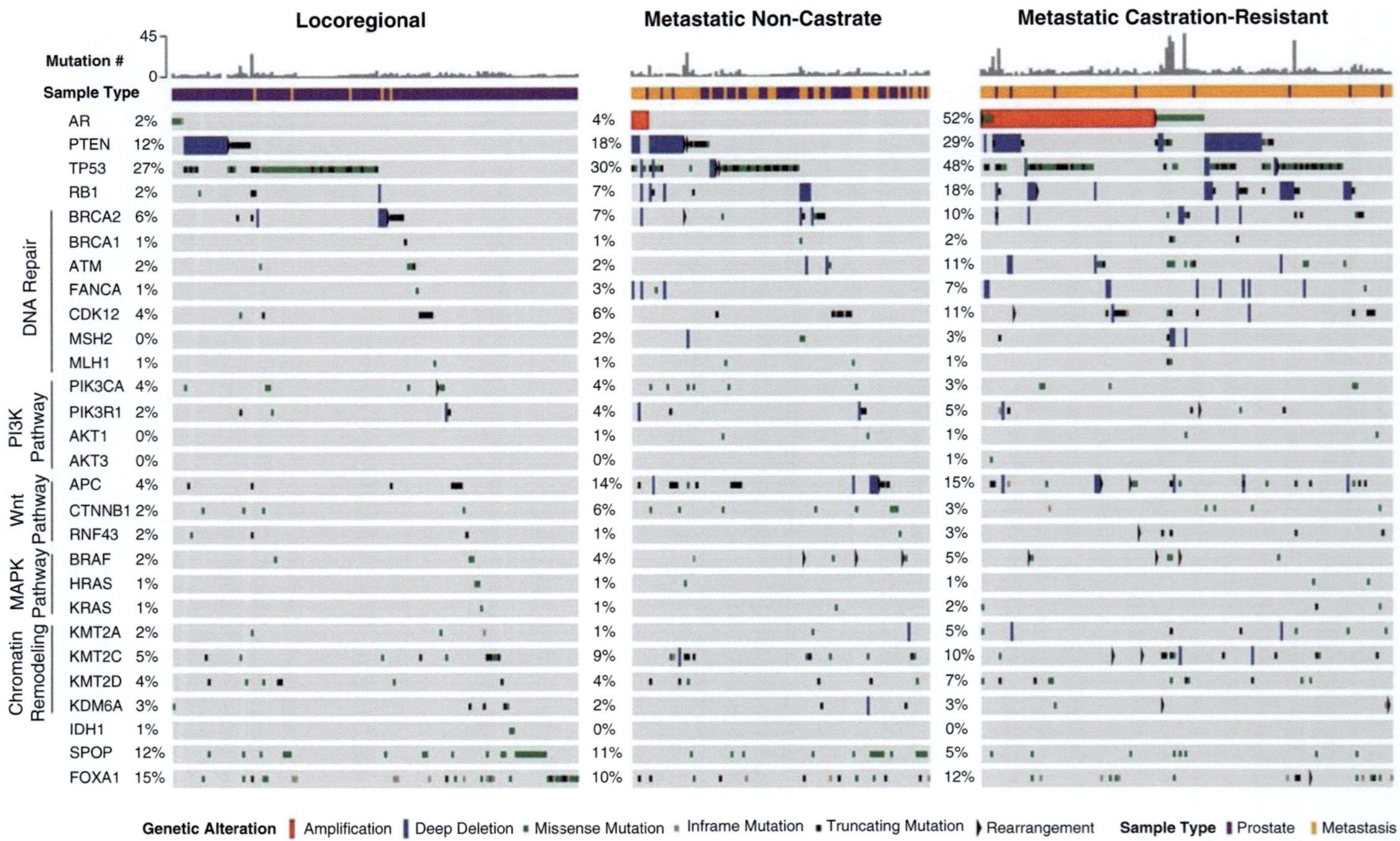

Fig. 9.2 Genomic alterations across disease states in the MSK-IMPACT dataset [14]. (Reprinted with permission of © 2017 American Society of Clinical Oncology. All rights reserved)

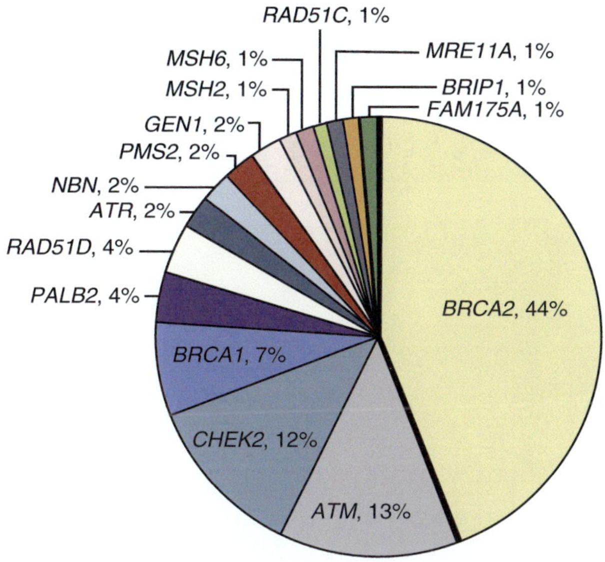

Fig. 9.3 Distribution of inherited DNA repair gene mutations in men with metastatic PCa [16]. (Reprinted with permission from Massachusetts Medical Society)

setting [25–27]. In patients with metastatic disease, treatment primarily involves chemotherapy and more recently immunotherapy with immune checkpoint inhibitors interfering in the PD-1/PD-L1 pathway [28–30]. Predictive biomarkers of response are under active investigation.

Diagnostic Assays

Noninvasive urine-based diagnostic approaches for early detection and surveillance of bladder cancer are being investigated. The current NCCN guidelines recommend consideration of such markers during follow-up for high-risk NMIBC. Most commonly used and promising urine-based assays are shown in Table 9.2.

Genomic Taxonomy, Targets of Therapy, and Predictive Markers

Two TCGA studies of bladder cancer have been completed that support a novel molecular taxonomy for MIBC with two major subclasses of luminal and basal/squamous tumors. Luminal tumors are characterized by KRT20, GATA3, and FOXA1 positivity, while basal/squamous tumors are typically positive for KRT5/6/14 and negative for GATA3 and FOXA1. These two subclasses can be further stratified based on genetic, epigenetic, and proteomic signature into four molecular subclasses: luminal-papillary (35%), luminal-infiltrated (19%), luminal (6%), and basal/squamous (35%). A fifth group of tumors (neuronal) is now also recognized accounting for 5% of MIBC (see Fig. 9.4).

Table 9.2 Urine-based assays

Assay (manufacturer)	Marker	Specimen	Assay platform	Sensitivity (%)	Specificity (%)	FDA approval
Cytology [31]	Tumor cells	Voided urine,	Microscopy	11–76	>90	
BTA-Stat® (Polymedco) [32, 33]	Complement factor H-related protein (and complement factor H)	Voided urine	Dipstick enzyme immunoassay	65%	74%	For bladder cancer detection and surveillance [34]
BTA-TRAK® (Polymedco) [33]	Complement factor H-related protein (and complement factor H)	Voided urine	ELISA	64%	77%	For bladder cancer detection and surveillance [34]
NMP-22® ELISA (Abcott Inc.) [33, 35]	Nuclear mitotic apparatus protein 1	Voided urine	ELISA	69%	77%	For bladder cancer detection and surveillance [34]
NMP22® BladderChek® (Abcott Inc.) [36]	Nuclear mitotic apparatus protein 1	Voided urine	Immunochromatographic assay	56%	88%	For bladder cancer detection and surveillance [34]
ImmunoCyt/uCyt+™ (Scimedx Inc.) [37]	Carcinoembryonic antigen (19A211), 2 bladder tumor cell–associated mucins (LDQ10 and M344)	Exfoliated cells	Immunocytochemistry	78%	78%	Surveillance [34]
UroVysion (Abcott Inc.) [33, 38]	Alterations in chromosomes 3, 7, 17, and 9p21	Exfoliated cells	Multicolored, multiprobe FISH	63%	87%	For bladder cancer detection and surveillance [34]
UroMark [39]	150 CpG loci biomarker panel	Urinary sediment DNA	Next-generation bisulfide sequencing	95%	96%	
Cxbladder [33, 35, 40]	*CDC2, HOXA13, MDK*, and *IGFBP5, CXCR2*	Voided urine	Reverse transcriptase PCR of 5 mRNA	82%	85%	
UroSEEK and Cytology [41]	*TERT, FGFR3, TP53, CDKN2A, ERBB2, HRAS, KRAS, PIK3CA, MET, VHL, and MLL*, aneuploidy Tumor cells (cytology)	Urinary cells from voided urine	Multiplex PCR, aneuploidy analysis, analysis of TERT promoter region Microscopy	Early detection: 95% Surveillance: 71%	Early detection: 93% Surveillance: 80%	

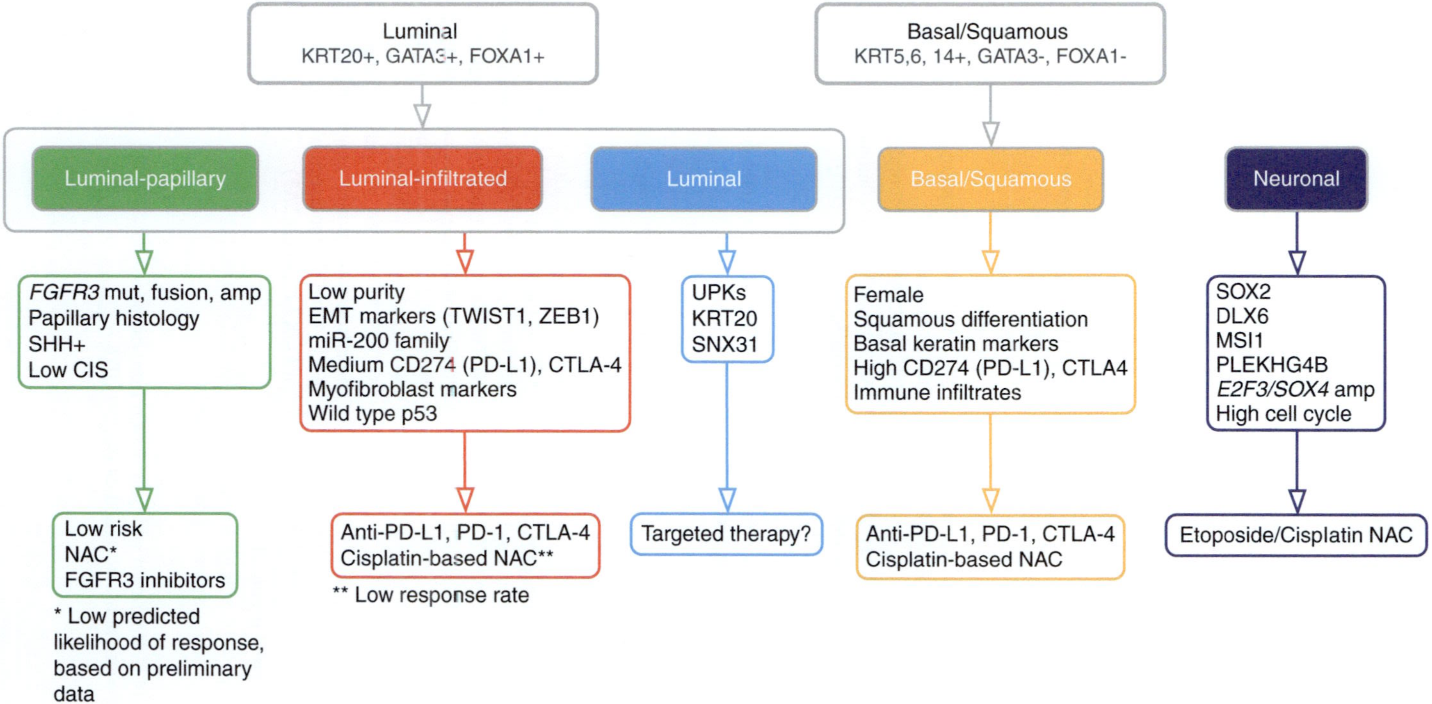

Fig. 9.4 Proposed TCGA molecular subtypes of muscle-invasive bladder cancer with prognostic and therapeutic implications [42]. (Reprinted with permission from Elsevier)

Table 9.3 Pathway alterations and targets of therapy

Altered gene/ protein	Drug category	Drug examples	Clinical trials examples (phase)
RTK/RAS pathway			
FGFR1, FGFR2, FGFR3	Pan-FGFR inhibitor	BAY1163877; dovitinib	NCT01976741 (1) NCT01732107 (2) (completed)
	FGFR 3 inhibitor	B-701	NCT02401542 (1b/2) NCT03123055 (1b/2) (combined with prembrolizumab)
ERBB2, ERBB3	ERBB2 inhibitor	Trastuzumab; lapatinib; DN24–02; T-DM1	NCT00238420 (1/2) NCT01245660 (1) (completed) NCT02342587 (2) (completed) NCT01353222 (2) (terminated) NCT01953926 (2)
PI3K/AKT/mTOR pathway			
PIK3CA, AKT1, AKT3, TSC1, TSC2, PTEN	mTOR inhibitor	Sapanisertib; Everolimus; AZD2014	NCT03047213 (2) NCT00805129 (2) (not recruiting) NCT02546661 (1) NCT01259063 (1) (completed)
	pan-PI3K inhibitor	BKM120 (buparlisib); BYL719	NCT01470209 (1) (combined with everolimus) (completed)
Immune modulators			
CTLA4	Anti-CTLA4	Ipilimumab; tremelimumab	NCT02812420 (1) (combined with durvalumab) NCT03150836 (1/2) (combined with durvalumab) NCT03234153 (2) (combined with durvalumab) NCT03601455 (2) (combined with durvalumab and radiation therapy)
PD-L1 (CD274) PD-1	Anti-PDL1 Anti-PD1	Atezolizumab; pembrolizumab (MK-3475)	NCT02450331 (3) NCT02108652 (2) (active not recruiting) NCT02302807 (3) (active not recruiting) NCT02256436 (3) (active not recruiting) NCT02853305 (3) (active not recruiting) NCT02625961 (2) NCT03577132 (NA) for patients with basal/squamous tumors (high KRT5/6 and KRT14 and low/undetectable expression of FOXA1 and GATA3)
Treatment based on genetic profile of the tumor			
MATCH screening trial		Drugs based on genetic profile of the tumor	NCT02465060 (2)

From Netto and Tafe [43]. Reprinted with permission from Elsevier
https://clinicaltrials.gov/ct2/home Accessed 24 August 2018

The luminal-infiltrated and the basal/squamous subtypes show high levels of immune-expression signature and therefore tend to benefit most from treatment with checkpoint inhibitors like antibodies against PD-1, PD-L1, and CTLA4. The luminal-papillary subtype displays *FGFR3* activation (mutations, amplifications, or overexpression) in 44% of the cases making them a target for treatment with FGFR3 inhibitors. While the luminal-papillary and luminal-infiltrated subclass tend to be resistant to chemotherapy, patients with tumors of the basal/squamous and neuronal subclass are more likely to benefit for neoadjuvant chemotherapy [42]. Additional targets of therapy are shown in Table 9.3.

References

1. Siegel RL, Miller KD, Jemal A. Cancer statistics, 2017. CA Cancer J Clin. 2017;67:7–30.
2. Weier C, Haffner MC, Mosbruger T, Esopi DM, Hicks J, Zheng Q, et al. Nucleotide resolution analysis of TMPRSS2 and ERG rearrangements in prostate cancer. J Pathol. 2013;230:174–83.
3. Netto GJ. Clinical applications of recent molecular advances in urologic malignancies: no longer chasing a "mirage"? Adv Anat Pathol. 2013;20:175–203.
4. Kote-Jarai Z, Mikropoulos C, Leongamornlert DA, Dadaev T, Tymrakiewicz M, Saunders EJ, et al. Prevalence of the HOXB13 G84E germline mutation in British men and correlation with prostate cancer risk, tumour characteristics and clinical outcomes. Ann Oncol. 2015;26:756–61.
5. Bryant HE. The clinical impact of BRCA2 loss in prostate cancer. Eur Urol. 2016;69:996–7.
6. Ryan S, Jenkins MA, Win AK. Risk of prostate cancer in Lynch syndrome: a systematic review and meta-analysis. Cancer Epidemiol Biomarkers Prev. 2014;23:437–49.
7. Network NCC. National Comprehensive Cancer Network (NCCN): prostate. Cancer. 2018. https://www.nccn.org/store/login/login.aspx?ReturnURL=https://www.nccn.org/professionals/physician_gls/pdf/prostate.pdf.
8. Cuzick J, Swanson GP, Fisher G, Brothman AR, Berney DM, Reid JE, et al. Prognostic value of an RNA expression signature derived from cell cycle proliferation genes in patients with prostate cancer: a retrospective study. Lancet Oncol. 2011;12:245–55.
9. Knezevic D, Goddard AD, Natraj N, Cherbavaz DB, Clark-Langone KM, Snable J, et al. Analytical validation of the Oncotype DX prostate cancer assay – a clinical RT-PCR assay optimized for prostate needle biopsies. BMC Genomics. 2013;14:690.
10. Erho N, Crisan A, Vergara IA, Mitra AP, Ghadessi M, Buerki C, et al. Discovery and validation of a prostate cancer genomic classifier that predicts early metastasis following radical prostatectomy. PLoS One. 2013;8:e66855.
11. Karnes RJ, Bergstralh EJ, Davicioni E, Ghadessi M, Buerki C, Mitra AP, et al. Validation of a genomic classifier that predicts metastasis following radical prostatectomy in an at risk patient population. J Urol. 2013;190:2047.
12. Blume-Jensen P, Berman DM, Rimm DL, Shipitsin M, Putzi M, Nifong TP, et al. Development and clinical validation of an in situ biopsy-based multimarker assay for risk stratification in prostate cancer. Clin Cancer Res. 2015;21:2591–600.
13. Network CGAR. The molecular taxonomy of primary prostate cancer. Cell. 2015;163:1011–25.
14. Abida W, Armenia J, Gopalan A, Brennan R, Walsh M, Barron D, et al. Prospective genomic profiling of prostate cancer across disease states reveals germline and somatic alterations that may affect clinical decision making. JCO Precis Oncol. 2017;2017 https://doi.org/10.1200/PO.17.00029.

15. Antonarakis ES, Lu C, Luber B, Liang C, Wang H, Chen Y, et al. Germline DNA-repair gene mutations and outcomes in men with metastatic castration-resistant prostate cancer receiving first-line abiraterone and enzalutamide. Eur Urol. 2018;74:218–25.
16. Pritchard CC, Mateo J, Walsh MF, De Sarkar N, Abida W, Beltran H, et al. Inherited DNA-repair gene mutations in men with metastatic prostate cancer. N Engl J Med. 2016;375:443–53.
17. Robinson D, Van Allen EM, Wu YM, Schultz N, Lonigro RJ, Mosquera JM, et al. Integrative clinical genomics of advanced prostate cancer. Cell. 2015;162:454.
18. Kaufman B, Shapira-Frommer R, Schmutzler RK, Audeh MW, Friedlander M, Balmana J, et al. Olaparib monotherapy in patients with advanced cancer and a germline BRCA1/2 mutation. J Clin Oncol. 2015;33:244–50.
19. Le DT, Durham JN, Smith KN, Wang H, Bartlett BR, Aulakh LK, et al. Mismatch repair deficiency predicts response of solid tumors to PD-1 blockade. Science. 2017;357:409–13.
20. Imyanitov EN, Moiseyenko VM. Drug therapy for hereditary cancers. Hered Cancer Clin Pract. 2011;9:5.
21. Chamie K, Litwin MS, Bassett JC, Daskivich TJ, Lai J, Hanley JM, et al. Recurrence of high-risk bladder cancer: a population-based analysis. Cancer. 2013;119:3219–27.
22. Millan-Rodriguez F, Chechile-Toniolo G, Salvador-Bayarri J, Palou J, Algaba F, Vicente-Rodriguez J. Primary superficial bladder cancer risk groups according to progression, mortality and recurrence. J Urol. 2000;164:680–4.
23. Babjuk M, Bohle A, Burger M, Capoun O, Cohen D, Comperat EM, et al. EAU guidelines on non-muscle-invasive urothelial carcinoma of the bladder: update 2016. Eur Urol. 2017;71:447–61.
24. Chang SS, Boorjian SA, Chou R, Clark PE, Daneshmand S, Konety BR, Pruthi R, Quale DZ, Ritch CR, Seigne JD, Skinner EC, Smith ND, McKiernan JM. Diagnosis and treatment of non-muscle invasive bladder cancer: AUA/SUO Joint Guideline. 2016. http://www.auanet.org/guidelines/bladder-cancer-non-muscle-invasive-(2016).
25. Network NCC. NCCN Clinical Practice Guidelines in Oncology. Bladder Cancer. 2018. https://www.nccn.org/store/login/login.aspx?ReturnURL=https://www.nccn.org/professionals/physician_gls/PDF/bladder.pdf.
26. Chang SS, Bochner BH, Chou R, Dreicer R, Kamat AM, Lerner SP, Lotan Y, Meeks JJ, Michalski JM, Morgan TM, Quale DZ, Rosenberg JE, Zietman AL, Holzbeierlein JM. Treatment of non-metastatic muscle-invasive bladder cancer: AUA/ASCO/ASTRO/SUO Guideline. 2017. http://www.auanet.org/guidelines/bladder-cancer-non-metastatic-muscle-invasive-(2017).
27. Witjes JA (Chair), Bruins M, Compérat E, Cowan NC, Gakis G, Hernández V, Lebret T, Lorch A, Ribal MJ (Vice-chair), van der Heijden AG, Veskimäe E. European Association of Urology (EAU) Guideline: muscle-invasive and metastatic bladder cancer. 2018. http://uroweb.org/guideline/bladder-cancer-muscle-invasive-and-metastatic/.
28. Bellmunt J, de Wit R, Vaughn DJ, Fradet Y, Lee JL, Fong L, et al. Pembrolizumab as second-line therapy for advanced urothelial carcinoma. New Engl J Med. 2017;376:1015–26.
29. Balar AV, Galsky MD, Rosenberg JE, Powles T, Petrylak DP, Bellmunt J, et al. Atezolizumab as first-line treatment in cisplatin-ineligible patients with locally advanced and metastatic urothelial carcinoma: a single-arm, multicentre, phase 2 trial. Lancet. 2017;389:67–76.
30. Balar AV, Castellano D, O'Donnell PH, Grivas P, Vuky J, Powles T, et al. First-line pembrolizumab in cisplatin-ineligible patients with locally advanced and unresectable or metastatic urothelial cancer (KEYNOTE-052): a multicentre, single-arm, phase 2 study. Lancet Oncol. 2017;18:1483–92.
31. Lokeshwar VB, Habuchi T, Grossman HB, Murphy WM, Hautmann SH, Hemstreet GP 3rd, et al. Bladder tumor markers beyond cytology: International Consensus Panel on bladder tumor markers. Urology. 2005;66:35–63.
32. Guo A, Wang X, Gao L, Shi J, Sun C, Wan Z. Bladder tumour antigen (BTA stat) test compared to the urine cytology in the diagnosis of bladder cancer: a meta-analysis. Can Urol Assoc J. 2014;8:E347–52.

33. Chou R, Gore JL, Buckley D, Fu R, Gustafson K, Griffin JC, et al. Urinary biomarkers for diagnosis of bladder cancer: a systematic review and meta-analysis. Ann Intern Med. 2015;163:922–31.
34. Smith ZL, Guzzo TJ. Urinary markers for bladder cancer. F1000Prime Rep. 2013;5:21.
35. O'Sullivan P, Sharples K, Dalphin M, Davidson P, Gilling P, Cambridge L, et al. A multi-gene urine test for the detection and stratification of bladder cancer in patients presenting with hematuria. J Urol. 2012;188:741–7.
36. Wang Z, Que H, Suo C, Han Z, Tao J, Huang Z, et al. Evaluation of the NMP22 BladderChek test for detecting bladder cancer: a systematic review and meta-analysis. Oncotarget. 2017;8:100648–56.
37. He H, Han C, Hao L, Zang G. ImmunoCyt test compared to cytology in the diagnosis of bladder cancer: a meta-analysis. Oncol Lett. 2016;12:83–8.
38. Lavery HJ, Zaharieva B, McFaddin A, Heerema N, Pohar KS. A prospective comparison of UroVysion FISH and urine cytology in bladder cancer detection. BMC Cancer. 2017;17:247.
39. Feber A, Dhami P, Dong L, de Winter P, Tan WS, Martinez-Fernandez M, et al. UroMark-a urinary biomarker assay for the detection of bladder cancer. Clin Epigenetics. 2017;9:8.
40. Lotan Y, O'Sullivan P, Raman JD, Shariat SF, Kavalieris L, Frampton C, et al. Clinical comparison of noninvasive urine tests for ruling out recurrent urothelial carcinoma. Urol Oncol. 2017;35:531.e15–22.
41. Springer SU, Chen CH, Rodriguez Pena MDC, Li L, Douville C, Wang Y, et al. Non-invasive detection of urothelial cancer through the analysis of driver gene mutations and aneuploidy. Elife. 2018;7. pii: e32143.
42. Robertson AG, Kim J, Al-Ahmadie H, Bellmunt J, Guo G, Cherniack AD, et al. Comprehensive molecular characterization of muscle-invasive bladder cancer. Cell. 2017;171:540–56 e25.
43. Netto GJ, Tafe LJ. Emerging bladder cancer biomarkers and targets of therapy. Urol Clin North Am. 2016;43:63–76.

Chapter 10
Gynecologic Malignancies

Jessica L. Dillon and Laura J. Tafe

Key Points

- Gynecologic malignancies are a histologically and molecularly heterogeneous group of tumors comprising tumors of epithelial, mesenchymal, germ cell, and sex cord origins.
- Molecular diagnostics of gynecological malignancies is becoming a more valuable tool for diagnosis, prognosis, and prediction of response to therapies.
- Recurrent genetic alterations can now define rare subtypes of tumors that share a similar clinical course.

Key Online Resources

- Ovary NCCN: https://www.nccn.org/patients/guidelines/ovarian/files/assets/common/downloads/files/ovarian.pdf
- Endometrial cancer NCCN: https://www.nccn.org/professionals/physician_gls/pdf/uterine.pdf
- Uterine mesenchymal tumors NCCN: https://www.nccn.org/professionals/physician_gls/pdf/uterine.pdf

J. L. Dillon · L. J. Tafe (✉)
Department of Pathology and Laboratory Medicine, Dartmouth-Hitchcock Medical Center, Lebanon, NH, USA

Geisel School of Medicine at Dartmouth, Hanover, NH, USA
e-mail: Jessica.L.Dillon@hitchcock.org; Laura.J.Tafe@hitchcock.org

L. J. Tafe, M. E. Arcila (eds.), *Genomic Medicine*,
https://doi.org/10.1007/978-3-030-22922-1_10

Introduction

In recent years, large-scale genomic efforts, like The Cancer Genome Atlas (TCGA) project have produced a wealth of genomic information and provided new frameworks in which to view and classify the morphologic heterogeneity of gynecologic neoplasms. For some tumors, new classification systems further define the stepwise progression of tumorigenesis. In others, like endometrial cancers, grouping tumors into molecular classifications correlate with patient prognosis. Identification of germline mutations in genes associated with inherited syndromes, such as hereditary breast and ovarian cancer syndrome and Lynch syndrome has allowed for early detection of precursor lesions in risk-reducing prophylactic surgeries and genetic counseling for families with germline mutations. In addition, somatic and germline alterations in these same genes have implications for eligibility for therapy with PARP inhibitors or immunotherapies, respectively. Molecular characterization of gynecologic tumors complements standard histology assessment and can inform the diagnosis, prognosis, and selection of therapeutic approaches.

Ovary

Epithelial ovarian tumors are the most common primary ovarian malignancies, accounting for 90% of newly diagnosed cases of ovarian cancer [1, 2]. Broadly, epithelial ovarian tumors can be divided into two categories, Type I and Type II. Type I tumors, such as low-grade serous carcinoma (LGSC), develop from precursor lesions (i.e., atypical proliferative serous tumors) and are typically present at an earlier clinical stage [2–5]. Activating mutations in *KRAS* and *BRAF* are potential biomarkers identified in the development of low-grade serous carcinomas that lead to aberrant signaling in the RAS-MAPK (mitogen-activated protein kinase) pathway (Table 10.1) [1, 2, 5–7]. The stepwise, indolent growth pattern of LGSC is problematic for treatment, as many patients recur despite surgery and/or hormonal therapy [6]. Clinical trials are evaluating MEK inhibitors for targeted therapy of low-grade serous carcinoma, particularly in patients with resistance to cytotoxic chemotherapy and protracted or recurrent disease [2, 7].

Type II epithelial ovarian tumors, including high-grade serous carcinoma (HGSC), carcinosarcoma (MMMT), and undifferentiated carcinomas, are genetically unstable, are typically present in older women, and are highly aggressive [1–4]. Although once thought to originate from the surface epithelium of the ovary, intraepithelial lesions in the fallopian tube (i.e., serous tubal intraepithelial lesion) are now thought to be precursors of high-grade serous carcinoma [2, 6]. In contrast to the activating *KRAS* and *BRAF* mutations in LGSC, many HGSC harbor *TP53* mutations or lose the integrity of BRCA1 and BRCA2 functionality [1–6, 8]. *TP53* mutations in HGSC can often be identified immunohistochemically by an aberrant (mutant) nuclear overexpression or a complete loss (null pattern) of p53 expression

Table 10.1 Mutations commonly identified in epithelial ovarian tumors [1–16]

Tumor type	Gene	Mutation type/specific mutation	% of cases with mutation/genetic alteration	Clinical implication
Low-grade serous carcinoma (LGSC)	*BRAF (RAS-MAPK pathway)*	Activating mutation	2–5%	RAS/RAF/MEK/ERK pathway inhibitor
	RAS (KRAS, NRAS, HRAS) (RAS-MAPK pathway)	Activating mutation	16–19%	RAS/RAF/MEK/ERK pathway inhibitor
High-grade serous carcinoma (HGSC)	*TP53*	Missense (>50%) Frameshift/splicing junctions/nonsense (39%)	96%	Advanced stage at presentation, poor 5-year survival, early relapse, broad chemoresistance
	BRCA1 *BRCA2*	Germline LOH (hereditary breast and ovarian cancer syndrome) Somatic (6%) Hypermethylation of the *BRCA1* promoter	47%	Eligibility for PARP inhibitor therapy
Clear cell carcinoma	*ARID1A*	Aberrant chromatin remodeling	46–57%	High resistance to platinum-based therapy
	PIK3CA	Exons 9 and 20 Kinase activation of p110α	33%	Small molecular inhibitors, targeting PI3K
	TERT	Promoter gain-of-function mutation C228T C250T	15.9%	Mutually exclusive with loss of *ARID1A* and *PIK3CA*
Endometrioid carcinoma	*CTNNB1*	Missense mutation	16–54%	Frequently lower grade, more favorable prognosis (BELL)
	MLH1, PMS2, MSH2, MSH6	Germline mutation Somatic mutation (including *MLH1* promoter hypermethylation)	12–19%	Microsatellite instability; Lynch and Lynch-like syndrome
	PTEN	LOH	20%	Mutations and LOH have been identified in adjacent endometriotic cysts Germline mutation: Cowden syndrome
Mucinous tumors	*KRAS*	Activating mutation	33–86%	
Brenner tumor	*KRAS*	Mutation		
	CCND1	Amplification		
	MYC	Amplification		

and a concomitant elevation in the Ki-67 proliferation index (Table 10.1) [6]. Treatment of HGSC can be challenging given the genetic instability, highly aggressive nature of these tumors, and development of chemoresistance [3, 8–11]. Also, patients often present with an advanced stage of disease at the time of clinical presentation. Novel treatment options for somatic and germline mutations in *BRCA1/2* genes, including eligibility for poly (ADP-ribose) polymerase (PARP) inhibitors, are showing promising results, and several of these agents are now FDA approved [10, 11]. Mutation in *BRCA1/2* genes is one mechanism leading to homologous repair deficiency (HRD) in tumor cells. Tumors with HRD are sensitized to PARP inhibition, which blocks the base excision repair pathway. The combination of HRD and PARP inhibition leads to DNA damage and death of tumor cells and also has less adverse treatment side effects than standard chemotherapies [10, 11].

Endometrioid carcinomas of the ovary can be categorized as either Type I (low-grade endometrioid carcinoma) or Type II (high-grade endometrioid carcinoma) epithelial ovarian tumors and most commonly harbor genetic mutations in *CTNNB1* and *PTEN* [1]. Similar to endometrial carcinomas, germline mutations in DNA mismatch repair genes *MLH-1, PMS2, MSH2*, and *MSH6* are associated with Lynch syndrome, imparting an increased lifetime risk for ovarian cancer in susceptible patients (Table 10.1) [1].

The discovery of similar mutational profiles in endometriotic lesions with adjacent endometrioid or clear cell carcinomas strongly suggests endometriosis as a precursor for endometrioid and clear cell carcinomas of the ovary [1, 12–14]. Clear cell carcinoma typically presents as a lower stage, like Type I tumors; however, the clinical course is often more aggressive with a worse prognosis and poor response to platinum-based agents, similar to Type II tumors [3, 12–16]. The tumor suppressor gene, *ARID1A*, is the most commonly altered gene in clear cell carcinoma [12–16].

Sex cord tumors with annular tubules (SCTAT) are exceedingly rare ovarian tumors that can present as a result of sporadic or germline mutations in *STK11/LKB1* [17, 18]. Sporadic tumors tend to be symptomatic as a result of larger, unilateral tumors and have a greater propensity to behave aggressively. Conversely, SCTAT tumors in patients with Peutz-Jeghers syndrome are less likely to present with clinical symptoms, behave in a benign manner, and are commonly identified in both ovaries on microscopic examination [17]. Additional alterations in sex cord-stromal tumors are shown in Table 10.2 [17–19].

Small cell carcinoma of the ovary of hypercalcemic type (SCCOHT) characteristically contains a somatic or germline mutation in the *SMARCA4 (BRG1)* gene located on chromosome 19p [20]. The deleterious mutation leads to aberrant functioning of the SWI/SNF chromatin remodeling [21] complex and results in a highly aggressive ovarian tumor. SCCOHT is most commonly diagnosed in the second decade of life with hypercalcemia identified in 30–66% of all tested patients [22]. Mutations in the *SMARCB1* gene associated with the SWI/SNF chromatin remodel-

Table 10.2 Mutations identified in sex cord-stromal tumors of the ovary [17–22]

Tumor type	Gene	Mutation type/ specific mutation	% of cases with mutation/genetic alteration	Clinical implication
Adult granulosa cell tumor	*FOXL2*	p.C134W (c.402C>G)	61–97%	Reportedly worse disease-free and overall survival
	TERT	Promoter gain-of-function mutation C228T C250T	22% (primary) 41% (recurrent)	
Sertoli-Leydig cell tumors	*DICER1*	Germline Somatic mutations p.D1709N (c.5125G>A) (38%) p.E1705K (c.5113G>A) (80%)	0–62.5%	Well-differentiated SLCTs do not appear to harbor *DICER1* mutations
Sex cord tumor with annular tubules (SCTAT)	*STK11/ LKB1*	Germline mutation, LOH		Peutz-Jeghers syndrome (PJS), tumors are often small and bilateral

ing pathway are also found in pediatric rhabdoid tumors (i.e., atypical teratoid rhabdoid tumor (ATRT) and malignant rhabdoid tumors of the kidney) [22]. SCCOHT have a poor prognosis due to the increased frequency of extraovarian spread at the time of diagnosis [17, 22]. Despite attempts to further subclassify this tumor, the cell of origin remains unclear and the undifferentiated nature is problematic for determining the best course of treatment [21].

Endometrial Cancer

Uterine carcinomas are divided into Type I, endometrioid carcinomas (typically grades 1–2), and Type II, other carcinomas (serous, clear cell, and some grade 3 endometroid carcinomas). Type I tumors are more common in perimenopausal and menopausal women with an elevated body mass index (BMI) and hyperestrogenic state and tend to be lower grade and stage at diagnosis [23]. The most common gene alterations identified in Type I endometrioid carcinomas include *PTEN, CTNNB1 (β-catenin),* DNA mismatch repair genes, *KRAS, PIK3CA*, and *POLE* (Table 10.3) [24, 25]. Some tumors are thought to arise through a stepwise progression from

Table 10.3 Clinically significant mutations in endometrial tumors [23–30]

Tumor type	Gene	Mutation type/specific mutation	% of cases with mutation/ genetic alteration	Clinical implication
Endometrioid	*PTEN*	Loss of heterozygosity (LOH); Somatic mutation	LOH: (40%) Somatic: (37–61%)	Associated with hyperestrogenic state, found in endometrial hyperplasia
	POLE (DNA polymerase epsilon)	Mutation in exons 9–14 (exonuclease domain)		Ultramutated
	MLH1, PMS2, MSH2, MSH6	Germline or somatic mutations (including *MLH1* promoter hypermethylation)		Lynch syndrome, Lynch-like syndrome, MSI
	CTNNB1	Exon 3 mutation (nuclear accumulation)	14–44%	
	KRAS	*RAS-RAF-MEK-ERK* signaling pathway aberrations	10–30%	
	PIK3CA	Helical (exon 9) and kinase (exon 20) activating mutation	36%	Small molecular inhibitors, targeting PI3K, can coexist with PTEN mutations
Serous carcinoma	*TP53*	Mutation or wild type	90%	Copy number high (p53abn) Copy number low (p53wt)
	CDKN2A	Deletion; promoter hypermethylation	40%	
	CDH1	LOH; promoter hypermethylation	80–90%	
	ERBB2	Amplification	17–80% 17–68%	Overexpression associated with significantly shorter survival time, often seen in African American women, and +/– history of breast cancer
Clear cell carcinoma	*TERT*	Gain-of-function mutation; aberration in telomere length	21%	
Uterine carcinosarcoma	*TP53*	Mutation	70–90%	
	Chromatin remodeling genes (e.g. *ARID1A*) and histone genes		Up to 75%	

precursor hyperplastic lesions, as evidenced by the discovery of *PTEN* mutations in nonatypical and atypical endometrial hyperplasia associated with endometrioid carcinomas arising in a hyperestrogenic state [23]. Women with endometrial carcinomas associated with Lynch syndrome have germline mutations in the DNA mismatch repair genes *MLH-1, PMS2, MSH2, and MSH6*, whereas tumors with sporadic mismatch repair deficiency and microsatellite instability can result from somatic mutations in these same genes or, most frequently, *MLH1* promoter hypermethylation [25, 26]. Women affected by Lynch syndrome present with endometrial tumors nearly a decade earlier than sporadic cases and occasionally harbor synchronous or metachronous tumors in extrauterine organs, including the ovaries and lower gastrointestinal tract at the time of diagnosis.

Type II carcinomas, including serous, clear cell, and some grade 3 endometrioid carcinomas, are high-grade cancers that more frequently develop in postmenopausal women. Serous carcinomas typically arise from atrophic endometrium or endometrial polyps and are not associated with unopposed estrogen or endometrial hyperplasia. The tumors are highly aggressive, frequently displaying chromosomal instability, aneuploidy, and loss of heterozygosity (Table 10.3). Nearly all serous carcinomas are associated with mutations in *TP53*, identified through immunohistochemical staining as an aberrant diffuse nuclear overexpression or "null" phenotype with complete loss of expression of p53 [23].

The ProMisE (Proactive Molecular Risk Classifier for Endometrial Cancer) is a proposed method for subclassifying endometrial carcinomas into four distinct groups based on the clinicopathologic and molecular analysis of more than 400 endometrial tumors [27]. Using immunohistochemistry, and *POLE* mutation analysis, endometrial tumors are divided into mismatch repair deficient (MMR-D, hypermutated), *POLE* (ultramutated), copy number high (p53 abnormal), and copy number low (p53 wild-type) tumors, the same four categories delineated by the Endometrial TCGA studies [27, 28]. Application of this algorithm assists clinicians with therapeutic management and potential clinical trial entry by subclassifying the endometrial tumors into prognostically significant groups [27, 28].

Uterine Mesenchymal Tumors

With the application of next-generation sequencing technologies, an increasing number of recurrent genetic alterations have been identified in a very challenging category of gynecologic tumors, the mesenchymal derived tumors (Table 10.4) [29–38]. In some instances, such as the high-grade endometrial stromal sarcoma, recurrent fusions define tumors with distinct morphology, immunohistochemical phenotype, and clinical course [32].

Table 10.4 Clinically significant molecular alterations in uterine mesenchymal tumors [31–38]

Tumor type	Gene	Mutation type/ specific mutation	% of cases with mutation/ genetic alteration	Clinical implication
Leiomyoma	*Fumarate hydratase*	Biallelic inactivation	1.6–37%	Germline mutation: hereditary leiomyomatosis and renal cell cancer syndrome (HLRCC)
Endometrial stromal nodule/low-grade endometrial stromal sarcoma	*JAZF1-SUZ12* *PHF1-JAZF1* *EPC1-PHF1* *MEAF6-PHF1*	t(7, 17) t(6;7)(p21;p15) t(6;10)(p21;p11) t(1;6)(p34;p21)	50%	
High-grade endometrial stromal sarcoma	*YWHAE-NUTM2*	t(10;17)		
	ZC3H7B-BCOR	t(X;22) (p11.4;q13.2)		Histologic mimic of myxoid leiomyosarcoma; aggressive behavior
Leiomyosarcoma	*MED12*			Marker for identifying LMS arising from LM More favorable prognosis
Inflammatory myofibroblastic (IMT)	*ALK* (also *ROS1, RET, and NTRK3* described in other anatomic sites)	Rearrangements	Up to 50% with *ALK* rearrangement	Crizotinib therapy
SMARCA4-deficient undifferentiated uterine sarcoma	*SMARCA4*			

References

1. Bell D. Origins and molecular pathology of ovarian cancer. Mod Pathol. 2005;18:S19–32.
2. Cho KR, IeM S. Ovarian cancer. Annu Rev Pathol. 2009;4:287–313.
3. Jones PM, Drapkin R. Modeling high-grade serous carcinoma: how converging insights into pathogenesis and genetics are driving better experimental platforms. Front Oncol. 2013;3:217.
4. Vang R, Shih I, Kurman RJ. Fallopian tube precursors of ovarian low- and high-grade serous neoplasms. Histopathology. 2013;62(1):44–58.
5. Singer GS, Oldt R, Cohen Y, Wang BG, Sidransky D, Kurman RJ, Shih IE. Mutations in BRAF and KRAS characterize the development of low-grade ovarian serous carcinoma. J Natl Cancer Inst. 2003;95(6):484–6.

6. Kaldawy A, Segev Y, Lavie O, Auslender R, Sopik V, Narod SA. Low-grade serous ovarian cancer: a review. Gynecol Oncol. 2016;143(2):433–8.
7. Han C, Bellone S, Zammataro L, Schwartz PE, Santin AD. Binimetinib (MEK 162) in recurrent low-grade serous ovarian cancer resistant to chemotherapy and hormonal treatment. Gynecol Oncol Rep. 2018;25:41–4.
8. Ahmed AA, Etemadmoghadam D, Temple J, Lynch AG, Riad M, Sharma R, Stewart C, Fereday S, Caldas C, Defazio A, Bowtell D, Brenton JD. Driver mutations in TP53 are ubiquitous in high grade serous carcinoma of the ovary. J Pathol. 2010;221(1):49–56.
9. Han C, Bellone S, Schwartz PE, Govindan SV, Sharkey RM, Goldenberg DM, Santin AD. Sacituzumab Govitecan (IMMU-132) in treatment-resistant uterine serous carcinoma: a case report. Gynecol Oncol Rep. 2018;25:37–40.
10. Helleday T. The underlying mechanism for the PARP and BRCA synthetic lethality: clearing up the misunderstandings. Mol Oncol. 2011;5(4):387–93.
11. Fong PC, Boss DS, Yap TA, Tutt A, Wu P, Mergui-Roelvink M, Mortimer P, Swaisland H, Lau A, O'Connor MJ, Ashworth A, Carmichael J, Kaye SB, Schellens JH, de Bono JS. Inhibition of poly (ADP-ribose) polymerase in tumors from BRCA mutation carriers. N Engl J Med. 2009;361(2):123–34.
12. Wiegand KC, Shah SP, Al-Agha OM, Zhao Y, Tse K, Zeng T, Senz J, McConechy MK, Anglesio MS, Kalloger SE, Yang W, Heravi-Moussavi A, Giuliany R, Chow C, Fee J, Zayed A, Prentice L, Melnyk N, Turashvili G, Delaney AD, Madore J, Yip S, McPherson AW, Ha G, Bell L, Fereday S, Tam A, Galletta L, Tonin PN, Provencher D, Miller D, Jones SJ, Moore RA, Morin GB, Oloumi A, Boyd N, Aparicio SA, Shih I, Mes-Masson AM, Bowtell DD, Hirst M, Gilks B, Marra MA, Huntsman DG. ARID1A mutations in endometriosis-associated ovarian carcinomas. N Engl J Med. 2010;363(16):1532–43.
13. Berns K, Caumanns JJ, Hijmans EM, et al. ARID1A mutation sensitizes most ovarian clear cell carcinomas to BET inhibitors. Oncogene. 2018;37(33):4611–25.
14. Sato E, Nahayama K, Razia S, Nakamura K, Ishikawa M, Minamoto T, Ishibashi T, Yamashita H, Iida K, Kyo S. ARID1B as a potential therapeutic target for ARID1A-mutant ovarian clear cell carcinoma. Int J Mol Sci. 2018;19(6):E1710.
15. Kuo KT, Mao TL, Jones S, et al. Frequent activating mutations of PIK3CA in ovarian clear cell carcinoma. Am J Pathol. 2009;174(5):1597–601.
16. Wu RC, Ayhan A, Maeda D, Kim KR, Clarke BA, Shaw P, Chui MH, Rosen B, Shih I, Wang TL. Frequent somatic mutations of the telomerase reverse transcriptase promoter in ovarian clear cell carcinoma but not in other major types of gynaecological malignancy. J Pathol. 2014;232(4):473–81.
17. Connolly DC, Katabuchi H, Cliby WA, Cho KR. Somatic mutations in the STK11/LKB1 gene are uncommon in rare gynecological tumor types associated with Peutz-Jeghers syndrome. Am J Pathol. 2000;156(1):339–45.
18. Fuller P, Leung D, Chu S. Genetics and genomics of ovarian sex cord-stromal tumors. Clin Genet. 2017;91:285–91.
19. Pilsworth JA, Cochrane DR, Xia Z, Aubert G, Färkkilä AEM, Horlings HM, Yanagida S, Yang W, Lim JLP, Wang YK, Bashashati A, Keul J, Wong A, Norris K, Brucker SY, Taran FA, Krämer B, Staebler A, van Meurs H, Oliva E, Shah SP, Kommoss S, Kommoss F, Gilks CB, Baird DM, Huntsman DG. TERT promoter mutation in adult granulosa cell tumor of the ovary. Mod Pathol. 2018;31(7):1107–15.
20. Foulkes WD, Gore M, McCluggage WG. Rare non-epithelial ovarian neoplasms: pathology, genetics and treatment. Gynecol Oncol. 2016;142:190–8.
21. Jelinic P, Schlappe BA, Conlon N, Tseng J, Olvera N, Dao F, Mueller Y, Soslow RA, Levine DA. Concomitant loss of SMARCA2 and SMARCA4 expression in small cell carcinoma of the ovary, hypercalcemic type. Mod Pathol. 2016;29(1):60–6.
22. Fahiminiya S, Witkowski L, Carrot-Zhang J, Albrecht S, Hamel N, Tomiak E, Grynspan D, Saloustros E, Nadaf J, Rivera B, Gilpin C, Castellsagué E, Silva-Smith R, Plourde F, Wu M, Saskin A, Arseneault M, Karabakhtsian RG, Reilly EA, Ueland FR, Margiolaki A, Pavlakis K, Castellino SM, Lamovec J, Mackay HJ, Roth LM, Ulbright TM, Bender TA, Georgoulias V, Longy M, Berchuck A, Tischkowitz M, Nagel I, Siebert R, Stewart CJ, Arseneau J, McCluggage

WG, Clarke BA, Riazalhosseini Y, Hasselblatt M, Majewski J, Foulkes WD. Germline and somatic SMARCA4 mutations characterize small cell carcinoma of the ovary, hypercalcemic type. Nat Genet. 2014;46(5):438–43.
23. Kurman RJ. Endometrial carcinoma. In: Kurman RJ, Ellenson LH, Ronnett BM, editors. Blaustein's pathology of the female genital tract. New York: Springer; 2011. p. 394–411.
24. O'Hara AJ, Bell DW. The genomics and genetics of endometrial cancer. Adv Genomics Genet. 2012;2012(2):33–47.
25. Llobet D, Pallares J, Yeramian A, Santacana M, Eritja N, Velasco A, Dolcet X, Matias-Guiu X. Molecular pathology of endometrial carcinoma: practical aspects from the diagnostic and therapeutic viewpoints. J Clin Pathol. 2009;62(9):777–85.
26. Mills AM, Longacre TA. Lynch syndrome screening in the gynecologic tract: current state of the art. Am J Surg Pathol. 2016;40(4):e35–44.
27. Kommoss S, McConechy MK, Kommoss F, Leung S, Bunz A, Magrill J, Britton H, Kommoss F, Grevenkamp F, Karnezis A, Yang W, Lum A, Krämer B, Taran F, Staebler A, Lax S, Brucker SY, Huntsman DG, Gilks CB, McAlpine JN, Talhouk A. Final validation of the ProMisE molecular classifier for endometrial carcinoma in a large population-based case series. Ann Oncol. 2018;29(5):1180–8.
28. Cancer Genome Atlas Research Network, Kandoth C, Schultz N, et al. Integrated genomic characterization of endometrial carcinoma. Nature. 2013;497(7447):67–73.
29. Cherniack AD, Shen H, Walter V, Stewart C, Murray BA, Bowlby R, Hu X, Ling S, Soslow RA, Broaddus RR, Zuna RE, Robertson G, Laird PW, Kucherlapati R, Mills GB; Cancer Genome Atlas Research Network, Weinstein JN, Zhang J, Akbani R, Levine DA. Integrated molecular characterization of uterine carcinosarcoma. Cancer Cell. 2017;31(3):411–23.
30. Zhao S, Bellone S, Lopez S, Thakral D, Schwab C, English DP, Black J, Cocco E, Choi J, Zammataro L, Predolini F, Bonazzoli E, Bi M, Buza N, Hui P, Wong S, Abu-Khalaf M, Ravaggi A, Bignotti E, Bandiera E, Romani C, Todeschini P, Tassi R, Zanotti L, Odicino F, Pecorelli S, Donzelli C, Ardighieri L, Facchetti F, Falchetti M, Silasi DA, Ratner E, Azodi M, Schwartz PE, Mane S, Angioli R, Terranova C, Quick CM, Edraki B, Bilgüvar K, Lee M, Choi M, Stiegler AL, Boggon TJ, Schlessinger J, Lifton RP, Santin AD. Mutational landscape of uterine and ovarian carcinosarcomas implicates histone genes in epithelial-mesenchymal transition. Proc Natl Acad Sci U S A. 2016;113(43):12238–43.
31. Kurihara S, Oda Y, Ohishi Y, et al. Endometrial stromal sarcomas and related high-grade sarcomas: immunohistochemical and molecular genetic study of 31 cases. Am J Surg Pathol. 2008;32:1228–38.
32. Micci F, Gorunova L, Gatius S, Matias-Guiu X, Davidson B, Heim S, Panagopoulos I. MEAF6/PHF1 is a recurrent gene fusion in endometrial stromal sarcoma. Cancer Lett. 2014;347(1):75–8.
33. Miettinen M, Felisiak-Golabek A, Wasag B, et al. Fumarase-deficient uterine leiomyomas: an immunohistochemical, molecular genetic, and clinicopathologic study of 86 cases. Am J Surg Pathol. 2016;40(12):1661–9.
34. Hoang LN, Aneja A, Conlon N, et al. Novel high-grade endometrial stromal sarcoma: a morphologic mimicker of myxoid leiomyosarcoma. Am J Surg Pathol. 2017;41(1):12–24.
35. Hodge JC, Bedroske PP, Pearce KE, Sukov WR. Molecular cytogenetic analysis of JAZF1, PHF1, and YWHAE in endometrial stromal tumors: discovery of genetic complexity by fluorescence in situ hybridization. J Mol Diagn. 2016;18(4):516–26.
36. Koontz JI, Soreng AL, Nucci M, et al. Frequent fusion of the JAZF1 and JJAZ1 genes in endometrial stromal tumors. Proc Natl Acad Sci. 2001;98:6348–53.
37. Nucci MR, Harburger D, Koontz J, et al. Molecular analysis of the JAZF1-JJAZ1 gene fusion by RT-PCR and fluorescence in situ hybridization in endometrial stromal neoplasms. Am J Surg Pathol. 2007;31:65–70.
38. Kolin DL, Dong F, Baltay M, Lindeman N, MacConaill L, Nucci MR, Crum CP, Howitt BE. SMARCA4-deficient undifferentiated uterine sarcoma (malignant rhabdoid tumor of the uterus): a clinicopathologic entity distinct from undifferentiated carcinoma. Mod Pathol. 2018;31(9):1442–56.

Chapter 11
Sarcomas

Konstantinos Linos

Key Points

- Soft tissue tumors constitute a rare, heterogeneous group of mesenchymal neoplasms exhibiting a spectrum of morphologies.
- Soft tissue tumors are categorized in 12 groups according to the 2013 World Health Organization (WHO) classification.
- Approximately one-third of sarcomas are associated with translocations, whereas the remaining 70% of sarcomas are of complex karyotype.
- The identification of reciprocal chromosomal translocations, fusion genes, and activating or inactivating mutations of select oncogenes or tumor suppressor genes with potential implications in the pathogenesis, diagnosis, and treatment has been revolutionary

Key Online Resources

- http://www.cbioportal.org/
- Soft Tissue Sarcoma, Version 2.2018, NCCN Clinical Practice Guidelines in Oncology: https://jnccn.org/view/journals/jnccn/16/5/article-p536.xml
- World Sarcoma Network: http://www.worldsarcomanetwork.com/
- NIH U.S National Library of Medicine: https://clinicaltrials.gov/ct2/home

K. Linos (✉)
Dartmouth-Hitchcock Medical Center, Department of Pathology and Laboratory Medicine, Lebanon, NH, USA

Geisel School of Medicine at Dartmouth, Hanover, NH, USA
e-mail: konstantinos.linos@hitchcock.org

L. J. Tafe, M. E. Arcila (eds.), *Genomic Medicine*,
https://doi.org/10.1007/978-3-030-22922-1_11

Introduction

Soft tissue tumors constitute a rare, heterogeneous group of mesenchymal neoplasms exhibiting a spectrum of morphologies. There are more than 100 histologic subtypes, and sarcomas collectively account for 1% of adult and 15% of pediatric malignancies. During the last two decades, considerable progress in the understanding and application of molecular techniques has been achieved in refining our current understanding beyond the limits of traditional approaches.

The development of novel therapies has been slow due to the inherent genetic heterogeneity of these tumors and the difficulty conducting large clinical trials. Although treatment continues to be based on cytotoxic chemotherapy regimens, the identification of reciprocal chromosomal translocations, fusion genes, and activating or inactivating mutations of select oncogenes or tumor suppressor genes with potential implications in the pathogenesis, diagnosis, and treatment has been revolutionary. The era of molecular targeted therapy presents an opportunity for biomarker discovery and meaningful treatment options for patients who do not respond to traditional therapies.

- Soft tissue tumors are categorized in 12 groups according to the 2013 World Health Organization (WHO) classification:
  - Adipocytic
  - Fibroblastic/myofibroblastic
  - Fibrohisitocytic
  - Smooth muscle
  - Pericytic (perivascular)
  - Skeletal muscle
  - Vascular
  - Chondro-osseous
  - Gastrointestinal stromal
  - Nerve sheath
  - Uncertain differentiation
  - Undifferentiated/unclassified
- Tumor behavior is classified as benign, intermediate (locally aggressive, rarely metastasizing), and malignant.
- Approximately one-third of sarcomas are associated with translocations [1–3].
  - These are mainly balanced, reciprocal with generally simple karyotype.
  - Common methods of detection is fluorescence in situ hybridization (FISH), RT-PCR, and next-generation sequencing (NGS).
  - They frequently involve tyrosine kinases and can cause constitutive activation and tumor proliferation.
- The remaining 70% of sarcomas are of complex karyotype.

Sarcomas with Recurrent Translocations (*Table 11.1*)

Table 11.1 Recurrent translocations and clinically relevant genetic abnormalities in selected sarcomas

Soft tissue tumor	Chromosomal abnormality	Gene fusion	Approximate prevalence	Comment(s)
Alveolar Rhabdomyo-sarcoma	t(2;13)(q35;q14) t(1;13)(p36;q14) Other t with 2q35	*PAX3-FOXO1* *PAX7-FOXO1* *PAX3 (FOXO4, NCOA1, NCOA2, AFX)*	75% 20% 5%	
Alveolar soft part sarcoma	t(X;17)(p11.2;q25)	*ASPSCR1-TFE3*	>95%	
Angiomatoid fibrous histiocytoma	t(2;22)(q34;q12) t(2;22)(q34;q12) t(12;16)(q13;p11)	*EWSR1-CREB1* *EWSR1-ATF1* *FUS-ATF1* *EWSR1-CREM*	72% 21% 7% Rare	*EWSR1-ATF1* especially in unusual sites
Angiosarcoma, radiation associated [4]	MYC amplification			
Angiosarcoma, sporadic		*ROS1-GOPC/FIG*		Preliminary data; one recent case of hepatic angiosarcoma. Potentially targetable with crizotinib
		EWSR1-ATF1		One case reported in the salivary gland
Atypical lipomatous tumor/ well-differentiated liposarcoma	12q rings and giant markers	*NA*	Most	*HMGIC*, *CDK4*, and *MDM2* amplification
Biphenotypic sinonasal Sarcoma [5, 6]		*PAX3-MAML3* *PAX3-FOXO1* *PAX3-NCOA1* *PAX3-NCOA2* *PAX3-WWTR1* *PAX3* with unknown partner *MAML3* without *PAX3*	*PAX3-MAML3* most common	
Clear cell sarcoma of soft parts	t(12;22)(q13;q12) t(2;22)(q34;q12)	*EWSR1-ATF1* *EWSR1-CREB1* *EWSR1-CREM*	90% 10% Rare	
Clear cell sarcoma of the kidney (CCSK)		*BCOR* internal tandem duplication	Most cases	Overlap with renal sarcomas harboring *BCOR-CCNB3* or *YWAAE-NUTM2B*
Dermatofibro-sarcoma protuberans/giant cell fibroblastoma [7, 8]	+ring/marker chromosome from t(17;22)(q22;q13)	*COL1A1-PDGFB*	95%	
		COL6A3- PDGFD *EMILIN2-PDGFD*		

(continued)

Table 11.1 (continued)

Soft tissue tumor	Chromosomal abnormality	Gene fusion	Approximate prevalence	Comment(s)
Desmoplastic small round cell tumor	t(11;22)(p13;q12)	*EWSR1-WT1*	>95%	
Endometrial stromal cell sarcoma [9]	t(7;17)	*JAZF1-SUZ12*	Low grade	
		JAZF1-PHF1		
		JAZF1-BCORL1		
		EPC1-PHF1		
		MEAF6-PHF1		
		BRD8-PHF1		
		MBTD1-CXorf67		
	t(10:17)(q22;p13)	*KDM2B-CREBBP*	High grade	
	t(X;22)(p11.4;q13.2)	*YWHAE-NUTM2A and/or NUTM2B*		
		ZC3H7B-BCOR		
Epithelioid hemangioendothelioma [10–13]	t(7;9)(q22;q13) t(X;11)(p11.2;q22.1)	*WWTR1-CAMTA1* *TFE3-YAP1*	85% NA	
Ewing sarcoma/PNET/Ewing family of tumors [14]	t(11;22)(q24;q12) t(21;22)(q22;q12) t(7;22)(q22;q12) t(17;22)(q21;q12) t(2;22)(q36;q12) inv(22)(q12q12) t(2;22)(q31;q12) t(20;22)(q13;q12) t(4;22)(q31;12) t(6;22)(p21;q12) t(16;21)(p11;q22) t(2;16)(q36;p11)	*EWSR1-FLI1* *EWSR1-ERG* *EWSR1-ETV1* *EWSR1-ETV4* *EWSR1-FEV* *EWSR1-PATZ1* *EWSR1-SP3* *EWSR1-NFATC2* *EWSR1-SMARCA5* *EWSR1-POU5F1* *FUS-ERG* *FUS-FEV*	90% 5% <1% <1% <1% <1% <1% <1% <1% <1% <1% <1%	
Extraskeletal myxoid chondrosarcoma	t(9;22)(q22;q12) t(9;17)(q22;q12) t(9;15)(q22;q21) t(3;9)(q12;q22)	*EWSR1-NR4A3* *TAF15-NR4A3* *TCF12-NR4A3* *TFG-NR4A3* *HSPA8-NR4A3* *NR4A3-FUS*	75% 15% <1% <1% Very rare Very rare	
Infantile fibrosarcoma	t(12;15)(p13;q25)	*ETV6-NTRK3* *EML4-NTRK3* *BRAF* gene fusions	>95% Rare Rare	*BRAF* intragenic deletion, *TPM3-NTRK1, LMNA-NTRK1, SQSTM1-NTRK1*, and *TFG-MET* have been reported in pediatric sarcomas resembling infantile fibrosarcoma

Table 11.1 (continued)

Soft tissue tumor	Chromosomal abnormality	Gene fusion	Approximate prevalence	Comment(s)
Inflammatory myofibroblastic tumor [15]	t with 2p23	*ALK* fusion with various partners (*TPM3/4, CLTC, RANBP2, CARS, ATIC, SEC31L1, SEC31A, IGFB5, THBS1, PPF1BP1, DCTN1, EML4, PRKAR1A, LMNA, TFG, FN1, DES, A2M, NUMA1, HNRNPA1*), *ALK* amplification *ROS, RET, ETV6, PDGFRb, NTRK3* fusions with various partners	75%	
Leiomyosarcoma, epithelioid, uterine	t(9;11)(q22.3;q22.1)	*NRA4A3-PGR* *PGR* rearrangements	A subset of epithelioid leiomyo-sarcomas	
Leiomyosarcoma, myxoid, uterine [16]		*TRPS1-PLAG1* *RAD51B-PLAG1*		
Low-grade fibromyxoid sarcoma	t(7;16)(q33;p11) t(11;16)(p11;p11)	*FUS-CRE3L2* *FUS-CREB3L1* *EWSR1-CREB3L1*	>95% <5%	
Malignant tenosynovial giant cell tumor	t(1;2)(p13;q37) Subset without t(1;2)	*CSF1-COL6A3*	Most	*CSF1* overexpression
Mesenchymal chondrosarcoma	del(8)(q13.3q21.1)	*HEY1-NCOA2*	>90%	
Myoepithelial tumor, soft tissue [17, 18]	t(6;22)(p21;q12) t(19;22)(q13;q12) t(1;22)(q23;q12) t with 16p11	*EWSR1-POU5F1* *EWSR1-ZNF444* *EWSR1-PBX1* *EWSR1-PBX3* *EWSR1-KLF17* *EWSR1-ATF1* *FUS*		*EWSR1-POU5F1* and *EWSR1-PBX1* are the most common fusions
Myxoid liposarcoma	t(12;16)(q13;p11) t(12;22)(q13;q12)	*FUS-DDIT3* *EWSR1-DDIT3*	>90% <10%	
Myxoinflammatory fibroblastic sarcoma/hemosiderotic fibrolipomatous tumor/pleomorphic hyalinizing angiectatic tumor [19, 20]	Der(10)t(1;10)(p22;q24)	*TGFBR3-MGEA5*		
		BRAF rearrangements		Only in myxoinflammatory fibroblastic tumor

(continued)

Table 11.1 (continued)

Soft tissue tumor	Chromosomal abnormality	Gene fusion	Approximate prevalence	Comment(s)
Ossifying fibromyxoid tumor [21–23]	t with 6p21	*MEAF6-PHF1*		
		EPC1-PHF1		
		EP400-PHF1		
		PHF1-TFE3		
	t(X;22)(p11.4;q13.2)	*ZC3H7B-BCOR*		
		CREBBP-BCORL1		
		KDM2A-WWTR1		
Perivascular epithelioid cell tumor (PEComa) [24, 25]		*TSC2* mutation *PSF-TFE3* *DVL2-TFE3* *NONO-TFE3* *RAD51B-RRAGB/OPHN1* *HTR4-ST3GALI* *RASSF1-PDZRN3* *SLC4A10-ROS1* *ROS1-NETO1* *RBMX-TFE3*		*TFE3* rearranged-PEComas lack *TSC2* mutations indicating alternative pathways
PRDM10-rearranged Soft tissue tumor		*CITED2-PRDM10* *MED12-PRMD10*		Provisional data. Pleomorphic morphology and low mitotic count. Overlap with superficial CD34+ fibroblastic tumor
Pseudomyogenic hemangioendothelioma [26, 27]	t(7;19)(q22;q13)	*SERPINE1-FOSB* *ACTB-FOSB*	50% 50%	
Primary pulmonary myxoid sarcoma	t(2;22)(q34;q12)	*EWSR1-CREB1*		
Sclerosing epithelioid fibrosarcoma [28]		*EWSR1-CREB2L2*		
		EWSR1-CREB2L1		
		EWSR1- CREB3L3		
		FUS-CREB3L2	Minority of cases	
Solitary fibrous tumor [29]	inv(12)(q13q13)	*NAB2-STAT6*	>95%	
Spindle/sclerosing cell rhabdomyosarcoma [30–33]	t with 8q13	*VGLL2-CITED2* *NCOA2* fusion with SRF(6p21), *TEAD1*(11p15), *VGLL2*	Most common	Tumors with fusion present at birth or within 1 year and have favorable outcome
	MyoD1 (L122R) mutation			Tumors with *MyoD1* mutations have aggressive clinical course in children or adults

Table 11.1 (continued)

Soft tissue tumor	Chromosomal abnormality	Gene fusion	Approximate prevalence	Comment(s)
Synovial sarcoma [34]	t(X;18)(p11.2;q11.2)	*SS18-SSX1*	65%	
		SS18-SSX2	35%	
		SS18-SSX4	<1%	
	t(X;20)(p11.2;q13.3)	*SS18L1-SSX1*	Rare	
Undifferentiated small round cell sarcomas [35–41]	t(4;19)(q35;q13) t(10;19)(q26.3;q13) inv(X)(p11.4p11.22)	*CIC-DUX4* *CIC-DUX4L* *CIC-FOXO4* *CIC-NUTM1* *NUTM2A-CIC* *BCOR-CCNB3* *BCOR-MAML3* *BCOR* internal tandem duplications *CRTC1-SS18*		
Undifferentiated spindle cell sarcoma [42]		*MEIS-NCOA2*	2 cases reported	Provisional entity reported in the kidney
Undifferentiated soft tissue and/or visceral tumors [40, 43–45]		*BRD3-NUTM1* *BRD4-NUTM1* *BCORL1-NUTM1* *MXD1-NUTM1* *MXD4-NUTM1* *MGA-NUTM1*		The relationship of *NUT*-associated tumors in soft tissue and/or viscera and conventional *NUT* carcinoma remains to be elucidated.
Uterine sarcoma with features of fibrosarcoma [46]		*TPM3-NTRK1* *LMNA-NTRK1* *RBPMS-NTRK3* *TPR-NTRK1*		Provisional findings, 4 cases reported
Uterine sarcoma with variable sex-cord differentiation		*GREB1* rearrangements *(NCOA1, NCOA2, CTNNB1, NR4A3, SS18)*		
Uterine tumor resembling Ovarian sex cord tumor (UTROSCT)		*ESR1-NCOA2* *ESR1-NCOA3* *GREB1-NCOA2*		

Benign Mesenchymal Neoplasms with Recurrent Translocations (Table 11.2)

Adipocytic Neoplasms (Tables 11.3 and 11.4)

- *MDM2* gene maps to chromosome band 12q13 and encodes a p53-binding protein which may result in functional inactivation of p53.
- Molecular deregulation of MDM2 is not specific for well-differentiated/dedifferentiated liposarcoma.
- It has also been reported in leiomyosarcoma, rhabdomyosarcoma, and Ewing sarcoma [58–61].

Table 11.2 Recurrent translocations and clinically relevant genetic abnormalities in selected benign mesenchymal neoplasms

Tumor type	Translocation	Gene fusion		
Acral fibroblastic spindle cell neoplasm [47, 48]	t(15;22)(q22.33;12.2)	*EWSR1-SMAD3*		
"Aggressive," deep angiomyxoma	12q15 rearrangements	*HMGA2*		
Aneurysmal bone cyst, primary		*USP6* with various partners (*CDH11*[most common], *SEC31A, EIF1, FOSL2, RUNX2, PAFAH1B1, CTNNB1, STAT3, ZNF9, TRAP150, SPARC THRAP3, CNBP, OMD, COL1A1,USP9X*)	Can also arise exclusively in soft tissue locations. *COL1A1* is a common partner of *USP6* in these cases. Giant cell reparative granulomas of the hands and feet harbor *USP6* gene rearrangements and should be classified as aneurysmal bone cysts	
Angiofibroma of soft tissue [49]	t(5;8)(p15;q13) t(7;8;14)(q11;q13;q31)	*AHRR-NCOA2* *GTF2I-NCOA2* *GAB1-ABL1* *TBCK-P4HA2* *P4HA2-TBCK* *NCOA2-ETV4* *ETV4-AHRR*	AHRR-NCOA2 is the most frequent recurrent fusion	NA
Calcifying aponeurotic fibroma	ins(2;4)(q35;q25)	*FN1-EGF*		
Chondroblastoma			*H3F3B* (K36M) mutations	
Chondromyxoid fibroma		*COL12A1-GRM1* *TBL1XR1-GRM1* *BCLAF1-GRM1*	Several 5′ partner genes which represent strong promoters	

Table 11.2 (continued)

Tumor type	Translocation	Gene fusion		
Cranial fasciitis		*USP6* rearrangements		
Cutaneous non-neural granular cell tumor		*SQSTM1-ALK* *DCTM1-ALK*	Potential for regional lymph node spread. *ALK* rearrangements in a subset of cases	
Desmoid tumor	NA	*NA*	*CTNNB1* (sporadic) or *APC* (somatic) mutations	
Desmoplastic fibroblastoma	t(2;11)(q31;q12)	Unknown	NA	
Ectomesenchymal chondromyxoid tumor [50]		*RREB1-MKL2* *EWSR1* rearrangements		
Epithelioid fibrous histiocytoma [51]		*ALK* fusion with various partners		
Fibroma of tendon sheath	t(2;11) (q31-32;q12)	Unknown		
Fibro-osseous pseudotumor of the digits [52]		*USP6* rearrangements		
Fibrous dysplasia	NA	NA	*GNAS* mutations	
Fibrous hamartoma of infancy		*EGFR* internal tandem duplications		
Hibernoma	11q13-21 rearrangements	Unknown		
Gastroblastoma		*MALAT1-GLI1*		
Giant cell tumor of bone			*H3F3A* mutations Majority of cases with *H3F3A* G34W/V mutations Minority of cases with *H3F3A* G34L and G34R mutations	
Lipoblastoma	t with 8q11-13, 8 gain	*PLAG1* fusions with various partners(*HAS2, COL1A2, RAD51L1, COL3A1, RAB2A*)	80%	
Lipofibromatosis		*HBEGF-RBM27* *EGR1-GRIA1* *TPR-ROS* *SPARC-PDGFRB* *VCL-RET* *EGFR-BRAF*	*FN1-TGFA* and *FN1-EGF* most likely early calcifying aponeurotic fibroma	
Lipofibromatosis-like neural tumor [53]		*NTRK1*-related gene fusions	Common gene partners include *LMNA*, *TPR*, and *TPM3*	

(continued)

Table 11.2 (continued)

Tumor type	Translocation	Gene fusion		
Lipoma, ordinary	t with 12q14.3 t with 6p21	*HMGA2* fusions *HMGA1* fusions	30% 10%	
Lipoma, chondroid	t(11;16) (q13;p13)	*C11orf95-MKL2*	NA	
Spindle cell lipoma/ pleomorphic lipoma, mammary-type myofibroblastoma, cellular angiofibroma	16q13-qter rearrangement/ loss, monosomy 13 or partial del [13]q			
Myofibroma, cellular [54]		*SRF-RELA*	A subset	
Myopericytoma/ myofibroma [55]		*PDGFRB* mutations		
Myositis ossificans		*USP6* rearrangements	Genetically related to nodular fasciitis, aneurysmal bone cyst, and fibro-osseous pseudotumor of the digits	
Myxoma	NA	NA	Activating Gs-a mutations in *GNAS* gene	
Nodular fasciitis	t(17;22) (p13;q13.1)	*MYH9-USP6* (most common) *USP6* with various partners including *RRBP1, CALU, CTNNB1, MIR22HG, SPARC, THBS2, COL6A2*	90%	
Pericytoma	t(7;12) (7p22;q13)	*ACTB-GLI1*		
Phosphaturic mesenchymal tumor	t(2;8)(q35;p11)	*FN1-FGFR1*		
Plexiform fibromyxoma		*MALAT1-GLI1*		
Osteoblastoma/ osteoid osteoma [56]		*FOS* and *FOSB* rearrangements		
Schwannoma	22q12 loss		*NF2* loss	
Synovial chondromatosis		*FN1-ACVR2A and ACVR2A-FN1*	These alterations are present in the benign and malignant forms	
Tenosynovial giant cell tumor	t(1;2)(p13;q37) other t with 1p13	*CSF1-COL6A3*		

Table 11.3 *MDM2* amplification in liposarcomas and other soft tissue and bone sarcomas

Tumor type	Comment
ALT/WDL[a]	
Dedifferentiated liposarcoma	
Low-grade central osteosarcoma	
Conventional osteosarcoma	~10% of cases
Intimal sarcoma [57]	
Parosteal osteosarcoma	>85% of cases
Undifferentiated high-grade pleomorphic sarcoma of bone	~20% of cases
Rhabdomyosarcomas	Rare

[a]ALT/WDL: Atypical lipomatous tumor/well-differentiated liposarcoma

Table 11.4 Chromosomal aberrations in benign and malignant adipocytic neoplasms

Tumor type	Common cytogenetic aberrations
Ordinary lipoma	Translocations involving 12q13-15 Rearrangements of 13q Rearrangements involving 6p21-33
Spindle cell/pleomorphic lipoma	Monosomy 13 or partial loss of 13q in association with losses of 16q
Lipoblastoma/ lipoblastomatosis	Rearrangement involving 8q11-13 (*PLAG*)
Hibernoma	Rearrangements involving 11q13
Chondroid lipoma	t(11;16)(q13;p13) *C11orf95-MKL2*
Angiolipoma	Normal karyotype
ALT/WDL	Ring chromosomes and long marker chromosomes from 12q13-15
Dedifferentiated liposarcoma	Ring chromosomes and long marker chromosomes from 12q13-15; additional complex aberrations
Myxoid liposarcoma	t(12;16)(q13;p11) *FUS-DDIT3* t(12;22)(q13;q12) *EWSR1-DDIT3*
Pleomorphic liposarcoma	Complex rearrangements
Spindle cell liposarcoma [62]	A recent case with *TRIO-TERT* fusion of unclear significance

Vascular Tumors (Table 11.5)

- Alterations in the Gaq family (*GNAQ, GNA11, GNA14*) appears to be a common pathway in the pathogenesis of benign small vessel lesions [68]
  - Hot spot mutations in the above genes has been shown to disrupt GTPase activity of the mitogen-activated protein (MAP) kinase pathway.
- *FOS* (14q24.3) and *FOSB* (19q13) genes belong to the Fos gene family which also includes *FOSL1* and *FOSL2*.
  - They encode a transcription factor that dimerizes with members of the Jun family (c-Jun, JunB, and JunD), constituting the major components of the activating protein-1 (AP-1) complex.

Table 11.5 Chromosomal aberrations and relevant genetic abnormalities in vascular tumors

Tumor type	Chromosomal aberrations/relevant genetic abnormalities	Comment
Anastomosing hemangioma [63, 64]	*GNAQ*, *GNA11* and *GNA14* mutations	
Capillary malformation (nevus flammeus)	*GNAQ* mutations	
Cherry hemangioma	*GNAQ, GNA11*, *GNA14*, *KRAS* and *HRAS* mutations	
Congenital hemangioma (rapidly involuting/RICH or non-involuting/NICH)	*GNAQ* and *GNA11* mutations	
Epithelioid hemangioma [65, 66]	*FOSB-ZFP36* *FOSB-WWTR1* (rare) *FOSB-ACTB* (rare)	Often associated with worrisome histologic features (cellularity, pleomorphism, necrosis)
	FOS with a variety of partners including *LMNA* and *VIM*	
Epithelioid Hemangioendothelioma	*WWTR1-CAMTA1* *TFE3-YAP1*	85% of cases Unknown but rare
Hepatic small vessel neoplasm [67]	*GNAQ* and *GNA14*	
Kaposiform Hemangioendothelioma	*GNA14 mutations*	
Lobular capillary hemangioma (pyogenic granuloma)	*GNA11 GNA14, BRAF, NRAS and KRAS mutations*	*BRAF* c.1799T>A (Val600Glu) appears to paly a pivotal role in the pathogenesis of sporadic and particularly secondary lobular capillary hemangiomas.
Pseudomyogenic Hemangioendothelioma	*SERPINE1-FOSB* *ACTB-FOSB*	~50% of cases ~50% of cases
Tufted angioma	*GNA14 mutations*	

Tumors with Recurrent Gene Fusions (Including EWSR1*) and Other Alterations (Tables 11.6, 11.7, 11.8, 11.9, 11.10, 11.11, and 11.12)*

- The Ewing sarcoma breakpoint region 1 gene (*EWSR1*) is located on chromosome 22q12.
- It encodes a ubiquitously expressed RNA-binding protein.
- It is a member of the *TET* gene family which includes other related genes such as *FUS* and *TAF15*.
- It is a "promiscuous" gene with rearrangements (involving a number of different partners) detected in a variety of mesenchymal, epithelial, and hematolymphoid neoplasms.
- An emerging group of neoplasms are associated with *EWSR1-CREB1* and/or *EWSR1-ATF1* fusions; see Table below.

Table 11.6 Tumors with *EWSR1* rearrangements

Tumor type	Chromosomal aberrations	Comment
Acute leukemia	*EWSR1-ZNF384*	Acute lymphoblastic leukemia, biphenotypic leukemia
Acral fibroblastic spindle cell neoplasm	*EWSR1-SMAD3*	
Angiomatoid fibrous histiocytoma	*EWSR1-CREB1* *EWSR1-ATF1* *EWSR1-CREM*	*EWSR1-ATF1* especially in unusual sites
Angiosarcoma	*EWSR1-ATF1*	One case reported in the parotid gland
Clear cell sarcoma of soft parts	*EWSR1-ATF1* *EWSR1-CREB1* *EWSR1-CREM*	*EWSR1-ATF1* most common
Clear cell sarcoma-like of the gastrointestinal tract	*EWSR1-CREB1* *EWSR1-ATF1*	*EWSR1-CREB1* most common
Clear cell odontogenic Carcinoma	*EWSR1-ATF1*	
Desmoplastic small round cell tumor	*EWSR1-WT1*	
Ectomesenchymal Chondromyxoid tumor	*EWSR1* rearrangements	*RREB1-MKL2* fusions most common
Ewing sarcoma/PNET	*EWSR1-FLI1* *EWSR1-ERG* *EWSR1-ETV1* *EWSR1-ETV4* *EWSR1-FEV*	*EWSR1-FLI1* approximately 90% of cases
Ewing-like sarcomas	*EWSR1-PATZ1* *EWSR1-SP3* *EWSR1-NFATC2* *EWSR1-SMARCA5*	
Extraskeletal myxoid Chondrosarcoma	*EWSR1-NR4A3*	*EWSR1-NR4A3* ~ 75% of cases
Hyalinizing clear cell carcinoma of salivary gland	*EWSR1-ATF1* *EWSR1-CREM*	
Hidradenoma of the skin	*EWSR1-POU5F1*	
Malignant mesothelioma [69]	*EWSR1-ATF1* *EWSR1-YY1*	Predilection in young adults
Myoepithelial tumor, soft tissue	*EWSR1-POU5F1* *EWSR1-ZNF444* *EWSR1-PBX1* *EWSR1-PBX3* *EWSR1-KLF17* *EWSR1-ATF1*	*EWSR1-POU5F1* and *EWSR1-PBX1* are the most common fusions
Myxoid liposarcoma	*EWSR1-DDIT3*	~10%, *FUS* rearrangements most common
Low-grade fibromyxoid sarcoma	*EWSR1-CREB3L1*	Rare, *FUS* rearrangements most common

(continued)

Table 11.6 (continued)

Tumor type	Chromosomal aberrations	Comment
Primary pulmonary myxoid sarcoma [70]	*EWSR1-CREB1*	
Rhabdomyosarcoma (RMS) [71]	*EWSR1-DUX4*	Found in a case of embryonal rhabdomyosarcoma
	EWSR1/FUS-TFCP2	Provisional data, intraosseous location; hybrid spindle and epithelioid phenotype. Express ALK by immunohistochemistry
Sclerosing epithelioid Fibrosarcoma	*EWSR1-CREB2L2* *EWSR1-CREB2L1* *EWSR1- CREB3L3*	
Benign vascular tumor	*EWSR1-NFATC1*	One case of benign vascular tumor in bone

Table 11.7 Tumors with *EWSR1-CREB1* and *EWSR1-ATF1* fusions

Tumor type	Genetic fusion
Angiomatoid fibrous histiocytoma (AFH)	*EWSR1-CREB1>>EWSR1-ATF1, FUS-ATF1*
Clear cell sarcoma (CCS) of soft parts	*EWSR1-ATF1>>EWSR1-CREB1, EWSR1-CREM*
Primary pulmonary myxoid sarcoma (PPMS)	*EWSR1-CREB1*
Clear cell sarcoma-like tumor of the gastrointestinal tract	*EWSR1-CREB1>>EWSR1-ATF1*
Myoepithelial tumor of soft tissue	*EWSR1-ATF1*
Hyalinizing clear cell carcinoma	*EWSR1-ATF1*
Malignant mesothelioma*	*EWSR-ATF1, FUS-ATF1*
Clear cell odontogenic carcinoma (CCOC) [72]	*EWSR1-ATF1*

*Predilection in young adults

  - Recently another distinct group of myxoid mesenchymal neoplasm occurring in children or young adults with a predilection for intracranial locations was reported [74].
  - It harbors fusions involving *EWSR1* with one of the *CREB* family member (*ATF1, CREB*, or *CREM*)
  - It is debatable if it represents a myxoid variant of angiomatoid fibrous histiocytoma or a distinct entity.

- *NCOA2* (nuclear receptor co-activator 2) gene is located on chromosome 8q13.
  - Encodes for a nuclear hormone receptor transcriptional co-activator.
  - Interacts with ligand-bound receptors to recruit histone acetyltransferases and methyltransferases to facilitate chromatin remodeling and transcription.
  - Has been implicated as 3′ partner in gene fusions in leukemias and mesenchymal neoplasms.
    - C-terminal transcriptional activation domains 1 and 2 are retained in the fusion proteins.

Table 11.8 Tumors with *NCOA2* fusions

Tumor type	Genetic fusion	Comment
Acute myeloid leukemia	*MYST3-NCOA2, ETV6-NCOA2*	Occasional cases
Biphenotypic sinonasal sarcoma [6]	*PAX3-NCOA2*	Rare fusion
Mesenchymal chondrosarcoma	*HEY1-NCOA2*	
Congenital/infantile spindle cell rhabdomyosarcoma	*NCOA2* with various partners (*VGLL2, SRF, TEAD1*)	Favorable prognosis compared to older childhood and adult sclerosing cell rhabdomyosarcoma associated with *MYOD1* mutations
Alveolar rhabdomyosarcoma	*PAX3-NCOA2*	Rare cases
Soft tissue angiofibroma	*AHRR-NCOA2 >>GTF21-NCOA2, NCOA2-ETV4*	
Primitive spindle cell sarcoma of the kidney [42]	*MEIS-NCOA2*	Provisional entity, 2 cases reported
Intraosseous rhabdomyosarcoma [71]	*MEIS-NCOA2*	Provisional data, more primitive and fascicular spindle cell appearance
Uterine tumor resembling Ovarian sex cord tumor (UTROSCT) [73]	*ESR1-NCOA2* *ESR1-NCOA3* *GREB1-NCOA2*	
Uterine sarcoma with variable sex-cord differentiation	*GREB1-NCOA1* *GREB1-NCOA2*	Also with partners CTNNB1, NR4A3 and SS18

Table 11.9 Tumors with GLI1 fusions

Tumor type	Genetic fusion	Comment
Gastroblastoma	*MALAT1-GLI1*	
Gastric plexiform fibromyxoma [74]	*MALAT1-GLI1*	
Pericytoma	*ACTB-GLI1*	
"Malignant epithelioid neoplasm" [75]	*ACTB-GLI1* *MALAT-GLI1* *PTCH1-GLI1*	Provisional data, reported in soft tissue and occasionally bone neoplasms. Often epithelioid phenotype and strong S100-protein positivity by immunohistochemistry

- *GLI1* functions as an effector of the sonic hedgehog (SHH) pathway, inducing upregulation or downregulation of multiple downstream targets.
- *NTRK* 1, 2, and 3 genes encode the TRKA, TRKB, and TRKC neurotrophic tyrosine kinase receptors, respectively.
- Chromosomal translocations result in ligand-independent activation of the constitutively expressed kinase.
- Clinical trials have reported high response rates to TRK inhibition in patients with TRK fusion irrespectively of morphology.

Table 11.10 Selected tumors with TRK (*NTRK1, 2, 3*) fusions [76]

Tumor type	Genetic fusion	Comment
Infantile fibrosarcoma	*ETV6-NTRK3* *EML4-NTRK3*	*ETV6-NTRK3* most common *TPM3-NTRK1, LMNA-NTRK1*, and *SQSTM1-NTRK1* have been reported in pediatric sarcomas resembling infantile fibrosarcoma
Inflammatory myofibroblastic tumor (IMT)	*NTRK3* with various partners	
Lipofibromatosis-like neural tumor (LPF-NT)	*NTRK1* fusions with *LMNA, TPR* and *TPM3*	
Cellular congenital mesoblastic nephroma	*ETV6-NTKR3* *EML4-NTRK3* *LMNA-NTRK1*	*BRAF* intragenic deletions have also been described
Secretory breast cancer	*ETV6-NTRK3*	High frequency of *NTRK3*
Mammary analog secretory carcinoma of the salivary gland	*ETV6-NTRK3*	High frequency of *NTRK3*
Spitzoid melanocytic neoplasms	*MYO5A-NTRK3* *ETV6-NTRK3* *NTRK1* fusions	Across the whole spectrum of Spitz nevi, atypical Spitz tumor and Spitzoid melanoma
Metastatic papillary thyroid cancer	*ETV6-NTRK3* *TPR-NTRK1* *SQSTM1-NTRK3*	In approximately 25% of children
High-grade gliomas		Especially in tumors of children <3 years old, poor prognosis

Table 11.11 *SMARCB1* (*INI1*)-deficient mesenchymal neoplasms

Tumor type	% of cases with SMARCB1 loss
Malignant rhabdoid tumor	100%
Epithelioid sarcoma, classical (distal) type	90%
Epithelioid sarcoma, proximal type	100%
Epithelioid malignant peripheral nerve sheath tumor (MPNST)	50–60%
Synovial sarcoma	6–100%
Myoepithelial carcinoma	10–40%
Extraskeletal myxoid chondrosarcoma	16%
Poorly differentiated chordoma	100%
Osteosarcomas	0.7%
Ossifying fibromyxoid tumor	74% (mosaic pattern, hemizygous deletions)
Gastrointestinal stromal tumor (GIST)	Up to 70%, mosaic pattern

- The SWI/SNF chromatin-remodeling complex is composed of a set of highly conserved units to include: SMARCA4/BRG1, SMARCB1/INI1, SMARCC1/BAF155, and SMARCC2/BAF170.
- The complex utilizes the energy of ATP hydrolysis to remodel nucleosomes and modulate transcription.
- It has a widespread role in tumor suppression as inactivating mutations in several subunits is seen in high frequencies in various cancers.
- Identical gene fusions can be found in clinically, morphologically, and immunohistochemically entirely different tumors [77, 78].
- Other factors beyond the fusion type such as specific gene breakpoints, the cell type, tissue type/microenvironment, epigenetic changes, and others play significant role in the development of specific tumors.

Table 11.12 Other selected tumors with identical fusion genes

Fusion gene	Tumor type
FUS-ERG	Ewing sarcoma t(16;21) acute myeloid/lymphoblastic leukemia
TMP3/4-ALK	Inflammatory myofibroblastic tumor Anaplastic large cell lymphoma Renal cell carcinoma
CLTC-ALK	Inflammatory myofibroblastic tumor Diffuse large cell lymphoma Extramedullary plasmacytoma
RANBP2-ALK	Inflammatory myofibroblastic tumor Diffuse large cell lymphoma Myeloid leukemia
ETV6-NTRK3	Infantile fibrosarcoma Inflammatory myofibroblastic tumor Congenital mesoblastic nephroma, cellular type Acute myeloid/lymphoblastic leukemia Secretory carcinoma (breast) Mammary analogue secretory carcinoma Pigmented spindle cell nevus of Reed/Spitz nevus Radiation-induced papillary thyroid carcinoma Gastrointestinal stromal tumor (GIST)
MEAF6-PHF1 *EPC1-PHF1* *EP400-PHF1* *ZC3H7B-BCOR* *PHF1-TFE3*	Endometrial stromal sarcoma Ossifying fibromyxoid tumor
ASPACR1-TFE3	Alveolar part sarcoma Renal cell carcinoma
MALAT1-GLI1	Gastroblastoma Plexiform fibromyxoma Malignant epithelioid neoplasm with GLI1 fusions and S100-protein expression (other GLI1 partners ACTB and PTCH1)
TGFBR3-MGEA5	Myxoinflammatory fibroblastic sarcoma Hemosiderotic lipomatous tumor Pleomorphic hyalinizing angiectatic tumor

Selected References

1. Smith SM, Coleman J, Bridge JA, Iwenofu OH. Molecular diagnostics in soft tissue sarcomas and gastrointestinal stromal tumors. J Surg Oncol. 2015r;111(5):520–31. https://doi.org/10.1002/jso.23882. Epub 2015 Mar 13. Review. PubMed PMID: 25772665.
2. Bridge JA. The role of cytogenetics and molecular diagnostics in the diagnosis of soft-tissue tumors. Mod Pathol. 2014;27(Suppl 1):S80–97. https://doi.org/10.1038/modpathol.2013.179. Review. PubMed PMID: 24384855.
3. Bridge JA, Cushman-Vokoun AM. Molecular diagnostics of soft tissue tumors. Arch Pathol Lab Med. 2011;135(5):588–601. https://doi.org/10.1043/2010-0594-RAIR.1. Review. PubMed PMID: 21526957.
4. Guo T, Zhang L, Chang NE, Singer S, Maki RG, Antonescu CR. Consistent MYC and FLT4 gene amplification in radiation-induced angiosarcoma but not in other radiation-associated atypical vascular lesions. Genes Chromosomes Cancer. 2011;50(1):25–33. https://doi.org/10.1002/gcc.20827. PubMed PMID: 20949568; PubMed Central PMCID: PMC3150534.
5. Huang SC, Ghossein RA, Bishop JA, Zhang L, Chen TC, Huang HY, Antonescu CR. Novel PAX3-NCOA1 fusions in biphenotypic sinonasal sarcoma with focal rhabdomyoblastic differentiation. Am J Surg Pathol. 2016;40(1):51–9. https://doi.org/10.1097/PAS.0000000000000492. PubMed PMID: 26371783; PubMed Central PMCID: PMC4679641.
6. Le Loarer F, Laffont S, Lesluyes T, Tirode F, Antonescu C, Baglin AC, Delespaul L, Soubeyran I, Hostein I, Pérot G, Chibon F, Baud J, Le Guellec S, Karanian M, Costes-Martineau V, Castain C, Eimer S, Le Bail B, Wassef M, Coindre JM. Clinicopathologic and molecular features of a series of 41 biphenotypic sinonasal sarcomas expanding their molecular spectrum. Am J Surg Pathol. 2019. https://doi.org/10.1097/PAS.0000000000001238. [Epub ahead of print] PubMed PMID: 30829729.
7. Dickson BC, Hornick JL, Fletcher CDM, Demicco EG, Howarth DJ, Swanson D, Zhang L, Sung YS, Antonescu CR. Dermatofibrosarcoma protuberans with a novel COL6A3-PDGFD fusion gene and apparent predilection for breast. Genes Chromosomes Cancer. 2018;57(9):437–45. https://doi.org/10.1002/gcc.22663. Epub 2018 Aug 14. PubMed PMID: 30014607.
8. Dadone-Montaudié B, Alberti L, Duc A, Delespaul L, Lesluyes T, Pérot G, Lançon A, Paindavoine S, Di Mauro I, Blay JY, de la Fouchardière A, Chibon F, Karanian M, MacGrogan G, Kubiniek V, Keslair F, Cardot-Leccia N, Michot A, Perrin V, Zekri Y, Coindre JM, Tirode F, Pedeutour F, Ranchère-Vince D, Le Loarer F, Pissaloux D. Alternative PDGFD rearrangements in dermatofibrosarcomas protuberans without PDGFB fusions. Mod Pathol. 2018;31(11):1683–93. Epub 2018 Jun 28. PubMed PMID: 29955147. https://doi.org/10.1038/s41379-018-0089-4.
9. Lewis N, Soslow RA, Delair DF, Park KJ, Murali R, Hollmann TJ, Davidson B, Micci F, Panagopoulos I, Hoang LN, Arias-Stella JA 3rd, Oliva E, Young RH, Hensley ML, Leitao MM Jr, Hameed M, Benayed R, Ladanyi M, Frosina D, Jungbluth AA, Antonescu CR, Chiang S. ZC3H7B-BCOR high-grade endometrial stromal sarcomas: a report of 17 cases of a newly defined entity. Mod Pathol. 2018;31(4):674–84. https://doi.org/10.1038/modpathol.2017.162. Epub 2017 Dec 1. PubMed PMID: 29192652.
10. Shah AA, Ohori NP, Yip L, Coyne C, Antonescu CR, Seethala RR. Epithelioid hemangioendothelioma: a rare primary thyroid tumor with confirmation of WWTR1 and CAMTA1 rearrangements. Endocr Pathol. 2016;27(2):147–52. https://doi.org/10.1007/s12022-016-9428-5. PubMed PMID: 27026033.
11. Anderson T, Zhang L, Hameed M, Rusch V, Travis WD, Antonescu CR. Thoracic epithelioid malignant vascular tumors: a clinicopathologic study of 52 cases with emphasis on pathologic grading and molecular studies of WWTR1-CAMTA1 fusions. Am J Surg Pathol. 2015;39(1):132–9. https://doi.org/10.1097/PAS.0000000000000346. PubMed PMID: 25353289; PubMed Central PMCID: PMC4268225.
12. Antonescu CR, Le Loarer F, Mosquera JM, Sboner A, Zhang L, Chen CL, Chen HW, Pathan N, Krausz T, Dickson BC, Weinreb I, Rubin MA, Hameed M, Fletcher CD. Novel YAP1-TFE3

fusion defines a distinct subset of epithelioid hemangioendothelioma. Genes Chromosomes Cancer. 2013;52(8):775–84. https://doi.org/10.1002/gcc.22073. Epub 2013 Jun 5. PubMed PMID: 23737213; PubMed Central PMCID: PMC4089994.
13. Errani C, Zhang L, Sung YS, Hajdu M, Singer S, Maki RG, Healey JH, Antonescu CR. A novel WWTR1-CAMTA1 gene fusion is a consistent abnormality in epithelioid hemangioendothelioma of different anatomic sites. Genes Chromosomes Cancer. 2011;50(8):644–53. https://doi.org/10.1002/gcc.20886. Epub 2011 May 16. PubMed PMID: 21584898; PubMed Central PMCID: PMC3264678.
14. Chen S, Deniz K, Sung YS, Zhang L, Dry S, Antonescu CR. Ewing sarcoma with ERG gene rearrangements: a molecular study focusing on the prevalence of FUS-ERG and common pitfalls in detecting EWSR1-ERG fusions by FISH. Genes Chromosomes Cancer. 2016;55(4):340–9. https://doi.org/10.1002/gcc.22336. Epub 2015 Dec 22. PubMed PMID: 26690869; PubMed Central PMCID: PMC5006947.
15. Lawrence B, Perez-Atayde A, Hibbard MK, Rubin BP, Dal Cin P, Pinkus JL, Pinkus GS, Xiao S, Yi ES, Fletcher CD, Fletcher JA. TPM3-ALK and TPM4-ALK oncogenes in inflammatory myofibroblastic tumors. Am J Pathol. 2000;157(2):377–84. PubMed PMID: 10934142; PubMed Central PMCID: PMC1850130.
16. Arias-Stella JA 3rd, Benayed R, Oliva E, Young RH, Hoang LN, Lee CH, Jungbluth AA, Frosina D, Soslow RA, Antonescu CR, Ladanyi M, Chiang S. Novel PLAG1 gene rearrangement distinguishes a subset of uterine myxoid leiomyosarcoma from other uterine myxoid mesenchymal tumors. Am J Surg Pathol. 2018. https://doi.org/10.1097/PAS.0000000000001196. [Epub ahead of print] PubMed PMID: 30489320.
17. Huang SC, Chen HW, Zhang L, Sung YS, Agaram NP, Davis M, Edelman M, Fletcher CD, Antonescu CR. Novel FUS-KLF17 and EWSR1-KLF17 fusions in myoepithelial tumors. Genes Chromosomes Cancer. 2015;54(5):267–75. https://doi.org/10.1002/gcc.22240. Epub 2015 Feb 23. PubMed PMID: 25706482; PubMed Central PMCID: PMC4376655.
18. Agaram NP, Chen HW, Zhang L, Sung YS, Panicek D, Healey JH, Nielsen GP, Fletcher CD, Antonescu CR. EWSR1-PBX3: a novel gene fusion in myoepithelial tumors. Genes Chromosomes Cancer. 2015;54(2):63–71. https://doi.org/10.1002/gcc.22216. Epub 2014 Sep 18. PubMed PMID: 25231231; PubMed Central PMCID: PMC4268355.
19. Kao YC, Ranucci V, Zhang L, Sung YS, Athanasian EA, Swanson D, Dickson BC, Antonescu CR. Recurrent BRAF gene rearrangements in myxoinflammatory fibroblastic sarcomas, but not hemosiderotic fibrolipomatous tumors. Am J Surg Pathol. 2017;41(11):1456–65. https://doi.org/10.1097/PAS.0000000000000899. PubMed PMID: 28692601; PubMed Central PMCID: PMC5636656.
20. Antonescu CR, Zhang L, Nielsen GP, Rosenberg AE, Dal Cin P, Fletcher CD. Consistent t(1;10) with rearrangements of TGFBR3 and MGEA5 in both myxoinflammatory fibroblastic sarcoma and hemosiderotic fibrolipomatous tumor. Genes Chromosomes Cancer. 2011;50(10):757–64. https://doi.org/10.1002/gcc.20897. Epub 2011 Jun 29. PubMed PMID: 21717526; PubMed Central PMCID: PMC3361892.
21. Suurmeijer AJ, Song W, Sung YS, Zhang L, Swanson D, Fletcher CD, Dickson BC, Antonescu CR. Novel recurrent PHF1-TFE3 fusions in ossifying fibromyxoid tumors. Genes Chromosomes Cancer. 2019. https://doi.org/10.1002/gcc.22755. [Epub ahead of print] PubMed PMID: 30920708.
22. Kao YC, Sung YS, Zhang L, Chen CL, Huang SC, Antonescu CR. Expanding the molecular signature of ossifying fibromyxoid tumors with two novel gene fusions: CREBBP-BCORL1 and KDM2A-WWTR1. Genes Chromosomes Cancer. 2017;56(1):42–50. https://doi.org/10.1002/gcc.22400. Epub 2016 Aug 26. PubMed PMID: 27537276; PubMed Central PMCID: PMC5570549.
23. Antonescu CR, Sung YS, Chen CL, Zhang L, Chen HW, Singer S, Agaram NP, Sboner A, Fletcher CD. Novel ZC3H7B-BCOR, MEAF6-PHF1, and EPC1-PHF1 fusions in ossifying fibromyxoid tumors--molecular characterization shows genetic overlap with endometrial stromal sarcoma. Genes Chromosomes Cancer. 2014;53(2):183–93. https://doi.org/10.1002/gcc.22132. Epub 2013 Nov 28. PubMed PMID: 24285434; PubMed Central.

24. Agaram NP, Sung YS, Zhang L, Chen CL, Chen HW, Singer S, Dickson MA, Berger MF, Antonescu CR. Dichotomy of genetic abnormalities in PEComas with therapeutic implications. Am J Surg Pathol. 2015;39(6):813–25. https://doi.org/10.1097/PAS.0000000000000389. PubMed PMID: 25651471; PubMed Central PMCID: PMC4431898.
25. McGregor SM, Alikhan MB, John RA, Kotler H, Bridge JA, Mujacic I, Kadri S, Segal J, Krausz T. Melanotic PEComa of the sinonasal mucosa with NONO-TFE3 fusion: an elusive mimic of sinonasal melanoma. Am J Surg Pathol. 2017;41(5):717–22. https://doi.org/10.1097/PAS.0000000000000778. PubMed PMID: 28009605.
26. Agaram NP, Zhang L, Cotzia P, Antonescu CR. Expanding the spectrum of genetic alterations in pseudomyogenic hemangioendothelioma with recurrent novel ACTB-FOSB gene fusions. Am J Surg Pathol. 2018;42(12):1653–61. https://doi.org/10.1097/PAS.0000000000001147. PubMed PMID: 30256258.
27. Zhu G, Benayed R, Ho C, Mullaney K, Sukhadia P, Rios K, Berry R, Rubin BP, Nafa K, Wang L, Klimstra DS, Ladanyi M, Hameed MR. Diagnosis of known sarcoma fusions and novel fusion partners by targeted RNA sequencing with identification of a recurrent ACTB-FOSB fusion in pseudomyogenic hemangioendothelioma. Mod Pathol. 2018. https://doi.org/10.1038/s41379-018-0175-7. [Epub ahead of print] PubMed PMID: 30459475.
28. Prieto-Granada C, Zhang L, Chen HW, Sung YS, Agaram NP, Jungbluth AA, Antonescu CR. A genetic dichotomy between pure sclerosing epithelioid fibrosarcoma (SEF) and hybrid SEF/low-grade fibromyxoid sarcoma: a pathologic and molecular study of 18 cases. Genes Chromosomes Cancer. 2015;54(1):28–38. https://doi.org/10.1002/gcc.22215. Epub 2014 Sep 18. PubMed PMID: 25231134; PubMed Central PMCID: PMC4232448.
29. Robinson DR, Wu YM, Kalyana-Sundaram S, Cao X, Lonigro RJ, Sung YS, Chen CL, Zhang L, Wang R, Su F, Iyer MK, Roychowdhury S, Siddiqui J, Pienta KJ, Kunju LP, Talpaz M, Mosquera JM, Singer S, Schuetze SM, Antonescu CR, Chinnaiyan AM. Identification of recurrent NAB2-STAT6 gene fusions in solitary fibrous tumor by integrative sequencing. Nat Genet. 2013;45(2):180–5. https://doi.org/10.1038/ng.2509. Epub 2013 Jan 13. PubMed PMID: 23313952; PubMed Central PMCID: PMC3654808.
30. Mosquera JM, Sboner A, Zhang L, Kitabayashi N, Chen CL, Sung YS, Wexler LH, LaQuaglia MP, Edelman M, Sreekantaiah C, Rubin MA, Antonescu CR. Recurrent NCOA2 gene rearrangements in congenital/infantile spindle cell rhabdomyosarcoma. Genes Chromosomes Cancer. 2013;52(6):538–50. https://doi.org/10.1002/gcc.22050. Epub 2013 Mar 5. PubMed PMID: 23463663; PubMed Central PMCID: PMC3734530.
31. Agaram NP, LaQuaglia MP, Alaggio R, Zhang L, Fujisawa Y, Ladanyi M, Wexler LH, Antonescu CR. MYOD1-mutant spindle cell and sclerosing rhabdomyosarcoma: an aggressive subtype irrespective of age. A reappraisal for molecular classification and risk stratification. Mod Pathol. 2018. https://doi.org/10.1038/s41379-018-0120-9. [Epub ahead of print] PubMed PMID: 30181563.
32. Alaggio R, Zhang L, Sung YS, Huang SC, Chen CL, Bisogno G, Zin A, Agaram NP, LaQuaglia MP, Wexler LH, Antonescu CR. A molecular study of pediatric spindle and sclerosing rhabdomyosarcoma: identification of novel and recurrent VGLL2-related fusions in infantile cases. Am J Surg Pathol. 2016;40(2):224–35. https://doi.org/10.1097/PAS.0000000000000538. PubMed PMID: 26501226; PubMed Central PMCID: PMC4712098.
33. Agaram NP, Chen CL, Zhang L, LaQuaglia MP, Wexler L, Antonescu CR. Recurrent MYOD1 mutations in pediatric and adult sclerosing and spindle cell rhabdomyosarcomas: evidence for a common pathogenesis. Genes Chromosomes Cancer. 2014;53(9):779–87. https://doi.org/10.1002/gcc.22187. Epub 2014 May 14. PubMed PMID: 24824843; PubMed Central PMCID: PMC4108340.
34. Alholle A, Karanian M, Brini AT, Morris MR, Kannappan V, Niada S, Niblett A, Ranchère-Vince D, Pissaloux D, Delfour C, Maran-Gonzalez A, Antonescu CR, Sumathi V, Tirode F, Latif F. Genetic analyses of undifferentiated small round cell sarcoma identifies a novel sarcoma subtype with a recurrent CRTC1-SS18 gene fusion. J Pathol. 2018;245(2):186–96. https://doi.org/10.1002/path.5071. Epub 2018 Apr 16. PubMed PMID: 29533464.

35. Kao YC, Owosho AA, Sung YS, Zhang L, Fujisawa Y, Lee JC, Wexler L, Argani P, Swanson D, Dickson BC, Fletcher CDM, Antonescu CR. BCOR-CCNB3 fusion positive sarcomas: a clinicopathologic and molecular analysis of 36 cases with comparison to morphologic spectrum and clinical behavior of other round cell sarcomas. Am J Surg Pathol. 2018;42(5):604–15. https://doi.org/10.1097/PAS.0000000000000965. PubMed PMID: 29300189; PubMed Central PMCID: PMC5893395.
36. Antonescu CR, Owosho AA, Zhang L, Chen S, Deniz K, Huryn JM, Kao YC, Huang SC, Singer S, Tap W, Schaefer IM, Fletcher CD. Sarcomas with CIC-rearrangements are a distinct pathologic entity with aggressive outcome: a clinicopathologic and molecular study of 115 cases. Am J Surg Pathol. 2017;41(7):941–9. https://doi.org/10.1097/PAS.0000000000000846. PubMed PMID: 28346326; PubMed Central PMCID: PMC5468475.
37. Yoshimoto T, Tanaka M, Homme M, Yamazaki Y, Takazawa Y, Antonescu CR, Nakamura T. CIC-DUX4 induces small round cell sarcomas distinct from Ewing sarcoma. Cancer Res. 2017;77(11):2927–37. https://doi.org/10.1158/0008-5472.CAN-16-3351. Epub 2017 Apr 12. PubMed PMID: 28404587; PubMed Central PMCID: PMC5488331.
38. Antonescu C. Round cell sarcomas beyond Ewing: emerging entities. Histopathology. 2014;64(1):26–37. https://doi.org/10.1111/his.12281. Epub 2013 Nov 12. Review. PubMed PMID: 24215322.
39. Koelsche C, Hartmann W, Schrimpf D, Stichel D, Jabar S, Ranft A, Reuss DE, Sahm F, Jones DTW, Bewerunge-Hudler M, Trautmann M, Klingebiel T, Vokuhl C, Gessler M, Wardelmann E, Petersen I, Baumhoer D, Flucke U, Antonescu C, Esteller M, Fröhling S, Kool M, Pfister SM, Mechtersheimer G, Dirksen U, von Deimling A. Array-based DNA-methylation profiling in sarcomas with small blue round cell histology provides valuable diagnostic information. Mod Pathol. 2018;31(8):1246–56. https://doi.org/10.1038/s41379-018-0045-3. Epub 2018 Mar 23. PubMed PMID: 29572501.
40. Schaefer IM, Dal Cin P, Landry LM, Fletcher CDM, Hanna GJ, French CA. CIC-NUTM1 fusion: a case which expands the spectrum of NUT-rearranged epithelioid malignancies. Genes Chromosomes Cancer. 2018;57(9):446–51. https://doi.org/10.1002/gcc.3. Epub 2018 Aug 14. PubMed PMID: 29700887.
41. Sugita S, Arai Y, Aoyama T, Asanuma H, Mukai W, Hama N, Emori M, Shibata T, Hasegawa T. NUTM2A-CIC fusion small round cell sarcoma: a genetically distinct variant of CIC-rearranged sarcoma. Hum Pathol. 2017;65:225–30. https://doi.org/10.1016/j.humpath.2017.01.012. Epub 2017 Feb 8. PubMed PMID: 28188754.
42. Argani P, Reuter VE, Kapur P, Brown JE, Sung YS, Zhang L, Williamson R, Francis G, Sommerville S, Swanson D, Dickson BC, Antonescu CR. Novel MEIS1-NCOA2 gene fusions define a distinct primitive spindle cell sarcoma of the kidney. Am J Surg Pathol. 2018;42(11):1562–70. https://doi.org/10.1097/PAS.0000000000001140. PubMed PMID: 30179902.
43. Dickson BC, Sung YS, Rosenblum MK, Reuter VE, Harb M, Wunder JS, Swanson D, Antonescu CR. NUTM1 gene fusions characterize a subset of undifferentiated soft tissue and visceral tumors. Am J Surg Pathol. 2018;42(5):636–45. https://doi.org/10.1097/PAS.0000000000001021. PubMed PMID: 29356724; PubMed Central PMCID: PMC5893407.
44. Diolaiti D, Dela Cruz FS, Gundem G, Bouvier N, Boulad M, Zhang Y, Chou AJ, Dunkel IJ, Sanghvi R, Shah M, Geiger H, Rahman S, Felice V, Wrzeszczynski KO, Darnell RB, Antonescu CR, French CA, Papaemmanuil E, Kung AL, Shukla N. A recurrent novel MGA-NUTM1 fusion identifies a new subtype of high-grade spindle cell sarcoma. Cold Spring Harb Mol Case Stud. 2018;4(6). pii: a003194. https://doi.org/10.1101/mcs.a003194. Print 2018 Dec. PubMed PMID: 30552129.
45. Tamura R, Nakaoka H, Yoshihara K, Mori Y, Yachida N, Nishikawa N, Motoyama T, Okuda S, Inoue I, Enomoto T. Novel MXD4-NUTM1 fusion transcript identified in primary ovarian undifferentiated small round cell sarcoma. Genes Chromosomes Cancer. 2018;57(11):557–63. https://doi.org/10.1002/gcc.22668. PubMed PMID: 30338611; PubMed Central PMCID: PMC6221051.

46. Chiang S, Cotzia P, Hyman DM, Drilon A, Tap WD, Zhang L, Hechtman JF, Frosina D, Jungbluth AA, Murali R, Park KJ, Soslow RA, Oliva E, Iafrate AJ, Benayed R, Ladanyi M, Antonescu CR. NTRK fusions define a novel uterine sarcoma subtype with features of fibrosarcoma. Am J Surg Pathol. 2018;42(6):791–8. https://doi.org/10.1097/PAS.0000000000001055. PubMed PMID: 29553955.
47. Michal M, Berry RS, Rubin BP, Kilpatrick SE, Agaimy A, Kazakov DV, Steiner P, Ptakova N, Martinek P, Hadravsky L, Michalova K, Szep Z, Michal M. EWSR1-SMAD3-rearranged fibroblastic tumor: an emerging entity in an increasingly more complex group of fibroblastic/myofibroblastic neoplasms. Am J Surg Pathol. 2018;42(10):1325–33. https://doi.org/10.1097/PAS.0000000000001109. PubMed PMID: 29957732.
48. Kao YC, Flucke U, Eijkelenboom A, Zhang L, Sung YS, Suurmeijer AJH, Antonescu CR. Novel EWSR1-SMAD3 gene fusions in a group of acral fibroblastic spindle cell neoplasms. Am J Surg Pathol. 2018;42(4):522–8. https://doi.org/10.1097/PAS.0000000000001002. PubMed PMID: 29309308; PubMed Central PMCID: PMC5844807.
49. Mariño-Enríquez A, Fletcher CD. Angiofibroma of soft tissue: clinicopathologic characterization of a distinctive benign fibrovascular neoplasm in a series of 37 cases. Am J Surg Pathol. 2012;36(4):500–8. https://doi.org/10.1097/PAS.0b013e31823defbe. PubMed PMID: 22301504.
50. Dickson BC, Antonescu CR, Argyris PP, Bilodeau EA, Bullock MJ, Freedman PD, Gnepp DR, Jordan RC, Koutlas IG, Lee CH, Leong I, Merzianu M, Purgina BM, Thompson LDR, Wehrli B, Wright JM, Swanson D, Zhang L, Bishop JA. Ectomesenchymal chondromyxoid tumor: a neoplasm characterized by recurrent RREB1-MKL2 fusions. Am J Surg Pathol. 2018;42(10):1297–305. https://doi.org/10.1097/PAS.0000000000001096. PubMed PMID: 29912715; PubMed Central PMCID: PMC6133728.
51. Doyle LA, Mariño-Enriquez A, Fletcher CD, Hornick JL. ALK rearrangement and overexpression in epithelioid fibrous histiocytoma. Mod Pathol. 2015;28(7):904–12. https://doi.org/10.1038/modpathol.2015.49. Epub 2015 Apr 10. PubMed PMID: 25857825.
52. Flucke U, Shepard SJ, Bekers EM, Tirabosco R, van Diest PJ, Creytens D, van Gorp JM. Fibro-osseous pseudotumor of digits - expanding the spectrum of clonal transient neoplasms harboring USP6 rearrangement. Ann Diagn Pathol. 2018;35:53–5. https://doi.org/10.1016/j.anndiagpath.2018.05.003. Epub 2018 May 12. PubMed PMID: 29787930.
53. Agaram NP, Zhang L, Sung YS, Chen CL, Chung CT, Antonescu CR, Fletcher CD. Recurrent NTRK1 gene fusions define a novel subset of locally aggressive lipofibromatosis-like neural tumors. Am J Surg Pathol. 2016;40(10):1407–16. https://doi.org/10.1097/PAS.0000000000000675. PubMed PMID: 27259011; PubMed Central PMCID: PMC5023452.
54. Antonescu CR, Sung YS, Zhang L, Agaram NP, Fletcher CD. Recurrent SRF-RELA fusions define a novel subset of cellular myofibroma/myopericytoma: a potential diagnostic pitfall with sarcomas with myogenic differentiation. Am J Surg Pathol. 2017;41(5):677–84. https://doi.org/10.1097/PAS.0000000000000811. PubMed PMID: 28248815; PubMed Central PMCID: PMC5391281.
55. Hung YP, Fletcher CDM. Myopericytomatosis: clinicopathologic analysis of 11 cases with molecular identification of recurrent PDGFRB alterations in myopericytomatosis and myopericytoma. Am J Surg Pathol. 2017;41(8):1034–44. https://doi.org/10.1097/PAS.0000000000000862. PubMed PMID: 28505006.
56. Fittall MW, Mifsud W, Pillay N, Ye H, Strobl AC, Verfaillie A, Demeulemeester J, Zhang L, Berisha F, Tarabichi M, Young MD, Miranda E, Tarpey PS, Tirabosco R, Amary F, Grigoriadis AE, Stratton MR, Van Loo P, Antonescu CR, Campbell PJ, Flanagan AM, Behjati S. Recurrent rearrangements of FOS and FOSB define osteoblastoma. Nat Commun. 2018;9(1):2150. https://doi.org/10.1038/s41467-018-04530-z. PubMed PMID: 29858576; PubMed Central PMCID: PMC5984627.
57. Barretina J, Taylor BS, Banerji S, Ramos AH, Lagos-Quintana M, Decarolis PL, Shah K, Socci ND, Weir BA, Ho A, Chiang DY, Reva B, Mermel CH, Getz G, Antipin Y, Beroukhim R, Major JE, Hatton C, Nicoletti R, Hanna M, Sharpe T, Fennell TJ, Cibulskis K, Onofrio RC, Saito T,

Shukla N, Lau C, Nelander S, Silver SJ, Sougnez C, Viale A, Winckler W, Maki RG, Garraway LA, Lash A, Greulich H, Root DE, Sellers WR, Schwartz GK, Antonescu CR, Lander ES, Varmus HE, Ladanyi M, Sander C, Meyerson M, Singer S. Subtype-specific genomic alterations define new targets for soft-tissue sarcoma therapy. Nat Genet. 2010;42(8):715–21. https://doi.org/10.1038/ng.619. Epub 2010 Jul 4. PubMed PMID: 20601955; PubMed Central PMCID: PMC2911503.

58. Ragazzini P, Gamberi G, Pazzaglia L, Serra M, Magagnoli G, Ponticelli F, Ferrari C, Ghinelli C, Alberghini M, Bertoni F, Picci P, Benassi MS. Amplification of CDK4, MDM2, SAS and GLI genes in leiomyosarcoma, alveolar and embryonal rhabdomyosarcoma. Histol Histopathol. 2004;19(2):401–11. https://doi.org/10.14670/HH-19.401. Erratum in: Histol Histopathol. 2004 Jul;19(3):1013. PubMed PMID: 15024701.
59. Anderson J, Gordon A, Pritchard-Jones K, Shipley J. Genes, chromosomes, and rhabdomyosarcoma. Genes Chromosomes Cancer. 1999;26(4):275–85. Review. PubMed PMID: 10534762.
60. Wunder JS, Eppert K, Burrow SR, Gokgoz N, Bell RS, Andrulis IL. Co-amplification and overexpression of CDK4, SAS and MDM2 occurs frequently in human parosteal osteosarcomas. Oncogene. 1999;18(3):783–8. Erratum in: Oncogene 2000 Mar 23;19(13):1734. Gogkoz N [corrected to Gokgoz N]. PubMed PMID: 9989829.
61. Ladanyi M, Lewis R, Jhanwar SC, Gerald W, Huvos AG, Healey JH. MDM2 and CDK4 gene amplification in Ewing's sarcoma. J Pathol. 1995;175(2):211–7. PubMed PMID: 7738717.
62. Suster DI, Deshpande V, Chebib I, Taylor MS, Mullen J, Bredella MA, Nielsen GP. Spindle cell liposarcoma with a TRIO-TERT fusion transcript. Virchows Arch. 2019. https://doi.org/10.1007/s00428-019-02545-5. [Epub ahead of print] PubMed PMID: 30793229.
63. Bean GR, Joseph NM, Folpe AL, Horvai AE, Umetsu SE. Recurrent GNA14 mutations in anastomosing haemangiomas. Histopathology. 2018;73(2):354–7. https://doi.org/10.1111/his.13519. Epub 2018 May 21. PubMed PMID: 29574926.
64. Bean GR, Joseph NM, Gill RM, Folpe AL, Horvai AE, Umetsu SE. Recurrent GNAQ mutations in anastomosing hemangiomas. Mod Pathol. 2017;30(5):722–7. https://doi.org/10.1038/modpathol.2016.234. Epub 2017 Jan 13. PubMed PMID: 28084343.
65. Huang SC, Zhang L, Sung YS, Chen CL, Krausz T, Dickson BC, Kao YC, Agaram NP, Fletcher CD, Antonescu CR. Frequent FOS gene rearrangements in epithelioid hemangioma: a molecular study of 58 cases with morphologic reappraisal. Am J Surg Pathol. 2015;39(10):1313–21. https://doi.org/10.1097/PAS.0000000000000469. PubMed PMID: 26135557; PubMed Central PMCID: PMC4567921.
66. Antonescu CR, Chen HW, Zhang L, Sung YS, Panicek D, Agaram NP, Dickson BC, Krausz T, Fletcher CD. ZFP36-FOSB fusion defines a subset of epithelioid hemangioma with atypical features. Genes Chromosomes Cancer. 2014;53(11):951–9. https://doi.org/10.1002/gcc.22206. Epub 2014 Jul 18. PubMed PMID: 25043949; PubMed Central PMCID: PMC4229947.
67. Joseph NM, Brunt EM, Marginean C, Nalbantoglu I, Snover DC, Thung SN, Yeh MM, Umetsu SE, Ferrell LD, Gill RM. Frequent GNAQ and GNA14 mutations in hepatic small vessel neoplasm. Am J Surg Pathol. 2018;42(9):1201–7. https://doi.org/10.1097/PAS.0000000000001110. PubMed PMID: 29975248.
68. Lim YH, Bacchiocchi A, Qiu J, Straub R, Bruckner A, Bercovitch L, Narayan D, Yale Center for Mendelian Genomics, McNiff J, Ko C, Robinson-Bostom L, Antaya R, Halaban R, Choate KA. GNA14 somatic mutation causes congenital and sporadic vascular tumors by MAPK activation. Am J Hum Genet. 2016;99(2):443–50. https://doi.org/10.1016/j.ajhg.2016.06.010. Epub 2016 Jul 28. PubMed PMID: 27476652; PubMed Central PMCID: PMC4974082.
69. Desmeules P, Joubert P, Zhang L, Al-Ahmadie HA, Fletcher CD, Vakiani E, Delair DF, Rekhtman N, Ladanyi M, Travis WD, Antonescu CR. A subset of malignant mesotheliomas in young adults are associated with recurrent EWSR1/FUS-ATF1 fusions. Am J Surg Pathol. 2017;41(7):980–8. https://doi.org/10.1097/PAS.0000000000000864. PubMed PMID: 28505004; PubMed Central PMCID: PMC5468482.

70. Prieto-Granada CN, Ganim RB, Zhang L, Antonescu C, Mueller J. Primary pulmonary myxoid sarcoma: a newly described entity-report of a case and review of the literature. Int J Surg Pathol. 2017;25(6):518–25. https://doi.org/10.1177/1066896917706413. Epub 2017 Apr 28. Review. PubMed PMID: 28449608.
71. Agaram NP, Zhang L, Sung YS, Cavalcanti MS, Torrence D, Wexler L, Francis G, Sommerville S, Swanson D, Dickson BC, Suurmeijer AJH, Williamson R, Antonescu CR. Expanding the spectrum of intraosseous rhabdomyosarcoma: correlation between 2 distinct gene fusions and phenotype. Am J Surg Pathol. 2019. https://doi.org/10.1097/PAS.0000000000001227. [Epub ahead of print] PubMed PMID: 30720533.
72. Yancoskie AE, Sreekantaiah C, Jacob J, Rosenberg A, Edelman M, Antonescu CR, Fantasia JE. EWSR1 and ATF1 rearrangements in clear cell odontogenic carcinoma: presentation of a case. Oral Surg Oral Med Oral Pathol Oral Radiol. 2014;118(4):e115–8. https://doi.org/10.1016/j.oooo.2014.02.004. Epub 2014 Feb 14. PubMed PMID: 24721473.
73. Dickson BC, Childs TJ, Colgan TJ, Sung YS, Swanson D, Zhang L, Antonescu CR. Uterine tumor resembling ovarian sex cord tumor: a distinct entity characterized by recurrent NCOA2/3 gene fusions. Am J Surg Pathol. 2019;43(2):178–86. https://doi.org/10.1097/PAS.0000000000001153. PubMed PMID: 30273195.
74. Kao YC, Sung YS, Zhang L, Chen CL, Vaiyapuri S, Rosenblum MK, Antonescu CR. EWSR1 fusions with CREB family transcription factors define a novel myxoid mesenchymal tumor with predilection for intracranial location. Am J Surg Pathol. 2017;41(4):482–90. https://doi.org/10.1097/PAS.0000000000000788. PubMed PMID: 280e09602; PubMed Central PMCID: PMC5350023.
75. Spans L, Fletcher CD, Antonescu CR, Rouquette A, Coindre JM, Sciot R, Debiec-Rychter M. Recurrent MALAT1-GLI1 oncogenic fusion and GLI1 up-regulation define a subset of plexiform fibromyxoma. J Pathol. 2016;239(3):335–43. https://doi.org/10.1002/path.4730. Epub 2016 May 20. PubMed PMID: 27101025; PubMed Central PMCID: PMC5586099.
76. Antonescu CR, Agaram NP, Sung YS, Zhang L, Swanson D, Dickson BC. A distinct malignant epithelioid neoplasm with GLI1 gene rearrangements, frequent S100 protein expression, and metastatic potential: expanding the spectrum of pathologic entities with ACTB/MALAT1/PTCH1-GLI1 fusions. Am J Surg Pathol. 2018;42(4):553–60. https://doi.org/10.1097/PAS.0000000000001010. PubMed PMID: 29309307; PubMed Central PMCID: PMC5844813.
77. Cocco E, Scaltriti M, Drilon A. NTRK fusion-positive cancers and TRK inhibitor therapy. Nat Rev Clin Oncol. 2018;15(12):731–47. https://doi.org/10.1038/s41571-018-0113-0. Review. PubMed PMID: 30333516.
78. Mertens F, Antonescu CR, Mitelman F. Gene fusions in soft tissue tumors: recurrent and overlapping pathogenetic themes. Genes Chromosomes Cancer. 2016;55(4):291–310. https://doi.org/10.1002/gcc.22335. Epub 2015 Dec 18. Review. PubMed PMID: 26684580; PubMed Central PMCID: PMC5012284.

Chapter 12
Salivary Gland Carcinomas

Snjezana Dogan

Key Points
- Detection of genetic alterations in salivary gland carcinomas is used to support the diagnosis and can help select patients for targeted therapy.
- *MAML2* rearrangements in mucoepidermoid carcinoma, *ETV6* in secretory carcinoma, and *MYB* in adenoid cystic carcinoma are most commonly used for diagnosis.
- Salivary gland carcinomas harboring *ETV6-NTRK3, ERBB2* amplification/mutations, or *EML4-ALK* fusion are most likely to be considered for targeted therapy.

Key Online Resource
- El-Naggar AK, Chan JKC, Grandis JR, Takata T, Slootweg PJ, editors. *WHO classification of head and neck tumours*, 4th ed.

Introduction

The majority of low- and intermediate-grade salivary gland carcinomas (SGC) are driven by recurrent genetic alterations, most commonly gene fusions. Among those that are present in the majority of cases and are the hallmark of disease are

S. Dogan (✉)
Department of Pathology, Memorial Sloan Kettering Cancer Center, New York, NY, USA
e-mail: dogans@mskcc.org

L. J. Tafe, M. E. Arcila (eds.), *Genomic Medicine*,
https://doi.org/10.1007/978-3-030-22922-1_12

MECT1-MAML2 and *CRTC3-MAML2* fusions in mucoepidermoid carcinoma and *MYB and MYBL1* rearrangements in adenoid cystic carcinoma. Similarly, *TGFBR3-PLAG1* rearrangement is specific for myoepithelial carcinoma but is present only in the minority of cases. Molecular markers that are of diagnostic value and present in the vast majority of cases include *PRKD1* E710D mutation and *PRKD1/3* rearrangments in polymorphous adenocarcinoma/cribriform adenocarcinoma of salivary gland, *EWSR1-ATF1* in clear cell carcinoma, and *ETV6-NTRK3* in secretory carcinoma, which also provides a molecular target for Trk-inhibitors. In contrast, salivary duct carcinoma, a prototype of a high-grade salivary gland cancer, is characterized by a heterogeneous molecular background but a relatively high proportion of potentially targetable mutations. These include frequent *ERBB2*, *PIK3CA*, and *HRAS* alterations and less commonly gene fusions such as *EML4-ALK, NCOA4-RET*, and *ETV6-NTRK3*.

Mucoepidermoid Carcinoma

Phenotype

Mucoepidermoid carcinoma (MEC) is the most common epithelial malignancy of salivary glands. It is comprised of epidermoid, mucin-producing, and intermediate cells arranged in cystic and solid growth patterns at variable proportions. MEC is histologically graded as low-, intermediate-, or high-grade [1]. Immunohistochemistry (IHC) for p63 and p40 is typically positive in epidermoid and intermediate cells, while mucicarmine special stain highlights mucin-producing cells. MEC is negative for S-100 protein.

Genetics and Clinical Utility

MECT1-MAML2 fusion is the most common recurrent genetic alteration in MEC [2] being detected in 70–80% of low-grade, 65–70% of intermediate-grade, and about 50% of high-grade tumors [3]. *CRTC3-MAML2* fusion occurs in about 5% of cases and is found in relatively younger patients [4, 5]. The two *MAML2* fusions are mutually exclusive and are both characteristic of MEC. Despite the controversies in published reports, *MECT1-MAML2* is unlikely to be a feature of Warthin tumor [6, 7]. Detection of *MECT1-MAML2* or *CRTC3-MAML2* can be helpful in diagnostically challenging cases. These include "very" low-grade tumors with cystic appearance, sometimes being interpreted as "benign salivary cysts," high-grade tumors with predominantly solid growth and inconspicuous mucin-producing cells, and/or tumors displaying high-grade cytological features with the differential diagnosis of adenosquamous carcinoma or acantholytic squamous carcinoma. *MAML2* fusions do not portend any prognostic significance [8] (Table 12.1).

Table 12.1 Clinical utility of genetic alterations in salivary gland carcinomas

Tumor type	Gene(s) involved	Alteration type	Frequency	Method(s) of detection	Clinical utility	Potential therapeutic agents	Immunohistochemistry (clone)
Mucoepidermoid carcinoma	*MECT1-MAML2*	t(11;19)(q21;p13)	50–80%	FISH, molecular assay (RNA-based)	Diagnostic	n/a	n/a
	CRTC3-MAML2	t(11;15)(q21;q26)	~5%		Diagnostic		
Adenoid cystic carcinoma[a]	*MYB-NFIB*	t(6;9)(q22-23;p23-24)	~65%	FISH, molecular assay (RNA-based)	Diagnostic		MYB (EP769Y)
	MYB-RAD51B		Rare				
	MYB-TGFBR3		Rare				
	MYBL1-NFIB	t(8;9)(q13;p22)	~10%	FISH, molecular assay (RNA-based)	Diagnostic		
	MYBL1-RAD51B	t(8;14)(q13;q24)	Rare				
	MYBL1-YTHDF3	t(8;8)(q12;q13)	Rare				
	MYB	Gain/amplification	n/a				MYB (EP769Y)
	NOTCH1	Missense, truncating	5–33%	Molecular assay (DNA-based)	Therapeutic, prognostic	NOTCH-inhibitor	
	PIK3CA	E542, E545, H1047 missense	Rare		Therapeutic	PI3K-inhibitor	
	FGFR1	Amplification	Rare	FISH, molecular assay (DNA-based)		Dovitinib	
	Chromosome arm 4q12	Gain/amplification	11%		Prognostic	Axitinib	

(continued)

Table 12.1 (continued)

Tumor type	Gene(s) involved	Alteration type	Frequency	Method(s) of detection	Clinical utility	Potential therapeutic agents	Immunohistochemistry (clone)
Secretory carcinoma	*ETV6-NTRK3*	t(12;15)(p13;q25)	>95%	FISH, molecular assay (RNA-based)	Diagnostic, therapeutic	Entrectinib, larotrectinib (for cases with secondary resistance mutation G623R)	pan-Trk (EPR17341)
	ETV6-RET		1–2%		Diagnostic, therapeutic (?)	RET-inhibitor	
	ETV6-MET		1–2%		Diagnostic		
Clear cell carcinoma	*EWSR1-ATF1*	t(12;22)(q13;q12)	80–90%	FISH, molecular assay (RNA-based)	Diagnostic	n/a	n/a
Myoepithelial carcinoma	*TGFBR3-PLAG1*		15%	FISH, molecular assay (RNA-based)	Diagnostic		
	MSN-ALK	t(X;2)(q11;p23)	2–3%		Therapeutic (?)		
	EWSR1-ATF1	t(12;22)(q13;q12)	~5%		Diagnostic		
Polymorphous adenocarcinoma/cribriform adenocarcinoma of minor salivary glands	*PRKD1*	E710D missense	~75%/<10%	Molecular assay (DNA-based)	Diagnostic	n/a	n/a
	ARID1A-PRKD1	t(1;14)(p36;q12)	<10%/~75%	FISH, molecular assay (RNA-based)			
	DDX3X-PRKD1	t(X;14)(p11;q12)					
	PRKD2/3	Rearrangement					

Salivary duct carcinoma	*PIK3CA*	E542, E545, H1047 missense	~30%	Molecular assay (DNA-based)	Therapeutic	PI3K/mTOR inhibitors	
	ERBB2	Amplification	~30%	FISH, molecular assay (DNA-based)		Trastuzumab	HER2
		E777, S310 missense	Rare	Molecular assay (DNA-based)		Trastuzumab, lapatinib, neratinib, afatinib	
	BRAF	V600E	Rare			Vemurafenib, MEK-inhibitor	BRAF V600E (VE-1)
	AKT1	E17K	Rare			AKT-inhibitor	
	HRAS	Q61, G13 missense	~20%			tipifarnib (?)	
	PTEN	Deletion	Rare	FISH, molecular assay (DNA-based)		mTOR inhibitors	PTEN
	FGFR1	Amplification	Rare			Dovitinib	
	ETV6-NTRK3	t(12;15)(p13;q25)	Rare	FISH, molecular assay (RNA-based)		Entrectinib, larotrectinib (for cases with secondary resistance mutation G623R)	pan-Trk (EPR17341)
	EML4-ALK	inv(2)(p21;p23)	Rare			Crizotinib	ALK (D5F3)
	HNRNPH3-ALK	t(2;10)(p23;q21)	Rare				
	NCOA4-RET	inv(10)(q11;q11)	Rare			RET-inhibitor	
Intraductal carcinoma	*NCOA4-RET*	inv(10)(q11;q11)	35%	FISH, molecular assay (RNA-based)	Diagnostic and/or therapeutic (?)	RET-inhibitor	n/a
	TRIM27-RET	t(6;10)(p22;q11)	12%				
Epithelial-myoepithelial carcinoma	*HRAS*	Q61, G13 missense	25%	Molecular assay (DNA-based)	n/a	n/a	n/a

FISH fluorescence in situ hybridization, *n/a* non-applicable or not available

[a]*MYB* and *MYBL1* abnormalities include fusions and gene activation due to proximity of strong enhancer elements of *NFIB*, *RAD51B*, and *TGFBR3*

Adenoid Cystic Carcinoma

Phenotype

Adenoid cystic carcinoma (AdCC) is a biphasic salivary gland tumor typically forming cribriform, tubular, and/or solid growth patterns. Myoepithelial markers such as p63 and S-100 protein are positive in the peripheral tumor cell layer. MYB IHC is of limited value due to relatively low specificity and sensitivity [9].

Genetics and Clinical Utility

The majority of AdCC are characterized by a tumor-specific fusion *MYB-NFIB*, which leads to activation of *MYB* [10]. Less frequently, *MYB* can be activated by duplication or by juxtaposition to enhancer elements of other genes such as *NFIB, RASD51B*, and *TGFBR3* [11]. In the minority of cases *MYBL1*, a gene closely related to *MYB* is fused to *NFIB* and results in *MYBL1-NFIB* fusion, which has similar biological consequences to *MYB-NFIB* [12, 13]. *MYB* and *MYBL1* gene fusions can be used as reliable diagnostic makers in diagnostically difficult cases such as AdCC with (predominantly) solid growth pattern and/or high-grade features or in a limited biopsy material. The genetic alterations with therapeutic implications include *NOTCH1* mutations detected in up to 10% of primary and 33% of recurrent/metastatic tumors, and less commonly *FGFR1* and *PIK3CA* alterations [14, 15]. *NOTCH1* variants in AdCC were also associated with poor prognosis [16]. Cases harboring 4q12 gain/amplification tend to respond better to targeted therapy with tyrosine kinase inhibitor axitinib [17] (Tablc 12.1).

Secretory Carcinoma of Salivary Gland

Phenotype

Secretory carcinoma (SC, also known as mammary analogue secretory carcinoma "MASC") is a salivary gland carcinoma morphologically and genetically resembling SC of breast and is characterized by papillary cystic growth pattern, multivacuolated tumor cells, typically lacking true zymogen granules. SC is usually positive for S-100 protein and mammaglobin IHC.

Genetics and Clinical Utility

Similar to its breast counterpart, the vast majority of SCs harbor *ETV6-NTRK3* fusion [18], and rare cases are positive for *ETV6-RET* [19] or *ETV6-MET* rearrangements [20]. *ETV6* encodes an ETS family transcription factor, and *NTRK3* is a member of the neurotrophic tyrosine receptor kinase (NTRK) family and encodes tropomyosin receptor kinase protein TrkC. *ETV6-NTRK3* fusion gene is detected in multiple different tumors [21]. In SC of salivary glands, *ETV6-NTRK3* portends important diagnostic and therapeutic implications. These tumors were reported to respond to Trk-inhibitor entrectinib, and to larotrectinib in the presence of secondary resistance variant G623R [22, 23]. In salivary glands, the *ETV6-NTRK3* fusion is not entirely specific for SC and was also reported in rare cases of salivary duct carcinoma [24]. However, in the context of appropriate morphology and immunophenotype, *ETV6-NTRK3* would be diagnostic of SC. Detection of *ETV6* rearrangement alone by FISH may be sufficient to support the diagnosis of SC but confirmation of *NTRK3* as the fusion partner would be necessary for treatment purposes with Trk-inhibitors. IHC by pan-Trk monoclonal antibody EPR17341 is of limited value as not all *ETV6-NTRK3* rearranged cases will be IHC positive [25]. In the head and neck region aside from salivary glands, SC can also arise in the thyroid gland [26, 27] (Table 12.1).

Clear Cell Carcinoma

Phenotype

Clear cell carcinoma (CCC, also known as hyalinizing clear cell carcinoma, "HCCC") is a low-grade malignancy arising mostly in minor salivary glands and is characterized by sheets and cords of clear tumor cells and intersecting dense hyalinized stroma. IHC for p63 and p40 are usually positive, while other (myoepithelial) markers such as S-100 protein, calponin, and SMA are typically negative.

Genetics and Clinical Utility

More than 90% of CCC harbor *EWSR1-ATF1* rearrangement [28]. This fusion can also be found in a variety of mesenchymal tumors [29]. In primary salivary gland tumors, the *EWSR1-ATF1* fusion can be used to confirm the diagnosis of CCC. However, a minor proportion of myoepithelial carcinomas (MECA) can also have *EWSR1-ATF1* fusion [30]. In such cases, confirmation of the myoepithelial phenotype by S-100, calponin, and/or SMA IHC is required for the diagnosis of *EWSR1-ATF1*-positive MECA. Aside from salivary gland tumors, clear cell odontogenic carcinoma is another tumor type arising in head and neck harboring *EWSR1-ATF1* translocation in more than 60% of cases [31] (Table 12.1).

Myoepithelial Carcinoma

Phenotype

Myoepithelial carcinoma (MECA) is an infiltrative salivary gland tumor comprised entirely of myoepithelial cells and is the second most common type of carcinoma arising in pre-existing pleomorphic adenoma (PA). MECA typically stains for CK5/6 and is variably positive for at least one myoepithelial marker including S-100 protein, SOX10, calponin, SMA, and vimentin.

Genetics and Clinical Utility

PLAG1 or *HMGA2* rearrangements typically seen in PA [32, 33] can be also detected in MECA ex-PA [34] with the exception of *FGFR1-PLAG1*, which in addition to PA is present in 18% of MECA arising *de novo*. In contrast, the *TGFBR3-PLAG1* rearrangement was detected exclusively in 15% of MECA and may be diagnostic of this tumor type [30] (Table 12.1).

Polymorphous Adenocarcinoma and Cribriform Adenocarcinoma of Minor Salivary Gland

Phenotype

Polymorphous adenocarcinoma (PAC), formerly known as polymorphous low-grade adenocarcinoma ("PLGA") typically arises in minor salivary glands of palate and is a monophasic tumor, comprised of one cell type with characteristic ovoid vesicular nuclei (papillary thyroid carcinoma-like). PAC shows a spectrum of tubular, fascicular, cribriform, papillary, or solid architecture and is commonly strongly positive for S-100 protein, variably positive for p63, and negative for p40 IHC. Cribriform adenocarcinoma of (minor) salivary gland (CAMSG) likely represents a variant of PAC that arises at the base of tongue. It shows a distinct papillary glomeruloid and cribriform architecture and has more pronounced cleared nuclei and a greater propensity for lymph node for metastasis, thus a relatively more aggressive biology than a garden variety of PACs [1].

Genetics and Clinical Utility

Classic PAC in ~75% of cases is found with *PRKD1* E710D somatic mutations, and <10% of cases were found with *PRKD1/3* rearrangements. In contrast,

PRKD1/3 rearrangements including *ARID1A-PRKD1* and *DDX3X-PRKD1* gene fusions are detected in ~75% of CAMSG, while single-nucleotide variants in *PRKD1* are far less common [35–37]. *PRKD1* E710 mutations define a subset of PAC and may be used to improve the diagnosis in this entity (Table 12.1).

Salivary Duct Carcinoma

Phenotype

Salivary duct carcinoma (SDC) is an aggressive, high-grade malignancy and the most common salivary gland carcinoma arising in pre-existing PA. Apocrine cytology, comedo-type necrosis, and CK7 and androgen receptor (AR) immunopositivity are characteristic features of SDC.

Genetics and Clinical Utility

More than 70% of SDCs harbor actionable somatic mutations including *ERBB2* amplification and *PIK3CA* and *HRAS* hotspot mutations, each being detected in ~20–30% of cases. A variety of potentially druggable genetic alterations occur at ~3–10% frequencies including *ERRB2* S310F, *BRAF* V600E, *AKT1* E17K, *ETV6-NTRK3, NCOA4-RET, EML4-ALK,* and *FGFR1* amplification and *PTEN* deletion/mutation [15, 24, 38–42]. Patients with *ERBB2* amplification-positive SDC can respond to trastuzumab [43, 44], and tumors with mutations in PI3K pathway can respond to PI3K/Akt/mTOR pathway inhibition [38, 39]. Mutational profiling of SDC by massive parallel sequencing assays would be an appropriate molecular approach to ensure detection of various clinically pertinent somatic mutations as certain proportions of SDC patients may be eligible for "basket" clinical trials (Table 12.1).

Intraductal Carcinoma

Phenotype

Intraductal carcinoma (IC), formerly known as "low-grade cribriform cystadenocarcinoma" or "low-grade salivary duct carcinoma," is a rare salivary gland tumor, characterized by intraductal or intracystic epithelial tumor cell growth [1]. Although typically noninvasive, foci of invasion are not uncommon in IC [45].

Genetics and Clinical Utility

About 35% of IC were recently reported to harbor *NCOA4-RET* fusion [45, 46], and a single study reported *TRIM27-RET* fusion in 12% of IC cases displaying apocrine features [46] (Table 12.1).

References

1. El-Naggar AK, Chan JKC, Grandis JR, Takata T, Slootweg PJ. World Health Organization classification of head and neck tumours. 4th ed. Lyon: International Agency for Research on Cancer (IARC); 2017.
2. Tonon G, Modi S, Wu L, Kubo A, Coxon AB, Komiya T, O'Neil K, Stover K, El-Naggar A, Griffin JD, Kirsch IR, Kaye FJ. t (11; 19)(q21; p13) translocation in mucoepidermoid carcinoma creates a novel fusion product that disrupts a Notch signaling pathway. Nat Genet. 2003;33:208–13.
3. Seethala RR, Dacic S, Cieply K, Kelly LM, Nikiforova MN. A reappraisal of the MECT1/MAML2 translocation in salivary mucoepidermoid carcinomas. Am J Surg Pathol. 2010;34:1106–21.
4. Fehr A, Röser K, Heidorn K, Hallas C, Löning T, Bullerdiek J. A new type of MAML2 fusion in mucoepidermoid carcinoma. Genes Chromosomes Cancer. 2008;47:203–6.
5. Nakayama T, Miyabe S, Okabe M, Sakuma H, Ijichi K, Hasegawa Y, Nagatsuka H, Shimozato K, Inagaki H. Clinicopathological significance of the CRTC3–MAML2 fusion transcript in mucoepidermoid carcinoma. Mod Pathol. 2009;22:1575–81.
6. Fehr A, Röser K, Belge G, Löning T, Bullerdiek J. A closer look at Warthin tumors and the t (11; 19). Cancer Genet Cytogenet. 2008;180:135–9.
7. Ishibashi K, Ito Y, Masaki A, Fujii K, Beppu S, Sakakibara T, Takino H, Takase H, Ijichi K, Shimozato K, Inagaki H. Warthin-like mucoepidermoid carcinoma. Am J Surg Pathol. 2015;39:1479–87.
8. Saade RE, Bell D, Garcia J, Roberts D, Weber R. Role of CRTC1/MAML2 translocation in the prognosis and clinical outcomes of mucoepidermoid carcinoma. JAMA Otolaryngol Head Neck Surg. 2016;142:234–40.
9. Xu B, Drill E, Ho A, Ho A, Dunn L, Prieto-Granada CN, Chan T, Ganly I, Ghossein R, Katabi N. Predictors of outcome in adenoid cystic carcinoma of salivary glands. Am J Surg Pathol. 2017;41:1422–32.
10. Persson M, Andrén Y, Mark J, Horlings HM, Persson F, Stenman G. Recurrent fusion of MYB and NFIB transcription factor genes in carcinomas of the breast and head and neck. Proc Natl Acad Sci U S A. 2009;106:18740–4.
11. Andersson MK, Stenman G. The landscape of gene fusions and somatic mutations in salivary gland neoplasms–implications for diagnosis and therapy. Oral Oncol. 2016;57:63–9.
12. Brayer KJ, Frerich CA, Kang H, Ness SA. Recurrent fusions in MYB and MYBL1 define a common, transcription factor–driven oncogenic pathway in salivary gland adenoid cystic carcinoma. Cancer Discov. 2015;6:176–87.
13. Mitani Y, Liu B, Rao P, Borra V, Zafereo M, Weber RS, Kies MS, Lozano G, Futreal A, Caulin C, El-Naggar AK. Novel MYBL1 gene rearrangements with recurrent MYBL1-NFIB fusions in salivary adenoid cystic carcinomas lacking t (6; 9) translocations. Clin Cancer Res. 2015;22:725–33.
14. Ho AS, Kannan K, Roy DM, Morris LG, Ganly I, Katabi N, Ramaswami D, Walsh LA, Eng S, Huse JT, Zhang J, Dolgalev I, Huberman K, Heguy A, Viale A, Drobnjak M, Leversha MA, Rice CE, Singh B, Iyer NG, Leemans CR, Bloemena E, Ferris RL, Seethala RR, Gross BE,

Liang Y, Sinha R, Peng L, Raphael BJ, Turcan S, Gong Y, Schultz N, Kim S, Chiosea S, Shah JP, Sander C, Lee W, Chan TA. The mutational landscape of adenoid cystic carcinoma. Nat Genet. 2013;45:791–8.
15. Morris LG, Chandramohan R, West L, Zehir A, Chakravarty D, Pfister DG, Wong RJ, Lee NY, Sherman EJ, Baxi SS, Ganly I, Singh B, Shah JP, Shaha AR, Boyle JO, Patel SG, Roman BR, Barker CA, McBride SM, Chan TA, Dogan S, Hyman DM, Berger MF, Solit DB, Riaz N, Ho AL. The molecular landscape of recurrent and metastatic head and neck cancers: insights from a precision oncology sequencing platform. JAMA Oncol. 2017;3:244–55.
16. Ferrarotto R, Mitani Y, Diao L, Guijarro I, Wang J, Zweidler-McKay P, Bell D, William WN Jr, Glisson BS, Wick MJ, Kapoun AM, Patnaik A, Eckhardt G, Munster P, Faoro L, Dupont J, Lee JJ, Futreal A, El-Naggar AK, Heymach JV. Activating NOTCH1 mutations define a distinct subgroup of patients with adenoid cystic carcinoma who have poor prognosis, propensity to bone and liver metastasis, and potential responsiveness to Notch1 inhibitors. J Clin Oncol. 2016;35:352–60.
17. Ho A, Dunn L, Sherman E, Fury M, Baxi S, Chandramohan R, Dogan S, Morris L, Cullen G, Haque S, Sima CS, Ni A, Antonescu CR, Katabi N, Pfister DG. A phase II study of axitinib (AG-013736) in patients with incurable adenoid cystic carcinoma. Ann Oncol. 2016;27:1902–8.
18. Skálová A, Vanecek T, Sima R, Laco J, Weinreb I, Perez-Ordonez B, Starek I, Geierova M, Simpson RH, Passador-Santos F, Ryska A, Leivo I, Kinkor Z, Michal M. Mammary analogue secretory carcinoma of salivary glands, containing the ETV6-NTRK3 fusion gene: a hitherto undescribed salivary gland tumor entity. Am J Surg Pathol. 2010;34:599–608.
19. Skalova A, Vanecek T, Martinek P, Weinreb I, Stevens TM, Simpson RH, Hyrcza M, Rupp NJ, Baneckova M, Michal M Jr, Slouka D, Svoboda T, Metelkova A, Etebarian A, Pavelka J, Potts SJ, Christiansen J, Steiner P, Michal M. Molecular profiling of mammary analog secretory carcinoma revealed a subset of tumors harboring a novel ETV6-RET translocation. Am J Surg Pathol. 2018;42:234–46.
20. Rooper LM, Karantanos T, Ning Y, Bishop JA, Gordon SW, Kang H. Salivary secretory carcinoma with a Novel ETV6-MET fusion: expanding the molecular spectrum of a recently described entity. Am J Surg Pathol. 2018;42:1121–6.
21. Stransky N, Cerami E, Schalm S, Kim JL, Lengauer C. The landscape of kinase fusions in cancer. Nat Commun. 2014;5:4846.
22. Drilon A, Li G, Dogan S, Gounder M, Shen R, Arcila M, Wang L, Hyman D, Hechtman J, Wei G, Cam NR, Christiansen J, Luo D, Maneval EC, Bauer T, Patel M, Liu SV, Ou SH, Farago A, Shaw A, Shoemaker RF, Lim J, Hornby Z, Multani P, Ladanyi M, Berger M, Katabi N, Ghossein R, Ho AL. What hides behind the MASC: clinical response and acquired resistance to entrectinib after ETV6-NTRK3 identification in a mammary analogue secretory carcinoma (MASC). Ann Oncol. 2016;27:920–6.
23. Drilon A, Nagasubramanian R, Blake JF, Ku N, Tuch BB, Ebata K, Smith S, Lauriault V, Kolakowski GR, Brandhuber BJ, Larsen PD, Bouhana KS, Winski SL, Hamor R, Wu WI, Parker A, Morales TH, Sullivan FX, DeWolf WE, Wollenberg LA, Gordon PR, Douglas-Lindsay DN, Scaltriti M, Benayed R, Raj S, Hanusch B, Schram AM, Jonsson P, Berger MF, Hechtman JF, Taylor BS, Andrews S, Rothenberg SM, Hyman DM. A next-generation TRK kinase inhibitor overcomes acquired resistance to prior TRK kinase inhibition in patients with TRK fusion–positive solid tumors. Cancer Discov. 2017;7:963–72.
24. Dalin MG, Desrichard A, Katabi N, Makarov V, Walsh LA, Lee KW, Wang Q, Armenia J, West L, Dogan S, Wang L, Ramaswami D, Ho AL, Ganly I, Solit DB, Berger MF, Schultz ND, Reis-Filho JS, Chan TA, Morris LG. Comprehensive molecular characterization of salivary duct carcinoma reveals actionable targets and similarity to apocrine breast cancer. Clin Cancer Res. 2016;22:4623–33.
25. Hechtman JF, Benayed R, Hyman DM, Drilon A, Zehir A, Frosina D, Arcila ME, Dogan S, Klimstra DS, Ladanyi M, Jungbluth AA. Pan-Trk immunohistochemistry is an efficient and reliable screen for the detection of NTRK fusions. Am J Surg Pathol. 2017;41:1547–51.

26. Dogan S, Wang L, Ptashkin RN, Dawson RR, Shah JP, Sherman EJ, Michael Tuttle R, Fagin JA, Klimstra DS, Katabi N, Ghossein RA. Mammary analog secretory carcinoma of the thyroid gland: a primary thyroid adenocarcinoma harboring ETV6–NTRK3 fusion. Mod Pathol. 2016;29:985–95.
27. Reynolds S, Shaheen M, Olson G, Barry M, Wu J, Bocklage T. A case of primary mammary analog secretory carcinoma (MASC) of the thyroid masquerading as papillary thyroid carcinoma: potentially more than a one off. Head Neck Pathol. 2016;10:405–13.
28. Antonescu CR, Katabi N, Zhang L, Sung YS, Seethala RR, Jordan RC, Perez-Ordoñez B, Have C, Asa SL, Leong IT, Bradley G, Klieb H, Weinreb I. EWSR1-ATF1 fusion is a novel and consistent finding in hyalinizing clear-cell carcinoma of salivary gland. Genes Chromosomes Cancer. 2011;50:559–70.
29. Thway K, Fisher C. Tumors with EWSR1-CREB1 and EWSR1-ATF1 fusions: the current status. Am J Surg Pathol. 2012;36:e1–e11.
30. Dalin MG, Katabi N, Persson M, Lee K-W, Makarov V, Desrichard A, Walsh LA, West L, Nadeem Z, Ramaswami D, Havel JJ, Kuo F, Chadalavada K, Nanjangud GJ, Ganly I, Riaz N, Ho AL, Antonescu CR, Ghossein R, Stenman G, Chan TA, Morris LGT. Multi-dimensional genomic analysis of myoepithelial carcinoma identifies prevalent oncogenic gene fusions. Nat Commun. 2017;8:1197.
31. Bilodeau EA, Weinreb I, Antonescu CR, Zhang L, Dacic S, Muller S, Barker B, Seethala RR. Clear cell odontogenic carcinomas show EWSR1 rearrangements: a novel finding and a biological link to salivary clear cell carcinomas. Am J Surg Pathol. 2013;37:1001–5.
32. Schoenmakers EF, Wanschura S, Mols R, Bullerdiek J, Van den Berghe H, Van de Ven WJ. Recurrent rearrangements in the high mobility group protein gene, HMGI-C, in benign mesenchymal tumours. Nat Genet. 1995;10:436–44.
33. Kas K, Voz ML, Röijer E, Åström A-K, Meyen E, Stenman G, Van de Ven WJ. Promoter swapping between the genes for a novel zinc finger protein and β-catenin in pleiomorphic adenomas with t(3; 8)(p21; q12) translocations. Nat Genet. 1997;15:170–4.
34. Katabi N, Ghossein R, Ho A, Dogan S, Zhang L, Sung Y-S, Antonescu CR. Consistent PLAG1 and HMGA2 abnormalities distinguish carcinoma ex-pleomorphic adenoma from its de novo counterparts. Hum Pathol. 2015;46:26–33.
35. Weinreb I, Piscuoglio S, Martelotto LG, Waggott D, Ng CK, Perez-Ordonez B, Harding NJ, Alfaro J, Chu KC, Viale A, Fusco N, da Cruz Paula A, Marchio C, Sakr RA, Lim R, Thompson LD, Chiosea SI, Seethala RR, Skalova A, Stelow EB, Fonseca I, Assaad A, How C, Wang J, de Borja R, Chan-Seng-Yue M, Howlett CJ, Nichols AC, Wen YH, Katabi N, Buchner N, Mullen L, Kislinger T, Wouters BG, Liu FF, Norton L, McPherson JD, Rubin BP, Clarke BA, Weigelt B, Boutros PC, Reis-Filho JS. Hotspot activating PRKD1 somatic mutations in polymorphous low-grade adenocarcinomas of the salivary glands. Nat Genet. 2014;46:1166–669.
36. Weinreb I, Zhang L, Tirunagari LM, Sung YS, Chen CL, Perez-Ordonez B, Clarke BA, Skalova A, Chiosea SI, Seethala RR, Waggott D, Boutros PC, How C, Liu FF, Irish JC, Goldstein DP, Gilbert R, Ud Din N, Assaad A, Hornick JL, Thompson LD. Antonescu CR: Novel PRKD gene rearrangements and variant fusions in cribriform adenocarcinoma of salivary gland origin. Genes Chromosomes Cancer. 2014;53:845–56.
37. Seethala RR, Stenman G. Update from the 4th Edition of the World Health Organization classification of head and neck tumours: tumors of the salivary gland. Head Neck Pathol. 2017;11:55–67.
38. Piha-Paul SA, Cohen PR, Kurzrock R. Salivary duct carcinoma: targeting the phosphatidylinositol 3-kinase pathway by blocking mammalian target of rapamycin with temsirolimus. J Clin Oncol. 2011;29:e727–e30.
39. Nardi V, Sadow PM, Juric D, Zhao D, Cosper AK, Bergethon K, Scialabba VL, Batten JM, Borger DR, Iafrate AJ, Heist RS, Lawrence DP, Flaherty KT, Bendell JC, Deschler D, Li Y, Wirth LJ, Dias-Santagata D. Detection of novel actionable genetic changes in salivary duct carcinoma helps direct patient treatment. Clin Cancer Res. 2013;19:480–90.

40. Chiosea SI, Williams L, Griffith CC, Thompson LD, Weinreb I, Bauman JE, Luvison A, Roy S, Seethala RR, Nikiforova MN. Molecular characterization of apocrine salivary duct carcinoma. Am J Surg Pathol. 2015;39:744–52.
41. Wang K, Russell JS, McDermott JD, Elvin JA, Khaira D, Johnson A, Jennings TA, Ali SM, Murray M, Marshall C, Oldham DS, Washburn D, Wong SJ, Chmielecki J, Yelensky R, Lipson D, Miller VA, Stephens PJ, Serracino HS, Ross JS, Bowles DW. Profiling of 149 salivary duct carcinomas, carcinoma ex pleomorphic adenomas, and adenocarcinomas, not otherwise specified reveals actionable genomic alterations. Clin Cancer Res. 2016;22:6061–8.
42. Dogan S, Ng CKY, Xu B, Kumar R, Wang LU, Edelweiss M, Scott SN, Zehir A, Drilon A, Morris LG, Lee NY, Antonescu CR, Ho A, Katabi N, Berger MF, Reis-Filho JS. The repertoire of genetic alterations in salivary duct carcinoma including a novel HNRNPH3-ALK rearrangement. Hum Pathol. 2019;88:66–77. https://doi.org/10.1016/j.humpath.2019.03.004. Epub 2019.
43. Nabili V, Tan JW, Bhuta S, Sercarz JA, Head CS. Salivary duct carcinoma: a clinical and histologic review with implications for trastuzumab therapy. Head Neck. 2007;29:907–12.
44. Nashed M, Casasola R. Biological therapy of salivary duct carcinoma. J Laryngol Otol. 2009;123:250–2.
45. Weinreb I, Bishop JA, Chiosea SI, Seethala RR, Perez-Ordonez B, Zhang L, Sung Y-S, Chen CL, Assaad A, Oliai BR, Antonescu CR. Recurrent RET gene rearrangements in intraductal carcinomas of salivary gland. Am J Surg Pathol. 2018;42:442–52.
46. Skálová A, Vanecek T, Uro-Coste E, Bishop JA, Weinreb I, Thompson LD, Schiavo-Lena M, Laco J, Badoual C, Santana TC, Ptáková N, Baněčkova M, Miesbauerová M, Michal M. Molecular profiling of salivary gland intraductal carcinoma revealed a subset of tumors harboring NCOA4-RET and novel TRIM27-RET fusions: a report of 17 cases. Am J Surg Pathol. 2018;42:1445–55.

Chapter 13
Sinonasal Carcinomas

Snjezana Dogan

Key Points

- *NUTM1* rearrangement in NUT carcinoma and *SMARCB1* deletion/mutation in SMARCB1-deficient carcinoma are genetic hallmarks of these entities, and both may indicate eligibility for targeted therapy.
- Hotspot mutations in *IDH2* R172 are detected in the vast majority of SNUC and sinonasal large cell neuroendocrine carcinoma (LCNEC), and in the minority of high-grade sinonasal carcinomas with glandular/acinar differentiation.
- IDH2 R172S/T (11C8B1) IHC can be used as an adjunct diagnostic marker of SNUC.

Key Online Resources

- El-Naggar AK, Chan JKC, Grandis JR, Takata T, Slootweg PJ, editors. WHO classification of head and neck tumours, 4th ed.

Introduction

Sinonasal carcinomas (SNC) comprise a diverse morphologic and genetic spectrum of tumors. NUT carcinoma, SMARCB1-deficient SNC, and sinonasal undifferentiated carcinoma (SNUC) are rare and biologically aggressive, and, although often

S. Dogan (✉)
Department of Pathology, Memorial Sloan Kettering Cancer Center, New York, NY, USA
e-mail: dogans@mskcc.org

L. J. Tafe, M. E. Arcila (eds.), *Genomic Medicine*,
https://doi.org/10.1007/978-3-030-22922-1_13

histologically remarkably similar, these three entities are genetically very distinct. An accurate molecular diagnosis portends a diagnostic value and can identify patients eligible for clinical trials with targeted therapies. Immunohistochemistry (IHC) for NUT and SMARCB1 (INI1) are useful surrogate diagnostic markers in all NUT and SMARCB1-deficient SNC, respectively. IDH2 R172S/T (11C8B1) IHC is a useful adjunct diagnostic marker in at least 70% SNUC.

NUT Carcinoma

Phenotype

NUT carcinoma (NC, also known as NUT midline carcinoma) is comprised of completely undifferentiated tumor cells with or without foci of mature squamous epithelium. About 35% cases occur in the head and neck and 65% of these arise in the sinonasal tract [1–4]. Most cases are positive for CK5/6, p63, and p40, and all cases are positive for NUT IHC.

Genetics and Clinical Utility

Molecular signature of NC is *NUTM1* fusion gene, most frequently *BRD4-NUTM1* and less commonly *BRD3-NUTM1*, while *NSD3-NUTM1* and other *NUTM1* variants are rare. *BRD4-NUT* fusion protein decreases transcription and blocks the differentiation of NC cells and thus maintains their proliferation and malignant growth through a potent chromatin-modifying mechanism [5, 6]. Detection of *NUTM1* rearrangement is both diagnostic and therapeutic. NUT immunohistochemistry is highly specific for this entity, and either detection of *NUTM1* rearrangement by FISH or molecular assay, or positive NUT IHC is sufficient for diagnosis and eligibility for targeted therapies. The latter includes bromodomain inhibitors and histone deacetylase inhibitors, which rendered promising results in NC patients [7] (Table 13.1).

SMARCB1-Deficient Sinonasal Carcinoma

Phenotype

SMARCB1-deficient SNC is most commonly comprised of undifferentiated tumor cells with or without rhabdoid features and in all cases there is a characteristic nuclear loss of SMARCB1 (INI1) protein [8, 9]. Although most SMARCB1-deficient SNC show basaloid morphology closely resembling

Table 13.1 Sinonasal carcinomas with recurrent genetic alterations

Tumor type	Gene(s) involved	Alteration type	Frequency	Method(s) of detection	Clinical utility	Potential therapeutic agents	Immunohistochemistry (clone)	Other tumors/sites with the same genetic alteration
NUT carcinoma	*BRD4-NUTM1*	t(15;19) (q14; p13)	70%	FISH, molecular assay (RNA-based)	Diagnostic, therapeutic	Bromo-domain inhibitors, histone deacetylase inhibitors	NUT (C52)	Adrenal gland, pancreas, bladder, lung, brain, kidney, soft tissue
	BRD3-NUTM1	t(9;15) (q34;q14)	6%					
	NSD3-NUTM1	t(8;15) (p12;q15)	rare					
	NUTM1 variants		rare	FISH				
SMARCB1-deficient sinonasal carcinoma	*SMARCB1*	Deletion	~80%	FISH, molecular assay (DNA-based)	Diagnostic, therapeutic	EZH2 inhibitors	INI1	Malignant rhabdoid tumor, rhabdoid tumor of the kidney, atypical teratoid rhabdoid tumor, renal medullary carcinoma, epithelioid sarcoma
	SMARCB1	Truncating mutation with LOH	~10%	Molecular assay (DNA-based)				
Sinonasal undifferentiated carcinoma	*IDH2*	R172 missense	>80%	Molecular assay (DNA-based)	Adjunct diagnostic, therapeutic (?)	IDH2 inhibitors	IDH2 R172S/T (11C8B1)	Intrahepatic cholangio-carcinoma, chondrosarcoma, angioimmunoblastic T-cell lymphoma, acute myeloid leukemia, solid papillary carcinoma with reverse polarity of the breast
Sinonasal large cell neuroendocrine carcinoma	*IDH2*	R172 missense	>70%					

(continued)

Table 13.1 (continued)

Tumor type	Gene(s) involved	Alteration type	Frequency	Method(s) of detection	Clinical utility	Potential therapeutic agents	Immunohistochemistry (clone)	Other tumors/sites with the same genetic alteration
Sinonasal non-intestinal-type adenocarcinoma	*ETV6-RET*		?	FISH, molecular assay (RNA-based)	Therapeutic (?)	RET inhibitors	n/a	Secretory carcinoma of salivary gland (rare)
Sinonasal intestinal-type adenocarcinoma	*KRAS*	G12, G13, G61 missense	6–40%	Molecular assay (DNA-based)	n/a	n/a	n/a	Adenocarcinomas of the lung, colon, pancreas, ovary (and others)
Sinonasal squamous cell carcinoma arising in oncocytic papilloma	*KRAS*	G12V, G12D missense	100%[a]		n/a	n/a	n/a	
Sinonasal squamous cell carcinoma arising in inverted papilloma	*EGFR*	Exon 20 insertion	~80%	Molecular assay (DNA-based)	(?)	(?)	n/a	Lung adenocarcinoma

FISH fluorescence *in situ* hybridization, *LOH* loss of heterozygosity, *n/a* non-applicable or not available

[a]Based on limited number of published cases

non-keratinizing squamous cell carcinoma, they can be histologically diverse and rather represent a morphologic and immunophenotypic spectrum of carcinomas arising in this location [10–12]. Pathologists should exercise caution and consider SMARCB1 (INI1) IHC in any unclassified high-grade SNC with or without rhabdoid cells.

Genetics and Clinical Utility

Loss of nuclear SMARCB1 (INI1) protein is the hallmark of SMARCB1-deficient SNC and in ~80% cases is the result of homozygous or heterozygous *SMARCB1* deletion, while in minor proportion of cases, *SMARCB1* can appear intact by FISH [10, 12]. Molecular profiling showed that in ~10%, a loss of INI1 protein could be due to pathogenic (truncating) *SMARCB1* mutation associated with loss of heterozygosity (LOH) [12]. Detection of *SMARCB1* abnormalities in SMARCB1-deficient SNC have both diagnostic and therapeutic value as these tumors may be amenable to targeted therapy with EZH2 inhibitor (tazemetostat) [13] (Table 13.1).

Sinonasal Undifferentiated Carcinoma and Large Cell Neuroendocrine Carcinoma

Phenotype

Sinonasal undifferentiated carcinoma (SNUC) is composed of entirely undifferentiated tumor cells and shows no evidence of squamous, glandular, or neuroendocrine differentiation. SNUC is typically positive for cytokeratin and negative for NUT IHC and has retained nuclear SMARCB1 (INI1) protein, and >70% are positive for IDH2 IHC (11C8B1) [14]. Large cell neuroendocrine carcinoma (LCNEC), is very rare and can be morphologically very similar to SNUC with the exception of the presence of substantial neuroendocrine differentiation [4]. LCNEC is also frequently positive for IDH2 IHC (11C8B1) [14].

Genetics and Clinical Utility

More than 80% of SNUC, >70% LCNEC, and a minor proportion of high-grade SNC with glandular/acinar differentiation harbor oncogenic *IDH2* R172 hotspot mutations [11, 15]. R172S and R172T are the most common variants (70%) [11, 15], and IDH2 (11C8B1) IHC can be used as a surrogate marker for *IDH2* R172S and R172T variant detection [14]. Given the virtual absence of *IDH2* R172, mutations in non-epithelial, i.e., other "small round cell tumors" in the sinonasal tract, 11C8B1 IHC can be used as an adjunct diagnostic marker of SNUC in tumors lacking any evidence of glandular/acinar or neuroendocrine differentiation [14]. In view of the rarity of *IDH2* R172 hotspot alterations in human tumors in general, positive 11C8B1 IHC in a metastasis/unknown primary high-grade/undifferentiated carcinoma would favor sinonasal primary. Similar to hematopoietic malignancies with the same genetic background, *IDH2*-mutated SNC may eventually become amenable to treatment with IDH2 inhibitors [16] (Table 13.1).

Sinonasal Squamous Cell Carcinomas and Adenocarcinomas with Genetic Signatures

Among sinonasal squamous cell carcinomas (SCC), highly recurrent somatic mutations include *EGFR* exon 20 insertions present in the vast majority of sinonasal SCC arising in inverted papilloma [17] and *KRAS* hotspot mutations in SCC arising in oncocytic papilloma [18]. Similar to their colonic counterpart, sinonasal intestinal-type adenocarcinomas (ITAC) can harbor *KRAS* variants [4, 19], while rare cases of sinonasal non-ITAC were reported to harbor *ETV6-RET* fusion [20] (Table 13.1). Sinonasal carcinomas of minor salivary gland origin will share the same genetic signature with their major salivary gland counterparts. (See Chap. 12).

References

1. French CA. NUT midline carcinoma. Cancer Genet Cytogenet. 2010;203:16–20.
2. Bishop JA, Westra WH. NUT midline carcinomas of the sinonasal tract. Am J Surg Pathol. 2012;36:1216–21.
3. Solomon LW, Magliocca KR, Cohen C, Müller S. Retrospective analysis of nuclear protein in testis (NUT) midline carcinoma in the upper aerodigestive tract and mediastinum. Oral Surg Oral Med Oral Pathol Oral Radiol. 2015;119:213–20.
4. El-Naggar AK, Chan JKC, Grandis JR, Takata T, Slootweg PJ. World Health Organization classification of head and neck tumours. 4th ed. Lyon: International Agency for Research on Cancer (IARC); 2017.
5. French CA, Miyoshi I, Kubonishi I, Grier HE, Perez-Atayde AR, Fletcher JA. BRD4-NUT fusion oncogene: a novel mechanism in aggressive carcinoma. Cancer Res. 2003;63:304–7.
6. French CA. Pathogenesis of NUT midline carcinoma. Annu Rev Pathol. 2012;7:247–65.
7. Stathis A, Zucca E, Bekradda M, Gomez-Roca C, Delord J-P, Rouge TLM, Uro-Coste E, de Braud F, Pelosi G, French CA. Clinical response of carcinomas harboring the BRD4-NUT oncoprotein to the targeted bromodomain inhibitor OTX015/MK-8628. Cancer Discov. 2016;6:492–500.
8. Agaimy A, Koch M, Lell M, Semrau S, Dudek W, Wachter DL, Knöll A, Iro H, Haller F, Hartmann A. SMARCB1 (INI1)-deficient sinonasal basaloid carcinoma: a novel member of the expanding family of SMARCB1-deficient neoplasms. Am J Surg Pathol. 2014;38:1274–81.
9. Bishop JA, Antonescu CR, Westra WH. SMARCB1 (INI-1) deficient carcinomas of the sinonasal tract. Am J Surg Pathol. 2014;38:1282–9.

10. Agaimy A, Hartmann A, Antonescu CR, Chiosea SI, El-Mofty SK, Geddert H, Iro H, Lewis JS, Märkl B, Mills SE, Reiner MO, Robertson T, Sandison A, Semrau S, Simpson RH, Stelow E, Westra WH, Bishop JA. SMARCB1 (INI-1)-deficient sinonasal carcinoma. Am J Surg Pathol. 2017;41:458–71.
11. Dogan S, Chute DJ, Xu B, Ptashkin RN, Chandramohan R, Casanova-Murphy J, Nafa K, Bishop JA, Chiosea SI, Stelow EB, Ganly I, Pfister DG, Katabi N, Ghossein RA, Berger MF. Frequent IDH2 R172 mutations in undifferentiated and poorly differentiated sinonasal carcinomas. J Pathol. 2017;242:400–8.
12. Cotzia P, Ptashkin R, Gounder M, Pfister DG, Berger MF, Ladanyi M, Ghossein RA, Antonescu CR, Dogan S. Genetic and histologic spectrum of SMARCB1-deficient carcinomas of the head and neck including sinonasal tract, thyroid and skin. Lab Invest. 2018;98:474–5.
13. Knutson SK, Warholic NM, Wigle TJ, Klaus CR, Allain CJ, Raimondi A, Scott MP, Chesworth R, Moyer MP, Copeland RA, Richon VM, Pollock RM, Kuntz KW, Keilhack H. Durable tumor regression in genetically altered malignant rhabdoid tumors by inhibition of methyltransferase EZH2. Proc Natl Acad Sci U S A. 2013;110:7922–7.
14. Dogan S, Frosina D, Fayad M, de Oliveira TB, Alemar B, Rosenblum M, Tang LH, Hameed M, Xu B, Ghossein RA, Chute DK, Wiegelt B, Jungbluth AA. The role of a monoclonal antibody 11C8B1 as a diagnostic marker of IDH2-mutated sinonasal undifferentiated carcinoma. Mod Pathol. 2019;32(2):205–15. https://doi.org/10.1038/s41379-018-0126-3.
15. Jo VY, Chau NG, Hornick JL, Krane JF, Sholl LM. Recurrent IDH2 R172X mutations in sinonasal undifferentiated carcinoma. Mod Pathol. 2017;30:650–9.
16. Stein EM, DiNardo CD, Pollyea DA, Fathi AT, Roboz GJ, Altman JK, Stone RM, DeAngelo DJ, Levine RL, Flinn IW, Kantarjian HM, Collins R, Patel MR, Frankel AE, Stein A, Sekeres MA, Swords RT, Medeiros BC, Willekens C, Vyas P, Tosolini A, Xu Q, Knight RD, Yen KE, Agresta S, de Botton S, Tallman MS. Enasidenib in mutant IDH2 relapsed or refractory acute myeloid leukemia. Blood. 2017;130:722–31.
17. Udager AM, Rolland DC, McHugh JB, Betz BL, Murga-Zamalloa C, Carey TE, Marentette LJ, Hermsen MA, DuRoss KE, Lim MS, Elenitoba-Johnson KSJ, Brown NA. High frequency targetable EGFR mutations in sinonasal squamous cell carcinomas arising from inverted sinonasal papilloma. Cancer Res. 2015;75:2600–6.
18. Udager AM, McHugh JB, Betz BL, Montone KT, Livolsi VA, Seethala RR, Yakirevich E, Iwenofu OH, Perez-Ordonez B, DuRoss KE, Weigelin HC, Lim MS, Elenitoba-Johnson KSJ, Brown NA. Activating KRAS mutations are characteristic of oncocytic sinonasal papilloma and associated sinonasal squamous cell carcinoma. J Pathol. 2016;239:394–8.
19. Saber AT, Nielsen LR, Dictor M, Hagmar L, Mikoczy Z, Wallin H. K-ras mutations in sinonasal adenocarcinomas in patients occupationally exposed to wood or leather dust. Cancer Lett. 1998;126:59–65.
20. Andreasen S, Kiss K, Melchior LC, Laco J. The ETV6-RET gene fusion is found in ETV6-rearranged low-grade sinonasal adenocarcinoma without NTRK3 involvement. Am J Surg Pathol. 2018;42:985–8.

Part III
Applications in Hematopathology

Chapter 14
Acute Myeloid Neoplasms

Eric Y. Loo

> **Key Points**
> - While acute myeloid leukemia is identifiable by morphologic assessment alone, characterization of the underlying genetic abnormalities is needed for definitive subclassification in most cases.
> - Current standard of care includes evaluating for selected gene sequence abnormalities (e.g., *FLT3*, *NPM1*, *CEBPA*, *KIT*, and others), in addition to traditional chromosome analysis and FISH studies.
> - Karyotype still represents the single most important prognostic factor in predicting remission rates, relapse risks, and overall survival outcomes in acute myeloid leukemia.
> - 40–50% of patients with de novo acute myeloid leukemia have a normal karyotype, and molecular profiling is quickly helping to better stratify this cohort with heterogeneous outcomes.

> **Key Online Resources**
> - National Comprehensive Cancer Network, Acute Myeloid Leukemia Guidelines: https://www.nccn.org/professionals/physician_gls/pdf/aml.pdf
> - National Cancer Institute, Adult Acute Myeloid Leukemia Treatment: https://www.cancer.gove/types/leukemia/hp/adult-aml-treatment-pdq

E. Y. Loo (✉)
Geisel School of Medicine at Dartmouth, Hanover, NH, USA

Department of Pathology and Laboratory Medicine, Dartmouth-Hitchcock Medical Center, Lebanon, NH, USA
e-mail: Eric.Y.Loo@Hitchcock.org

L. J. Tafe, M. E. Arcila (eds.), *Genomic Medicine*,
https://doi.org/10.1007/978-3-030-22922-1_14

Introduction

Acute myeloid leukemia (AML) represents a heterogeneous group of disease, but all subtypes are characterized by clonal proliferations of immature myeloid hematopoietic precursor cells. The first widely accepted subclassification system for AML, developed by the French-American-British (FAB) working group in 1972, was based solely on morphologic findings. This classification system was unfortunately found to lack clinical utility as the proposed disease subtypes were largely unable to provide meaningful prognostic stratification. While the terminology from the FAB classification system still persists in present-day medical vernacular, this system is considered obsolete.

Janet Rowley described the t(8;21)(q22;q22.1) translocation in 1973; this was the first recurrent genetic aberrancy reported in association with AML. As the cytogenetic profile for this disease was slowly elucidated over subsequent decades, a diagnostic paradigm shift occurred in the 2001 third edition of the World Health Organization (WHO) classification with inclusion of genetic abnormalities into the diagnostic algorithms for AML diagnosis. The importance of underlying cytogenetic aberrancies was recognized, as was secondary-AML arising from lower-grade myeloid neoplasms, prior cytotoxic therapies for unrelated malignancy, or disease arising in a background of multilineage dysplasia. These categories were expanded and refined further in 2008 and 2016. The 2016 WHO classification system is the most current AML classification system, and the use of prior less-specific terminology is discouraged [1].

The ability to risk-stratify cases of primary-AML was somewhat limited in first iteration of the WHO classification system. Recognized genetic defects were limited to chromosomal translocations at the time, and conventional cytogenetic testing modalities fail to detect aberrancies in a significant subset of cases (a disease subgroup often referred to as "normal karyotype AML"). The 2008 WHO revision broadened the scope of genetics in AML diagnosis, accepting that multiple types of genetic lesions could cooperate to create a leukemic process. More recent molecular sequencing studies have further characterized the genetic landscape of AML and have helped to close the knowledge gap. It is now understood that numerous cooperating mutations occur in AML [2]. While molecular profiling analysis is initially focused on normal karyotype AML, somatic sequence mutations appear to demonstrate prognostic importance across other genetic AML subtypes, and sequencing analysis appears to be indicated in all cases of AML [2, 3]. At present, most cases of primary/de novo AML can be genetically categorized, and several specific subtypes of AML can be diagnosed on the basis of underlying genetics without regard to blast cell count. The subgroup of AML, not otherwise specified, which has no distinct clinical, immunophenotypic, or genetic features is expected to continue to shrink as knowledge of AML pathogenesis accumulates (Fig. 14.1).

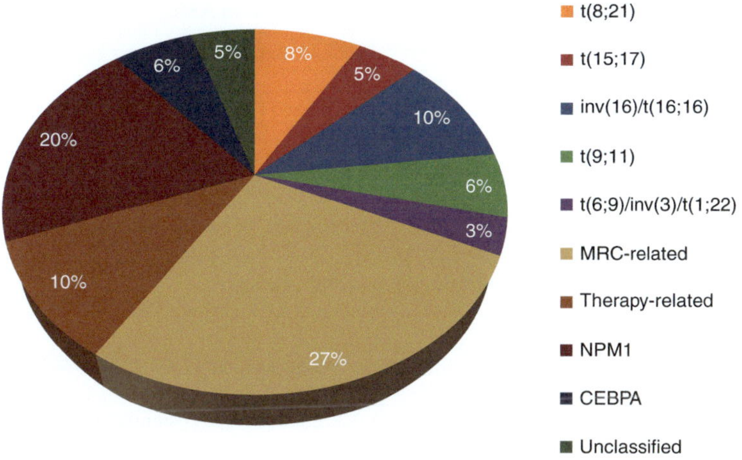

Fig. 14.1 General breakdown of AML subtypes by 2016 WHO classification

A Standard Genetic Workup

The specimen for evaluation (peripheral blood or bone marrow) should be obtained before initiation of any definitive therapy. At present, a standard workup for newly diagnosed AML should include:

- Complete karyotype and/or FISH analysis for subtype defining aberrancies
- *NPM1*, *CEBPA*, *RUNX1*, and *FLT3* somatic sequence mutation analysis
- *IDH1/2* mutation analysis for potential targeted therapy in relapsed/refractory disease
- *KIT* mutation analysis in all cases with t(8;21)(q22;q22.1) RUNX1-RUNX1T1 and AML with inv(16)(p13.1q22) or t(16;16)(p13.1;q22) CBFB-MYH11

Although detection of recurrent cytogenetic aberrancies generally provides the most significant prognostic information at diagnosis, nearly half of all adult AML cases will show no detectable abnormalities by karyotype. Molecular genetic analysis is quickly filling the knowledge gap. Many other gene mutations are also known to have prognostic significance or relevance for clinical trials in AML and may be readily evaluable by targeted next-generation sequencing gene mutation panels (a selection of these are found in Table 14.1).

AML with Recurrent Genetic Aberrancies

This category of acute myeloid leukemia includes entities that are defined by both by balanced chromosomal rearrangements and by specific gene sequence

Table 14.1 Genes with recurrent somatic sequence mutations in AML

Mutated gene	Prognostic significance in AML
ASXL1	Associated with worse DFS, EFS, RFS, and OS compared to cases with wt-*ASXL1*
CEBPA, biallelic	WHO AML subtype defining Better DFS, EFS, and OS compared to cases with single mutation or wt-CEBPA
DNMT3A	Conflicting reports regarding prognostic significance Concurrent mutation with mut-*NPM1* and *FLT3*-ITD appears to worsen EFS and OS
IDH1/2	Conflicting reports regarding prognostic significance Mut-*IDH1/2* qualifies for FDA-approved IDH inhibitor therapy in relapsed or refractory AML
FLT3-ITD	Significantly worse OS compared to those without *FLT3*-ITD, especially in persons <60 years old If present in the setting of AML with mutated *NPM1*, significantly worse EFS, RFS, DFS, and OS compared to cases with *NPM1* mutation alone 2017 ELN guidelines recognize increasingly worse RR and OS with increasing *FLT*-ITD mutant allele burden; ELN guidelines define *FLT3*-ITD^{low} as <0.5 and *FLT3*-ITD^{high} as ≥0.5 *FLT3*-ITD (and tyrosine kinase domain mutation) qualify for FDA-approved targeted therapy with Midostaurin
KIT	In t(8;21) AML, associated with shorter DFS, RFS, EFS, and OS compared to cases with wt-*KIT*
	In the setting of inv(16)/t(16;16) AML, no difference in EFS, RFS, PRS, or OS compared to cases with wt-*KIT* Some single studies report shorter RFS and OS compared to cases with wt-*KIT*
KMT2A-PTD	Among younger patients (<60 years), shorter OS than for patients without *KMT2A*-PTD
NPM1	WHO AML subtype defining In isolation, generally associated with good response to induction chemotherapy and a favorable prognosis If concurrent with *FLT3-ITD*, then EFS, RFS, DFS, and OS are significantly worsened
RUNX1	Potentially indicative of a WHO AML provisional subtype (in the absence of other subtype defining abnormalities) Shorter DFS, RFS, EFS, and OS compared to cases with wt-*RUNX1*
TET2	Conflicting reports regarding prognostic significance; some reports indicate no significant differences, whereas others report context-dependent worse EFS and OS
TP53, mut or loss	In the setting of a complex karyotype (≥3 abnormalities), associated with shorter RFS, EFS, and OS than for patients with wt-*TP53*
	In the setting of a complex karyotype (≥5 abnormalities), no significant difference in DFS or OS
	When associated with abnormalities of chromosomes, 5, 7, or 17, and/or a complex karyotype (≥5 abnormalities), associated with shorter OS than for patients with wt-*TP53*
WT1	Associated with worse RR and OS compared to cases with wt-*WT1* In the setting of pediatric AML, associated with worse treatment-resistant disease, EFS, and OS

DFS disease-free survival, *EFS* event-free survival, *ELN* European LeukemiaNet, *mut* mutant, *OS* overall survival, *PFS* progression-free survival, *PTD* partial tandem duplication, *RFS* relapse-free survival, *RR* risk of relapse, *wt* wild type mutations. The 2016 WHO classification system recognizes eight subtypes defining balanced chromosomal gene fusions and three subtypes related to specific somatic gene sequence mutations, each with distinctive clinicopathologic features and prognostic associations. Many other balanced gene rearrangements are known to recur in AML [4], but these are very rare and are not currently recognized to represent distinct diagnostic entities.

The diagnosis of AML typically requires demonstrating a myeloblast population that represents at least 20% of the peripheral blood or bone marrow cellularity. However, the WHO permits assigning an AML diagnosis without regard to blast count for three entities, based on the strength of associated underlying cytogenetic aberrancies. These entities are the two core binding factor AMLs associated with t(8;21) and inv(16)/t(16;16) and acute promyelocytic leukemia with *PML-RARA* fusion. The minimum threshold of 20% myeloblasts is still required for an AML diagnosis with the remaining recurrent genetic aberrancies.

Core Binding Factor AML *(Tables 14.2 and 14.3)*

AML with t(8;21)(q22;q22.1) results in the fusion of *RUNX1* (also known as core binding factor-α) and *RUNX1T1*, often presenting with large myeloblasts that have abundant basophilic cytoplasm, azurophilic granules, few large pseudo-Chédiak-Higashi granules, and perinuclear hoffs. AML with inv(16)(p13q22) or t(16;16)(p13;q22) *CBFB-MYH11* disrupts the beta subunit of core binding factor, often presenting with myelomonocytic blasts and abnormal background eosinophils, usually with large basophilic colored granules. These translocations disrupt the function of core binding factor, a crucial heterodimeric transcription factor that helps control stem cell development and normal hematopoiesis. Together these represent about 12–15% of acute myeloid leukemia cases in adults and are commonly referred to as the core binding factor (CBF) leukemias.

Table 14.2 General features of AML with t(8;21)(q22;q22.1)

Defining aberrancy	t(8;21)(q22;q22.1)
Genes involved	*RUNX1-RUNX1T1*
Frequency in adult AML	1–5%
Myeloblast requirement	Does not require 20% blast threshold for diagnosis of AML
Prognostic implication	Generally favorable
Prognostic modifier(s)	*KIT* gene mutation (20–30% of cases): higher risk of relapse and worse overall survival
2° cytogenetic abnormalities	Found in >70% of cases; more frequent findings include loss of a sex chromosome or del(9q)
Diagnostic testing	Karyotype and FISH PCR testing is available, but typically not used for diagnosis

Table 14.3 General features of AML with inv(16)(p13q22) or t(16;16)(p13;q22)

Defining aberrancy	inv(16)(p13q22) or t(16;16)(p13;q22)
Genes involved	*CBFB-MYH11*
Frequency in adult AML	5–8%
Myeloblast requirement	Does not require 20% blast threshold for diagnosis of AML
Prognostic implication	Generally favorable
Prognostic modifier(s)	Unfavorable: Trisomy 8 *KIT* gene mutation (30–40% of cases): higher risk of relapse and worse overall survival, effect not as severe as in cases with t(8;21) [1] *FLT3* mutations Favorable: Trisomy 22
2° cytogenetic abnormalities	Found in ~40% of cases; more frequent findings include gains of chromosomes 8, 21, and 22 and losses of 7q[1]
Diagnostic testing	Karyotype and FISH inv(16) is often subtle and may be missed on chromosome analysis; thus FISH testing may be preferred PCR testing is available, but typically not used for diagnosis

Most of these cases will also carry other cytogenetic aberrancies. Presence of secondary cytogenetic aberrations or complex karyotypes do not appear to affect clinical outcomes for patients with t(8;21) AML [5]. In AML with inv(16) or t(16;16), trisomy 8 is associated with a worse prognosis, and trisomy 22 has been associated with an improved prognosis [6]. Somatic sequence mutations in *KIT* exons 8 and 17 are associated with a worse prognosis [1], and patients may benefit from hematopoietic stem cell transplant at first remission. Sequence mutations in genes activating tyrosine kinase signaling are frequent in both subtypes of CBF-AML; genes involving the RTK/RAS signaling pathways are affected in nearly 30% of cases and may suggest shorter event-free survival [7]. Genes involved in chromatin modification of the cohesin complex are seen at high frequencies in t(8;21) AML (42% and 18%, respectively), but are generally absent in inv(16)/t(16;16) AML [8]. Similarly *ASXL2* mutations are seen in 20–25% of patients with t(8;21) AML, but are uncommon in inv(16)/t(16;16) disease [9]. RT-PCR targeted against fusion transcripts have been used for minimal residual disease (MRD) assessment in CBF-AML which appears to allow for identification of patients at high risk of relapse [10, 11]. MRD monitoring early after transplant may be more predictive of relapse risk than presence of *KIT* mutations [12].

Acute Promyelocytic Leukemia (APL) (Table 14.4)

APL presents with a predominance of abnormal promyelocytes and arises in the setting of fusion of the *PML* (a nuclear regulatory factor) and *RARA* (retinoic acid

Table 14.4 General features of APL with *PML-RARA*

Defining aberrancy	t(15;17)(q24.1;q21.2) The WHO no longer includes the karyotype in the disease name as the disease is defined by the gene fusion, even when cryptic
Genes involved	*PML-RARA*
Frequency in adult AML	5–8%
Myeloblast requirement	Does not require 20% blast threshold for diagnosis of AML
Prognostic implication	Has most favorable long-term outcomes of all AML subtypes, though significant complications may arise at disease onset
Prognostic modifier(s)	Secondary genetic abnormalities are of unclear prognostic relevance in the context of current therapy FLT3 mutations found in 30–40% of cases, internal tandem duplications are more frequent Alternate *RARA* translocations with *ZBTB16* and *STAT5B* show resistance to ATRA differentiation therapy
2° cytogenetic abnormalities	Found in ~40% of cases; gains of chromosomes 8 in ~10–15% of cases
Diagnostic testing	Karyotype and FISH FISH testing is preferred due to the shorter time to result PCR testing is available; while typically used for disease monitoring, it may be helpful for diagnostic confirmation in rare FISH cryptic cases

receptor alpha) genes. This fusion protein acts as a constitutive transcriptional repressor of RARα target-genes, but this repression may be alleviated by pharmacologic doses of tretinoin [13]. The leukemic blasts are highly sensitive to differentiating agents, tretinoin (also referred to as ATRA, all-*trans*-retinoic acid) and arsenic trioxide [14], as well as to anthracycline-based chemotherapy. APL is classically associated with the t(15;17)(q24.1;q21.2) translocation, but may arise from cryptic or variant *PML-RARA* fusions.

Three breakpoint cluster regions (bcr) are described in the *PML* gene; fusions involving bcr1 and bcr2 are of similar size and are together referred to as long (L) isoform, and those involving bcr3 result in a short (S) isoform [15]. Hypergranular/typical APL represents ~70% of all cases and is often associated with the long isoform. The short isoform is more common in the microgranular (also called hypogranular) variant APL. Both variants are associated with a high risk of disseminated intravascular coagulation, increased fibrinolysis, and significant coagulopathy associated with early death [16].

Secondary cytogenetic abnormalities are found in about 40% of cases. *FLT3* mutations are found in 30–40% of cases, and *FLT3*-ITD is associated with a higher WBC count, microgranular morphology, and involvement of the bcr3 breakpoint [17]. Variant *RARA* translocations also occur with gene partners other than *PML*. Described variant fusion partners include *ZBTB16* at 11q23.2, *NUMA1* at 11q13.4, *NPM1* at 5q35.1, and *STAT5B* at 17q11.2 [18]. Such cases should be diagnosed as "APL with a variant *RARA* translocation." The *ZBTB16-RARA* and *STAT5B-RARA* translocations demonstrate resistance to ATRA differentiation therapy [19].

Minimal residual disease (MRD) monitoring for *PML-RARA* transcripts by PCR is currently the best predictor of relapse-free survival [20]. Detection of *PML-RARA* by RT-PCR in the immediate post-treatment period does not impact the clinical outcome, as abnormal promyelocytes may persist for several weeks after initiating therapy. However, detection of fusion transcripts after achieving complete remission is strongly predictive of relapse, and early pre-emptive therapy may prevent overt clinical relapse [20, 21].

AML with t(9;11)(p21.3;q23.3), KMT2A-MLLT3 (Table 14.5)

This subtype accounts for about 2% of adult AML but represents 9–12% of pediatric cases. The leukemic blasts often show monocytic or myelomonocytic differentiation, and patients may present with disseminated intravascular coagulation, myeloid sarcoma, or soft tissue infiltration. *KMT2A* encodes a histone methyltransferase which participates in chromatin remodeling. While fusions involving *KMT2A* are seen in 5–10% of all AML, the WHO classification for this category is limited specifically to t(9;11)(p21.3;q23.3) [1].

Over 130 different translocations involving *KMT2A* have been described, including greater than 90 different gene fusion partners and at least 6 translocations with no obvious gene fusions [22]. Translocations with *MLLT3* are the most common of these (~30% of cases) and appear to define a more distinct pathologic entity [1, 22]. AML with other balanced translocations of 11q23.3 are classified as AML, not otherwise specified, though the translocation should also be stated in the diagnostic line (except in cases which meet criteria for therapy-related AML or AML with myelodysplasia-related changes).

Secondary cytogenetic aberrancies and complex karyotypes may be seen in t(9;11) AML, but do not appear to affect clinical outcomes for these patients [5]. Somatic sequence mutations of *NRAS* or *KRAS* are seen in 30–40% of cases, but

Table 14.5 General features of AML with t(9;11)(p21.3;q23.3)

Defining aberrancy	t(9;11)(p21.3;q23.3)
Genes involved	*KMT2A-MLLT3*
Frequency in adult AML	~2%
Myeloblast requirement	Requires ≥20% myeloblasts for AML diagnosis
Prognostic implication	Intermediate prognostic risk
Prognostic modifier(s)	Overexpression of *MECOM (EVI1)* associated with very poor prognosis
2° cytogenetic abnormalities	Varied, including trisomy 8 and complex karyotypes
Diagnostic testing	Karyotype and FISH

the incidence of *FLT3* mutations is low compared to other AML subtypes [23]. Overexpression of *MECOM* (previously known as *EVI1*) has been reported in about 40% of cases, and some reports suggest that t(9;11) AML positive for overexpression are biologically distinct from *MECOM*-negative cases [24]. Patients with de novo AML and t(9;11)(p21.3;q23.3) are at intermediate prognostic-risk but appear to have a relatively better survival than patients with other translocations at 11q23, who generally experience more adverse clinical outcomes [25]. Overexpression of *MECOM* in *KMT2A*-rearranged AML is associated with a very poor prognosis [24, 26].

AML with t(6;9)(p23;q34.1), DEK-NUP214 (Table 14.6)

This uncommon subtype accounts for 0.7–1.8% of all cases and often presents with basophilia (≥2% basophils), cytopenias, and multilineage dysplasia [1]. Despite the presence of multilineage dysplasia, the t(6;9) takes precedence over the less specific diagnosis of AML with myelodysplasia-related changes (AML-MRC). *NUP214* encodes the CAN nucleoporin. Fusion with the *DEK* oncogene results in abnormal transcription factor activity, most likely due to altered nuclear transport due to binding of soluble transport factors [27].

The *DEK-NUP214* fusion is the sole cytogenetic abnormality identified in nearly 90% of cases [28]. AML with t(6;9) has poor survival rates with conventional chemotherapy, and patients may benefit from allogeneic hematopoietic stem cell transplantation. Although the WHO requires ≥20% myeloblasts to diagnose this entity, this threshold requirement is controversial. *FLT3*-ITD mutation is found in 70–80% of cases, but the poor prognosis of this AML subtype is independent of *FLT3* mutation status [29, 30].

Table 14.6 General features of AML with t(6;9)(p23;q34.1)

Defining aberrancy	t(6;9)(p23;q34.1)
Genes involved	*DEK-NUP214*
Frequency in adult AML	0.7–1.8%
Myeloblast requirement	Requires ≥20% myeloblasts for AML diagnosis (controversial)
Prognostic implication	Poor prognostic risk
Prognostic modifier(s)	*FLT3* mutations found in 70–80% of cases, but finding does not appear to confer additional negative prognostic risk
2° cytogenetic abnormalities	Uncommon, though complex karyotypes have been described
Diagnostic testing	Karyotype and FISH

AML with inv(3)(q21.3q26.2) or t(3;3)(q21.3;q26.2); GATA2, MECOM (Table 14.7)

This uncommon subtype accounts for 1–2% of AML and often presents with normal to increased platelet counts and multilineage dysplasia, typically with prominent uni- or bi-lobed dwarf megakaryocytes [1]. Despite the presence of multilineage dysplasia, the presence of inv(3) or t(3;3) takes diagnostic precedence over the less specific diagnosis of AML-MRC. This rearrangement pairs the oncogene *MECOM* with a *GATA2* enhancer. No abnormal fusion transcript is generated by this gene rearrangement, but it contributes to leukemogenesis by both stimulating *MECOM* expression and causing *GATA2* insufficiency [31, 32]. Inappropriate expression of *MECOM* (previously known as *EVI1*) is seen in a variety of AMLs, and high expression is a poor prognostic indicator independent of 3q26.2 translocations [33]. While other aberrancies involving chromosome 3q26.2 and variant fusion partners for *MECOM* have been described, these are currently excluded by WHO from the AML with recurrent genetic abnormalities disease category [1].

Secondary cytogenetic aberrancies are found in most cases of AML with inv(3) or t(3;3) and are of the variety that are typically associated with myelodysplasia. Monosomy 7 can be found in up to 66% cases, and chromosome 5q deletions and complex karyotypes are also commonly described [34]. Activating mutations in genes affecting the RAS/receptor tyrosine kinase signaling pathways are found in about 98% of cases, including *NRAS, PTPN11, FLT3, KRAS, NF1, CBL,* and *KIT* [35]. Other commonly mutated genes include *GATA2*, *RUNX1*, and *SF3B1* [35, 36].

This subtype of AML is typically associated with an aggressive disease course, therapy resistance, and short survival. Although the WHO requires ≥20% myeloblasts to diagnose this entity, this threshold requirement is controversial as disease associated with inv(3) or t(3;3) and <20% blasts have an equally poor outlook, similar clinicopathologic features, and identical mutational patterns at the molecular genomic level [1]. A complex karyotype or concomitant monosomy 7 worsens the already adverse prognosis associated with this subtype [34].

Table 14.7 General features of AML with inv(3)(q21.3q26.2) or t(3;3)(q21.3;q26.2)

Defining aberrancy	inv(3)(q21.3q26.2) or t(3;3)(q21.3;q26.2)
Genes involved	*GATA2, MECOM*
Frequency in adult AML	1–2%
Myeloblast requirement	Requires ≥20% myeloblasts for AML diagnosis (controversial)
Prognostic implication	Poor prognostic risk
Prognostic modifier(s)	Monosomy 7 or complex karyotype associated with poorer prognosis
2° cytogenetic abnormalities	Seen in 75% of cases and are typically "MDS-related," including −5q, −7, and complex karyotypes
Diagnostic testing	FISH Chromosome 3q26.2 rearrangements may be cryptic to conventional chromosome analysis

Table 14.8 General features of AML with t(1;22)(p13.3;q13.1)

Defining aberrancy	t(1;22)(p13.3;q13.1)
Genes involved	*RBM15-MRTFA* (*MRTFA* previously known as *MKL1)*
Frequency in adult AML	<1%
Myeloblast requirement	Requires ≥20% myeloblasts for AML diagnosis
Prognostic implication	Intermediate prognostic risk
Prognostic modifier(s)	–
2° cytogenetic abnormalities	Uncommon, though additional abnormalities more frequently found in "older" patients (>6 months)
Diagnostic testing	Karyotype and FISH

AML (Megakaryoblastic) with t(1;22)(p13.3;q13.1), RBM15-MRTFA (Table 14.8)

This rare subtype with megakaryoblasts represents <1% of all AML cases. It presents almost exclusively in infants; 80% of diagnoses are made within the first year of life, and most occur within the first 6 months [1]. These children usually have marked hepatosplenomegaly, cytopenias, and a densely fibrotic marrow with bilateral periostitis or osteolytic lesions. The patient may also present with a soft tissue mass, mimicking other small round blue cell tumors. The translocation fuses *RBM15*, a RNA recognition motif-encoding gene, to *MRTFA* (previously known as *MLK1*), a protein with a DNA-binding motif involved in chromatin organization [37].

AML with t(1;22) represents only ~14% of the non-Down syndrome acute megakaryoblastic leukemias [38]. In most cases, the *RBM15-MRTFA* fusion is the sole cytogenetic aberrancy [1]. When compared to other de novo cases of non-Down syndrome acute megakaryoblastic leukemia, presence of the t(1;22) translocation appears to be associated with intermediate-risk disease and inferior event-free survival [38, 39].

AML with Mutated NPM1 (Table 14.9)

Mutations in *NPM1* are among the most frequent acquired genetic abnormalities in AML, occurring in 2–8% of childhood cases, 27–35% of adult cases, and 45–64% of adult normal karyotype (NK) AML [1]. The *NPM1* gene encodes nucleophosmin, a multifunctional chaperone protein which localizes to the nucleus, participates in the biogenesis of ribosomes, and helps regulate the ARF-TP53 tumor suppressor pathway [40, 41]. Mutations typically involve exon 12 and lead to a frameshift in the C-terminal protein region, with subsequent cytoplasmic displacement of the protein [42]. *NPM1* mutations are also considered late aberrancies in

Table 14.9 General features of AML with mutated *NPM1*

Defining aberrancy	*NPM1* exon 12 mutation
Genes involved	*NPM1*
Frequency in adult AML	27–35%
Myeloblast requirement	Requires ≥20% myeloblasts for AML diagnosis
Prognostic implication	Generally favorable
Prognostic modifier(s)	MDS-related cytogenetic abnormalities take diagnostic priority Concurrent *FLT3-ITD* mutation is associated with an intermediate prognostic risk Concurrent FLT3-ITD and DNMT3A mutation have particularly adverse impact on overall and event-free survival
2° cytogenetic abnormalities	Typically normal karyotype; 5–15% of cases may have a diagnostically nonspecific abnormality
Diagnostic testing	Molecular testing (sequencing, fragment size analysis, etc.) Cytoplasmic nucleophosmin staining by immunohistochemistry has been used as a surrogate method for detection of the gene mutation

leukemogenesis, following earlier somatic mutations in genes involved in epigenetic regulatory processes such as DNA methylation, histone modification, and chromatin looping [43, 44].

The leukemic blasts often have a monocytic or myelomonocytic phenotype.

NPM1 mutations are usually mutually exclusive of other recurrent AML-defining cytogenetic aberrancies and are typically associated with normal karyotypes [45]. A minority of cases (5–15%) will carry nonspecific chromosomal alterations such as +4, +8, −Y, del(9q), and +21; however these findings do not appear to alter the disease profile or survival outcomes, when compared to “normal-karyotype disease” [45]. Cytogenetic aberrancies typically associated with myelodysplasia are uncommon in this setting of *NPM1*-mutated AML [46], but morphologic dysplasia may be seen in up to a quarter of cases. However, AML-MRC-related cytogenetic abnormalities should take diagnostic precedence if detected. Other acquired sequence mutations are common, and commutated genes often include *FLT3, TET2, DNMT3A, IDH1/2,* and *KRAS/NRAS* and cohesin complex genes [47].

In NK-AML, *NPM1* mutation confers a favorable prognosis, similar to that of core binding factor AMLs [48]. A significant minority (~25%) of *NPM1*-mutated NK-AML may have multilineage dysplasia, but the finding does not impact the good prognosis associated with *NPM1* mutation unless myelodysplasia-associated cytogenetic aberrancies are also detected [49]. About 40% of *NPM1*-mutated AML will have concurrent *FLT3*-ITD mutations, and this abnormality appears to negate the favorable prognostic effect [50]. The relative allelic ratio of *FLT3*-ITD appears to have prognostic significance in this setting, and *NPM1*-mutated patients with a low-allelic burden of *FLT3*-ITD (i.e., <0.5) seem to retain favorable outcomes [51]. Regardless, patients with *NPM1* mutation appear to have a better prognosis than patients with *FLT3*-ITD and wild-type *NPM1*, especially in cases with a high *FLT3*-ITD allelic ratio (i.e., ≥0.5) [52, 53]. Concurrent mutations of *NPM1, FLT3*-ITD, and *DNMT3A* appear to have a particularly adverse impact on overall and event-free survival [54].

AML with Biallelic Mutations of CEBPA (Table 14.10)

Biallelic mutations of *CEBPA* may be seen in 4–9% of children with AML, at a lower frequency in adult disease, and are generally associated with a good prognosis similar to that seen in CBF-AML [1]. *CEBPA* encodes a protein called CCAAT enhancer-binding protein alpha, which serves multiple functions including as a hematopoiesis-associated transcription factor and also as a tumor suppressor gene. Biallelic gene mutation is required for diagnosis; the favorable prognostic association is linked to a specific gene expression profile that is not identified with single allele mutation [1, 55, 56]. Only sequence mutations of the *CEBPA* gene are taken into diagnostic consideration for this subtype, though there are many routes that can lead to *CEBPA* inactivation. This AML subtype does not have particularly distinctive morphologic features.

More than 70% of cases will be associated with a normal karyotype. Factors which might negatively impact the favorable prognostic risk include presence of cytogenetic aberrancies (i.e., an abnormal karyotype) and co-mutation with *FLT3*-ITD [57, 58], though this still requires additional clarification [1]. Concurrent *GATA1* and *WT1* mutations are relatively frequent in patients with biallelic *CEBPA* mutation, but *FLT3*-ITD, *NPM1, ASXL1,* and *RUNX1* mutations are uncommon and

Table 14.10 General features of AML with biallelic mutations of CEBPA

Defining aberrancy	Biallelic *CEBPA* mutations
Genes involved	*CEBPA*
Frequency in adult AML	~4–9% in children/young adults, likely less in adult disease
Myeloblast requirement	Requires ≥20% myeloblasts for AML diagnosis
Prognostic implication	Generally favorable
Prognostic modifier(s)	FLT3-ITD (5–9% of cases) and GATA2 mutations (~39% of cases) are described; currently have unclear significance Cytogenetic aberrancies; currently unclear significance Myelodysplasia-related abnormalities take diagnostic priority
2° cytogenetic abnormalities	Found in ~5–15% of cases; typically diagnostically nonspecific
Diagnostic testing	Molecular testing (gene sequencing) Sequencing CEBPA and confirmation of biallelic mutation is technically challenging due to high GC content and short sequence reads

Table 14.11 Cytogenetic abnormalities diagnostic[a] for AML-MRC

1. Complex karyotype (defined as three or more unrelated clonal abnormalities)	
2. Unbalanced abnormality	3. Balanced translocations
−7/del(7q)	t(11;16)(q23.3;p13.3)
del(5q)/t(5q)	t(3;21)(q26.2;q22.1)
i(17q)/t(17p)	t(1;3)(p26.3;q21.2)
−13/del(13q)	t(2;11)(p21;q23.3)
del(11q)	t(5;12)(q32;p13.2)
del(12p)/t(12p)	t(5;7)(q32;q11.2)
idic(x)(q13)	t(5;17)(q32;p13.2)
–	t(5;10)(q32;q21)
–	t(3;5)(q25.3;q35.1)

[a]Presence of any of these cytogenetic abnormalities is considered sufficiently specific to diagnose AML with MRC when there are ≥20% blood or marrow-based myeloblasts and prior therapy has been excluded

seen more frequently in *CEBPA* monoallelic cases [59]. Cytogenetic aberrancies typically associated with myelodysplasia are uncommon in this setting of biallelic *CEBPA* mutation, but morphologic dysplasia may be seen in about a quarter of cases [1, 60]. The finding of dysplasia alone does not influence the prognosis, but AML-MRC-related cytogenetic abnormalities should take diagnostic precedence if detected [1, 60] (see Table 14.11).

Germline mutation of *CEBPA* is also a described phenomenon and is well associated with predisposition to develop AML. Therefore, identification of biallelic *CEBPA* mutation in AML should prompt evaluation of possible germline inheritance, especially in patients presenting as children or young adults (see section "Myeloid Neoplasms with Germline Predisposition").

Provisional 2016 WHO AML with Recurrent Genetic Abnormality Subtypes

BCR-ABL1 fusion and *RUNX1* mutation define new provisional entities in the 2016 WHO AML classification system. AML with *BCR-ABL1* is a de novo AML with no evidence of chronic myeloid leukemia, both prior to and after therapy. This is a rare subtype, accounting for <1% of all cases of AML [1, 61]. Most cases demonstrate the p210 fusion, though a minority of reported cases had p190 transcripts. Most cases have additional cytogenetic abnormalities such as loss of chromosome 7, gain of chromosome 8, or complex karyotypes [61–63]. AML with *BCR-ABL1* is reported to be an aggressive disease with poor response to traditional AML therapy or tyrosine kinase inhibitor therapy alone.

RUNX1 mutations are reported to occur in 4–16% of AML, but can also be found in numerous other myeloid neoplasms. The diagnosis of AML with mutated *RUNX1* should not be made for cases that fulfill criteria for *any* of the other specific AML subtypes, including AML with recurrent genetic abnormalities, AML with myelodysplasia-related changes, and therapy-related myeloid neoplasms [1]. *RUNX1* mutations found in the setting of myelodysplasia (MDS) frequently coincide with additional gene mutations including *SRSF2, EZH2, STAG2,* and *ASXL1*, and this profile appears similar in AML with mutated *RUNX1* [64, 65]. Some studies have associated *RUNX1* mutations with worse overall survival in AML. Germline mutation of *RUNX1* is also described and is associated with an autosomal dominant thrombocytopenia and also increased risk for MDS/AML. When identified in AML, *RUNX1* mutation should prompt evaluation of family history and possible consideration for germline sequence analysis (see section "Myeloid Neoplasms with Germline Predisposition").

AML with Myelodysplasia-Related Changes

This diagnostic category represents 24–35% of AML and encompasses disease with ≥20% peripheral blood or bone marrow myeloblasts and (1) dysplasia in ≥50% of at least two cell lines, (2) a prior history of MDS or myelodysplastic/myeloproliferative neoplasm (MDS/MPN), or (3) underlying MDS-associated cytogenetic abnormalities [1]. Identifying an AML-associated recurrent cytogenetic aberrancy or history of cytotoxic/radiation therapy for unrelated disease would exclude this diagnostic category. The cytogenetic aberrancies associated with this category of AML are similar to those found in MDS and include complex karyotypes, unbalanced gains/losses of major chromosomal regions, and number of uncommon balanced translocations (Table 14.11). Some abnormalities that are common in MDS, such as trisomy 8, del(20q), and loss of chromosome Y, are not sufficiently specific in isolation to diagnose AML-MRC [1].

This category is generally associated with a poorer prognosis and lower rates of complete remission than other AML subtypes [66, 67]. There are generally no significant differences in survival between AMLs arising from myelodysplasia and de novo AMLs with multilineage dysplasia [67]. Some cases with a prior history of MDS, intermediate-risk cytogenetics, and relatively low blast counts (20–29%) may exhibit clinical behavior more similar to MDS [68], with response and survival benefit from hypomethylating agents. Cases with high-risk cytogenetics generally have no survival differences compared to AML cases with ≥30% blasts [68]. Of note, a significant minority of AML associated with *NPM1* or biallelic *CEBPA* mutations will show multilineage dysplasia. In the absence of MDS-specific cytogenetic aberrancies, these cases retain a good prognostic outlook, with similar behavior to cases without multilineage dysplasia [49, 60].

The 2016 WHO classification system does not recognize any somatic gene sequence mutations as being diagnostically specific for the AML-MRC category. However, acquired variants in some genes have frequent association with secondary AMLs arising from antecedent myeloid malignancy. Mutations in *SRSF2*, *SF3B1*,

U2AF1, *ZRSR2*, *ASXL1*, *EZH2*, *BCOR*, *STAG2*, *RUNX1*, and *TP53* are common in AML-MRC and occur at a higher frequency than in other forms of AML, NOS [69, 70]. Presence of *TP53* mutations is almost always associated with complex karyotypes and may suggest an even worse prognosis than other cases in this already poor prognostic group [69–72].

Therapy-Related Myeloid Neoplasms

Therapy-related myeloid neoplasms (t-MNs) arise as an uncommon late effect of chemotherapy and/or radiation therapy for an unrelated illness, usually another malignancy, solid organ transplant, or autoimmune disease. The morphologic presentation at diagnosis can be variable, and this category represents about 10–20% of all cases of AML, MDS, and MDS/MPN [1]. t-MNs are morphologically heterogeneous and can look like either MDS or AML, but the 2016 WHO classifies them collectively in a single category due to general behavioral similarities and extremely poor outcomes that are independent of blast counts [1]. The most common antecedent malignancies are breast, lung, and hematologic cancers, chiefly lymphomas and multiple myeloma [73, 74]. The leukemic blasts do not have diagnostically specific morphologic or immunophenotypic features.

The leukemic cells in t-MNs will demonstrate an abnormal karyotype in >90% of cases [75, 76]. Essentially all the balanced cytogenetic abnormalities associated with AML-MRC are also found in t-MNs; thus the clinical history is central to assigning a correct diagnosis. A positive history of cytotoxic therapy takes diagnostic precedence over morphologic dysplasia and MDS-associated cytogenetics. Two general subsets of t-MNs are clinically recognized, associated with either (1) alkylating agents and/or ionizing radiation therapy or (2) topoisomerase II inhibitor therapy (Table 14.12). However, as patients may undergo multiple therapeutic exposures, there can be overlap between the general archetypes [77]. The pathogenic effect of isolated limited-field radiation therapy is unclear, and the incidence of associated t-MNs associated with this form of therapy is uncertain [78].

The more common subtype arises after alkylating agent and/or radiation therapy (~70% of patients). There is usually latency period of 5–10 years, an MDS-like phase with dyspoiesis and cytopenias and rapid progression to overt AML with multilineage dysplasia. These cases are associated with unbalanced chromosomal losses (often involving chromosomes 5 and/or 7), complex karyotypes, and mutations or loss of *TP53*. Loss of 5q is often seen with additional chromosomal abnormalities in a complex karyotype, and up to 80% of patients with del(5q) will also have mutations or loss of *TP53* [1].

The second subtype arises after topoisomerase II inhibitor therapy, but may also be seen with radiation therapy alone. The latency period is shorter (1–5 years), patients usually do not have an MDS-phase, and overt leukemia is found on presentation. Balanced translocations are more frequent in this subgroup, often involving KMT2A at 11q23.3 or RUNX1 at 21q22.1. Category-specific balanced chromo-

Table 14.12 Major subtypes of therapy-related myeloid neoplasms

Class of prior therapy	Alkylating agent	Topoisomerase II inhibitor
Relative frequency	~70% of t-MNs	~30% of t-MNs
Latency to onset	5–10 years	1–5 years
MDS-phase preceding overt AML	Common	Uncommon
Common cytogenetic abnormalities	Unbalanced chromosomal losses; chromosomes 5 and/or 7 abnormalities, complex karyotypes, and mutations/ loss of TP53	Balanced translocations, KMT2A at 11q23.3 or RUNX1 at 21q22.1 frequently involved
Implicated medications	Alkylating agents Platinum-based therapy Antimetabolites	Topoisomerase II inhibitors Anthracyclines

The incidence of t-MNs due to limited-field radiation therapy is unknown
Antitubulin agents (vincristine, vinblastine, docetaxel, etc.) have been implicated, but usually in combination with other agents
Topoisomerase II inhibitors may also be associated with therapy-associated lymphoblastic leukemia

somal rearrangements have been described, such as the t(15;17) *PML-RARA* fusion associated with APL or the inv(16) *CBFB-MYH11* fusion associated with CBF-AML. The clinical behavior of these cases is still unresolved; some groups have reported comparable outcomes to de novo disease, while others have indicated worse overall and event-free survival [79, 80].

In general, the prognosis of this disease category is exceptionally poor with overall 5-year survival rates that are often reported at <10%. Cases with abnormalities of chromosome 5 and/or 7, *TP53* mutations, or complex karyotypes have a median survival time of <1 year regardless of presentation as overt t-AML or as t-MDS [1]. Somatic sequence mutations are frequently reported in the *TET2, PTPN11, IDH1/2, NRAS,* and *FLT3* genes, but the clinical significance of these findings is still undetermined [81, 82].

Myeloid Neoplasms with Germline Predisposition and AML in Children

Myeloid Neoplasms with Germline Predisposition

A number of germline abnormalities have been linked with an inherited predisposition toward myeloid malignancies, but only a few are specifically predisposing to AML. These are rare disorders which represent <1% of AMLs, but the relative frequency of subtypes within this diagnostic category has not been well established [1]. Patients present more frequently in childhood, though few subtypes with late-onset have been described, and recognition is important for the screening of family members. These disorders are quite rare but the few better-characterized entities fall into three groups within the 2016 WHO system, as summarized below:

- *Myeloid neoplasms with germline predisposition without a pre-existing disorder or organ dysfunction*
  - Acute myeloid leukemia with germline *CEBPA* mutation
  - Myeloid neoplasms with germline *DDX41* mutation
- *Myeloid neoplasms with germline predisposition and pre-existing platelet disorders*
  - Myeloid neoplasms with germline *RUNX1* mutation
  - Myeloid neoplasms with *ANKRD26* mutation
  - Myeloid neoplasms with *ETV6* mutation
- *Myeloid neoplasms with germline predisposition and other organ dysfunction*
  - Myeloid neoplasms with germline *GATA2* mutation
  - Myeloid neoplasms associated with bone marrow failure syndromes
  - Myeloid neoplasms associated with telomere biology disorders
  - Juvenile myelomonocytic leukemia associated with neurofibromatosis, Noonan syndrome, or Noonan syndrome-like disorders
  - Myeloid neoplasms associated with Down syndrome

AML may be seen associated with any of the germline predisposition entities, but a clinical picture dominated by either MDS or AML with no other significant organ dysfunction is primarily seen with the first group, including *CEBPA* and *DDX41* mutations. Disorders associated with germline *DDX41* mutation appear to have a longer latency period, with a median age of 62 years at malignancy onset [1]. An increased risk for lymphoid malignancies is also reported for the entities associated with *DDX41, RUNX1, ANKRD26,* and *ETV6* mutations and also with Down syndrome [1].

Transient Abnormal Myelopoiesis and Myeloid Leukemia Associated with Down Syndrome

Persons with Down syndrome have a 10- to 100-fold increased risk of developing acute leukemia than unaffected persons. About 70% of these cases have a megakaryoblastic phenotype, which is rare in non-Down syndrome associated AML [1]. Additionally, a significant minority of infants with Down syndrome may also present with a temporary clonal myeloid proliferation whose features can mimic and even meet criteria for AML. This unusual condition is referred to as transient abnormal myelopoiesis (TAM) associated with Down syndrome. The blasts found in the vast majority of TAM also exhibit a megakaryoblastic immunophenotype [1]. The unique clinical characteristics of both these myeloid proliferations were recognized by the WHO, resulting in a separate categorization in 2008, which has persisted into the 2016 update.

Trisomy 21 itself causes perturbation of fetal hematopoiesis with abnormal production in the liver, increases in the number of megakaryocyte-erythroid progenitors, and increases in the hematopoietic stem cell compartment [83]. These abnormalities are congenital and precede the acquisition of disease-associated somatic mutations [84]. Essentially all cases of Down syndrome-associated TAM and AML will acquire a subsequent mutation of *GATA1*, a hematopoietic transcription factor that regulates normal megakaryocyte and erythrocyte differentiation [83, 85, 86]. More than 95% of the pathologically significant variants are in exon 2 with the remainder in exon 3, with resultant N-terminal protein truncation [87]. Additionally, up to 25–30% of all neonates with Down syndrome may be found to carry these mutations, though the reason for the high frequency in this setting is unclear [88].

However, *GATA1* mutations are insufficient in isolation to cause myeloid leukemia associated with Down syndrome; 80–90% of patients with TAM will show spontaneous regression of the process within the first 3 months of life [1, 89, 90]. Patients with TAM who do progress to acute leukemia usually do so within the first 5 years of life, and acquisition of additional oncogenic mutations can usually be demonstrated. Trisomy 8 is common in this setting (13–44% of cases), but monosomy 7 is very rare [1, 91]. Whole genome or exome sequencing studies at progression to acute leukemia have shown about 50% of cases acquire mutations in cohesin complex genes (*RAD21*, *SMC1A*, *SMC3,* and *STAG2*), 45% will involve epigenetic regulators such as *EZH2* and *KANSL1*, and 20% will involve the transcription factor *CTCF* [89, 90]. Other signaling pathways such as JAK kinases, *MPL*, and RAS pathway genes (*NRAS, KRAS, CBL, PTPN11,* and *NF1*) were implicated in a smaller subset of cases [89, 90]. However, no specific genetic abnormalities can consistently predict transformation of TAM to acute leukemia at present.

Childhood AML

AML accounts for only 20% of pediatric acute leukemias, but is overtaking acute lymphoblastic leukemia as the leading cause of childhood leukemia-related mortality [92]. Both adult and childhood AML have a low overall mutation burden compared to other human cancers, with a broad spectrum of recurrently impacted but relatively infrequently affected genes [92]. However, the landscape of structural and sequence-related genomic aberrancies in pediatric AML shows significant differences from the adult cohort.

While there is some overlap of recurrent cytogenetic abnormalities seen in adult and childhood AML, the general types of balanced and unbalanced chromosomal abnormalities are different. Structural variants are disproportionately prevalent in younger patients, with a variety of uncommon recurrent balanced translocations and inversions beyond the specifically named entities in WHO classification system. A selection of these rare balanced rearrangements with higher prevalence in pediatric AML may be found in Table 14.13. Rearrangements involving *KMT2A* are the most common, seen in ~10–20% of children but in nearly half of affected infants [92, 93]. Similar to adult patients, AML associated with t(8;21), inv(16), and t(15;17) are

Table 14.13 Chromosomal translocations with a higher prevalence in pediatric AML

Translocation	Associated genes	Frequency in children	Frequency in adults	Age cohort bias	Prognosis
11q23 fusion family					
11q23.3	*KMT2A* translocated	25%	5–10%	Infants	Dependent on partner gene
t(9;11)(p21.3;q23.3)	*KMT2A-MLLT3*	9.5%	2%	Children	Intermediate
t(10;11)(p12;q23.3)	*KMT2A-MLLT10*	3.5%	1%	Children	Adverse
t(6;11)(q27;q23.3)	*KMT2A-AFDN*	ND	ND	Children	Adverse [97]
t(11;19)(q23.3;p13.11)	*KMT2A-ELL*	ND	ND	Infants, children	Adverse [98]
t(6;11)(q27;q23.3)	*KMT2A-AFDN*	2%	<0.5%	Children	Adverse
t(1;11)(q21;q23.3)	*KMT2A-MLLT11*	1%	<0.5%	Children	Favorable
NUP fusion family					
t(6;9)(p23;q34.1)	*DEK-NUP214*	1.7%	0.7–1.8%	Older children, rare in infants	Adverse
t(5;11)(q35.3;p15.5)[a]	*NUP98-NSD1*	7%	3%	Older children and young adults	Adverse
t(11;12)(p15.5;p13.5)[a]	*NUP98-KDM5A*	3%	0%	Children <5 years	Intermediate
ETS fusion family					
t(7;12)(q36.3;p13.2)	*MNX1-ETV6*	0.8%	<0.5%	Infants	Adverse
t(2;12)(q33.3;p13.2)	*ETV6-INO80D*	ND	ND	Infants	ND
t(16;21)(p11.2;q22.2)	*FUS-ERG*	ND	ND	Infants, children	ND
GLIS2 fusion family					
inv(16)(p13.3q24.3)[a]	*CBFA2T3-GLIS2*	3%	0%	Infants	Adverse
Others					
t(1;22)(p13.3;q13.1)	*RBM15-MRTFA*	0.8%	<0.5%	Infants, 95% of cases <2 years old	Intermediate
t(8;16)(p11.2;q13.3)	*KAT6A-CREBBP*	0.5%	<0.5%	Infants and children	Spontaneous regression reported in some infant cases, Intermediate risk in later childhood

ND not defined
[a]*Described as a cryptic translocation*

associated with superior outcomes, while complex karyotypes and monosomy 7 are associated with poor outcomes [92–94]. Monosomal karyotypes have also been described as an indicator of poor outcome [95, 96]. Recurrent focal deletions are other characteristic findings in pediatric AML. Copy number loss are more common in children, and the *ZEB2, MBNL1,* and *ELF1* genes are often affected; *ZEB2* and *MBNL1* co-deletion is a relatively frequent finding, and half of these are found accompanying *KMT2A-MLLT3* fusions [92]. *KMT2A* fusions were also commonly associated with RAS-related mutations (*KRAS, NRAS, PTPN1,* or *NF1*), and a subset of *KMT2A* fusions also showed recurrent mutation in post-transcriptional splicing genes (i.e., *SETD2, U2AF1,* and *DICER1*) as the sole additional abnormality [92].

Mutations of *WT1* appear to be mutually exclusive with those in *ASXL1* and *EZH2,* but *WT1* or *EZH2* variants are seen in about one-quarter of pediatric AML cases and may represent early clonal or near-clonal origin [92]. Widespread gene silencing by aberrant promoter methylation is enriched in younger patients with *WT1* mutations, and mutations of *WT1, ASXL1,* or *EZH2* are associated with induction failure [92]. Other recurrently mutated genes in pediatric AML include variants in *GATA2*, *CBL*, *MYC*-ITD, *NRAS*, and *KRAS*. *NRAS* and *WT1* are mutated more often in younger patients than adults; conversely, mutations in *DNMT3A, IDH1/2, RUNX1, NPM1,* and *TP53*, which are common in adults, are seen more often in older patients [92]. Given the ongoing discovery clarifying the genetics of pediatric AML, more robust classification systems for diagnosis and treatment of childhood AML will likely be forthcoming.

References

1. Swerdlow SH, Campo E, Harris NL, Jaffe ES, Pileri SA, Stein H, Thiele J, editors. WHO classification of tumours of haematopoietic and lymphoid tissues (Revised 4th edition). Lyon: IARC; 2017.
2. Cancer Genome Atlas Research Network. Genomic and epigenomic landscapes of adult de novo acute myeloid leukemia. N Engl J Med. 2013;368:2059–74.
3. Devillier R, Gelsi-Boyer V, Brecqueville M, Carbuccia N, Murati A, Vey N, et al. Acute myeloid leukemia with myelodysplasia-related changes are characterized by a specific molecular pattern with high frequency of ASXL1 mutations. Am J Hematol. 2012;87:659–62.
4. Grimwade D, Hills RK, Moorman AV, Walker H, Chatters S, Goldstone AH, et al. Refinement of cytogenetic classification in acute myeloid leukemia: determination of prognostic significance of rare recurring chromosomal abnormalities among 5876 younger adult patients treated in the United Kingdom Medical Research Council trials. Blood. 2010;116(3):354–65.
5. Byrd JC, Mrózek K, Dodge RK, Carroll AJ, Edwards CG, Arthur DC, et al. Pretreatment cytogenetic abnormalities are predictive of induction success, cumulative incidence of relapse, and overall survival in adult patients with de novo acute myeloid leukemia: results from Cancer and Leukemia Group B (CALGB 8461). Blood. 2002;100(13):4325–36.
6. Paschka P, Du J, Schlenk RF, Gaidzik VI, Bullinger L, Corbacioglu A, et al. Secondary genetic lesions in acute myeloid leukemia with inv(16) or t(16;16): a study of the German-Austrian AML Study Group (AMLSG). Blood. 2013;121(1):170–7.
7. Itzykson R, Duployez N, Fasan A, Decool G, Marceau-Renaut A, Meggendorfer M, et al. Clonal interference of signaling mutations holds prognostic relevance in core binding factor acute myeloid leukemia. Blood. 2018;132:187–96. Epub ahead of print. PMID: 29692343

8. Duployez N, Marceau-Renaut A, Boissel N, Petit A, Bucci M, Geffroy S, et al. Comprehensive mutational profiling of core binding factor acute myeloid leukemia. Blood. 2016;127(20):2451–9.
9. Micol JB, Duployez N, Boissel N, Petit A, Geffroy S, Nibourel O, et al. Frequent ASXL2 mutations in acute myeloid leukemia patients with t(8;21)/RUNX1-RUNX1T1 chromosomal translocations. Blood. 2014;124(9):1445–9.
10. Yin JA, O'Brien MA, Hills RK, Daly SB, Wheatley K, Burnett AK. Minimal residual disease monitoring by quantitative RT-PCR in core binding factor AML allows risk stratification and predicts relapse: results of the United Kingdom MRC AML-15 trial. Blood. 2012;120(14):2826–35.
11. Zhu HH, Zhang XH, Qin YZ, Liu DH, Jiang H, Chen H, et al. MRD-directed risk stratification treatment may improve outcomes of t(8;21) AML in the first complete remission: results from the AML05 multicenter trial. Blood. 2013;121(20):4056–62.
12. Wang Y, Wu DP, Liu QF, Qin YZ, Wang JB, Xu LP, et al. In adults with t(8;21)AML, posttransplant RUNX1/RUNX1T1-based MRD monitoring, rather than c-KIT mutations, allows further risk stratification. Blood. 2014;124(12):1880–6.
13. Pandolfi PP. In vivo analysis of the molecular genetics of acute promyelocytic leukemia. Oncogene. 2001;20:5726–35.
14. Shen ZX, Shi ZZ, Fang J, Gu W, Li JM, Zhu YM, et al. All-trans retinoic acid/As2O3 combination yields a high quality remission and survival in newly diagnosed acute promyelocytic leukemia. Proc Natl Acad Sci U S A. 2004;101(15):5328–35.
15. Lo-Coco F, Ammatuna E. The biology of acute promyelocytic leukemia and its impact on diagnosis and treatment. Hematology Am Soc Hematol Educ Program. 2006:156–61, 514. https://www.ncbi.nlm.nih.gov/pubmed/17124055.
16. Rahmé R, Thomas X, Recher C, Vey N, Delaunay J, Deconinck E, et al. Early death in acute promyelocytic leukemia (APL) in French centers: a multicenter study in 399 patients. Leukemia. 2014;28(12):2422–4.
17. Breccia M, Loglisci G, Loglisci MG, Ricci R, Diverio D, Latagliata R, et al. FLT3-ITD confers poor prognosis in patients with acute promyelocytic leukemia treated with AIDA protocols: long-term follow-up analysis. Haematologica. 2013;98(12):e161–3.
18. Zelent A, Guidez F, Melnick A, Waxman S, Licht JD. Translocations of the RARalpha gene in acute promyelocytic leukemia. Oncogene. 2001;20:7186–203.
19. Melnick A, Licht JD. Deconstructing a disease: RARalpha, its fusion partners, and their roles in the pathogenesis of acute promyelocytic leukemia. Blood. 1999;93:3167–215.
20. Grimwade D, Jovanovic JV, Hills RK, Nugent EA, Patel Y, Flora R, et al. Prospective minimal residual disease monitoring to predict relapse of acute promyelocytic leukemia and to direct pre-emptive arsenic trioxide therapy. J Clin Oncol. 2009;27:3650–8.
21. Esteve J, Escoda L, Martin G, Rubio V, Díaz-Mediavilla J, González M, et al. Outcome of patients with acute promyelocytic leukemia failing to front-line treatment with all-trans retinoic acid and anthracycline-based chemotherapy: benefit of an early intervention. Leukemia. 2007;21:446–52.
22. Meyer C, Burmeister T, Gröger D, Tsaur G, Fechina L, Renneville A, et al. The MLL recombinome of acute leukemias in 2017. Leukemia. 2018;32(2):273–84.
23. Chandra P, Luthra R, Zuo Z, Yao H, Ravandi F, Reddy N, et al. Acute myeloid leukemia with t(9;11)(p21-22;q23): common properties of dysregulated ras pathway signaling and genomic progression characterize de novo and therapy-related cases. Am J Clin Pathol. 2010;133(5):686–93.
24. Bindels EM, Havermans M, Lugthart S, Erpelinck C, Wocjtowicz E, Krivtsov AV, et al. EVI1 is critical for the pathogenesis of a subset of MLL-AF9-rearranged AMLs. Blood. 2012;119(24):5838–49.
25. Mrózek K, Heinonen K, Lawrence D, Carroll AJ, Koduru PR, Rao KW, et al. Adult patients with de novo acute myeloid leukemia and t(9;11)(p22;q23) have a superior outcome to patients with other translocations involving band 11q23: a Cancer and Leukemia Group B study. Blood. 1997;90:4532–8.
26. Gröschel S, Schlenk RF, Engelmann J, Rockova V, Teleanu V, Kühn MW, et al. Deregulated expression of EVI1 defines a poor prognostic subset of MLL-rearranged acute myeloid leuke-

mias: a study of the German-Austrian Acute Myeloid Leukemia Study Group and the Dutch-Belgian-Swiss HOVON/SAKK Cooperative Group. J Clin Oncol. 2013;31(1):95–103.
27. Scandura JM, Boccuni P, Cammenga J, Nimer SD. Transcription factor fusions in acute leukemia: variations on a theme. Oncogene. 2002;21(21):3422–44.
28. Slovak ML, Gundacker H, Bloomfield CD, Dewald G, Appelbaum FR, Larson RA, et al. A retrospective study of 69 patients with t(6;9)(p23;q34) AML emphasizes the need for a prospective, multicenter initiative for rare 'poor prognosis' myeloid malignancies. Leukemia. 2006;20(7):1295–7.
29. Oyarzo MP, Lin P, Glassman A, Bueso-Ramos CE, Luthra R, Medeiros LJ. Acute myeloid leukemia with t(6;9)(p23;q34) is associated with dysplasia and a high frequency of flt3 gene mutations. Am J Clin Pathol. 2004;122(3):348–58.
30. Tarlock K, Alonzo TA, Moraleda PP, Gerbing RB, Raimondi SC, Hirsch BA, et al. Acute myeloid leukaemia (AML) with t(6;9)(p23;q34) is associated with poor outcome in childhood AML regardless of FLT3-ITD status: a report from the Children's Oncology Group. Br J Haematol. 2014;166(2):254–9.
31. Gröschel S, Sanders MA, Hoogenboezem R, de Wit E, Bouwman BAM, Erpelinck C, et al. A single oncogenic enhancer rearrangement causes concomitant EVI1 and GATA2 deregulation in leukemia. Cell. 2014;157(2):369–81.
32. Yamazaki H, Suzuki M, Otsuki A, Shimizu R, Bresnick EH, Engel JD, et al. A remote GATA2 hematopoietic enhancer drives leukemogenesis in inv(3)(q21;q26) by activating EVI1 expression. Cancer Cell. 2014;25(4):415–27.
33. Nucifora G, Laricchia-Robbio L, Senyuk V. EVI1 and hematopoietic disorders: history and perspectives. Gene. 2006;368:1–11.
34. Lugthart S, Gröschel S, Beverloo HB, Kayser S, Valk PJ, van Zelderen-Bhola SL, et al. Clinical, molecular, and prognostic significance of WHO type inv(3)(q21q26.2)/t(3;3)(q21;q26.2) and various other 3q abnormalities in acute myeloid leukemia. J Clin Oncol. 2010;28(24):3890–8.
35. Gröschel S, Sanders MA, Hoogenboezem R, Zeilemaker A, Havermans M, Erpelinck C, et al. Mutational spectrum of myeloid malignancies with inv(3)/t(3;3) reveals a predominant involvement of RAS/RTK signaling pathways. Blood. 2015;125(1):133–9.
36. Haferlach C, Bacher U, Haferlach T, Dicker F, Alpermann T, Kern W, et al. The inv(3)(q21q26)/t(3;3)(q21;q26) is frequently accompanied by alterations of the RUNX1, KRAS and NRAS and NF1 genes and mediates adverse prognosis both in MDS and in AML: a study in 39 cases of MDS or AML. Leukemia. 2011;25(5):874–7.
37. Ma Z, Morris SW, Valentine V, Li M, Herbrick JA, Cui X, et al. Fusion of two novel genes, RBM15 and MKL1, in the t(1;22)(p13;q13) of acute megakaryoblastic leukemia. Nat Genet. 2001;28(3):220–1.
38. Inaba H, Zhou Y, Abla O, Adachi S, Auvrignon A, Beverloo HB, et al. Heterogeneous cytogenetic subgroups and outcomes in childhood acute megakaryoblastic leukemia: a retrospective international study. Blood. 2015;126(13):1575–84.
39. Schweitzer J, Zimmermann M, Rasche M, von Neuhoff C, Creutzig U, Dworzak M, et al. Improved outcome of pediatric patients with acute megakaryoblastic leukemia in the AML-BFM 04 trial. Ann Hematol. 2015;94(8):1327–36.
40. Lindström MS. NPM1/B23: a multifunctional chaperone in ribosome biogenesis and chromatin remodeling. Biochem Res Int. 2011;2011:195209.
41. Colombo E, Marine JC, Danovi D, Falini B, Pelicci PG. Nucleophosmin regulates the stability and transcriptional activity of p53. Nat Cell Biol. 2002;4:529–33.
42. Falini B, Mecucci C, Tiacci E, Alcalay M, Rosati R, Pasqualucci L, et al. Cytoplasmic nucleophosmin in acute myelogenous leukemia with a normal karyotype. N Engl J Med. 2005;352(3):254–66.
43. Corces-Zimmerman MR, Hong WJ, Weissman IL, Medeiros BC, Majeti R. Preleukemic mutations in human acute myeloid leukemia affect epigenetic regulators and persist in remission. Proc Natl Acad Sci U S A. 2014;111(7):2548–53.
44. Shlush LI, Zandi S, Mitchell A, Chen WC, Brandwein JM, Gupta V, et al. Identification of pre-leukaemic haematopoietic stem cells in acute leukaemia. Nature. 2014;506(7488):328–33.

45. Falini B, Mecucci C, Saglio G, Lo Coco F, Diverio D, Brown P, et al. NPM1 mutations and cytoplasmic nucleophosmin are mutually exclusive of recurrent genetic abnormalities: a comparative analysis of 2562 patients with acute myeloid leukemia. Haematologica. 2008;93(3):439–42.
46. Haferlach C, Mecucci C, Schnittger S, Kohlmann A, Mancini M, Cuneo A, et al. AML with mutated NPM1 carrying a normal or aberrant karyotype show overlapping biologic, pathologic, immunophenotypic, and prognostic features. Blood. 2009;114(14):3024–32.
47. Cancer Genome Atlas Research Network, Ley TJ, Miller C, Ding L, Raphael BJ, Mungall AJ, et al. Genomic and epigenomic landscapes of adult de novo acute myeloid leukemia. N Engl J Med. 2013;368(22):2059–74.
48. Döhner K, Schlenk RF, Habdank M, Scholl C, Rücker FG, Corbacioglu A, et al. Mutant nucleophosmin (NPM1) predicts favorable prognosis in younger adults with acute myeloid leukemia and normal cytogenetics: interaction with other gene mutations. Blood. 2005;106(12):3740–6.
49. Falini B, Macijewski K, Weiss T, Bacher U, Schnittger S, Kern W, et al. Multilineage dysplasia has no impact on biologic, clinicopathologic, and prognostic features of AML with mutated nucleophosmin (NPM1). Blood. 2010;115(18):3776–86.
50. Schlenk RF, Döhner K, Krauter J, Fröhling S, Corbacioglu A, Bullinger L, et al. Mutations and treatment outcome in cytogenetically normal acute myeloid leukemia. N Engl J Med. 2008;358(18):1909–18.
51. Pratcorona M, Brunet S, Nomdedéu J, Ribera JM, Tormo M, Duarte R, et al. Favorable outcome of patients with acute myeloid leukemia harboring a low-allelic burden FLT3-ITD mutation and concomitant NPM1 mutation: relevance to post-remission therapy. Blood. 2013;121(14):2734–8.
52. Gale RE, Green C, Allen C, Mead AJ, Burnett AK, Hills RK, et al. The impact of FLT3 internal tandem duplication mutant level, number, size, and interaction with NPM1 mutations in a large cohort of young adult patients with acute myeloid leukemia. Blood. 2008;111(5):2776–84.
53. Schlenk RF, Kayser S, Bullinger L, Kobbe G, Casper J, Ringhoffer M, et al. Differential impact of allelic ratio and insertion site in FLT3-ITD-positive AML with respect to allogeneic transplantation. Blood. 2014;124(23):3441–9.
54. Loghavi S, Zuo Z, Ravandi F, Kantarjian HM, Bueso-Ramos C, Zhang L, et al. Clinical features of de novo acute myeloid leukemia with concurrent DNMT3A, FLT3 and NPM1 mutations. J Hematol Oncol. 2014;7:74.
55. Wouters BJ, Löwenberg B, Erpelinck-Verschueren CA, van Putten WL, Valk PJ, Delwel R. Double CEBPA mutations, but not single CEBPA mutations, define a subgroup of acute myeloid leukemia with a distinctive gene expression profile that is uniquely associated with a favorable outcome. Blood. 2009;113(13):3088–91.
56. Taskesen E, Bullinger L, Corbacioglu A, Sanders MA, Erpelinck CA, Wouters BJ, et al. Prognostic impact, concurrent genetic mutations, and gene expression features of AML with CEBPA mutations in a cohort of 1182 cytogenetically normal AML patients: further evidence for CEBPA double mutant AML as a distinctive disease entity. Blood. 2011;117(8):2469–75.
57. Renneville A, Boissel N, Gachard N, Naguib D, Bastard C, de Botton S, et al. The favorable impact of CEBPA mutations in patients with acute myeloid leukemia is only observed in the absence of associated cytogenetic abnormalities and FLT3 internal duplication. Blood. 2009;113(21):5090–3.
58. Green CL, Koo KK, Hills RK, Burnett AK, Linch DC, Gale RE. Prognostic significance of CEBPA mutations in a large cohort of younger adult patients with acute myeloid leukemia: impact of double CEBPA mutations and the interaction with FLT3 and NPM1 mutations. J Clin Oncol. 2010;28(16):2739–47.
59. Fasan A, Haferlach C, Alpermann T, Jeromin S, Grossmann V, Eder C, et al. The role of different genetic subtypes of CEBPA mutated AML. Leukemia. 2014;28(4):794–803.
60. Bacher U, Schnittger S, Macijewski K, Grossmann V, Kohlmann A, Alpermann T, et al. Multilineage dysplasia does not influence prognosis in CEBPA-mutated AML, supporting the WHO proposal to classify these patients as a unique entity. Blood. 2012;119(20):4719–22.

61. Paietta E, Racevskis J, Bennett JM, Neuberg D, Cassileth PA, Rowe JM, et al. Biologic heterogeneity in Philadelphia chromosome-positive acute leukemia with myeloid morphology: the Eastern Cooperative Oncology Group experience. Leukemia. 1998;12(12):1881–5.
62. Soupir CP, Vergilio JA, Dal Cin P, Muzikansky A, Kantarjian H, Jones D, et al. Philadelphia chromosome-positive acute myeloid leukemia: a rare aggressive leukemia with clinicopathologic features distinct from chronic myeloid leukemia in myeloid blast crisis. Am J Clin Pathol. 2007;127(4):642–50.
63. Konoplev S, Yin CC, Kornblau SM, Kantarjian HM, Konopleva M, Andreeff M, et al. Molecular characterization of de novo Philadelphia chromosome-positive acute myeloid leukemia. Leuk Lymphoma. 2013;54(1):138–44.
64. Haferlach T, Nagata Y, Grossmann V, Okuno Y, Bacher U, Nagae G, et al. Landscape of genetic lesions in 944 patients with myelodysplastic syndromes. Leukemia. 2014;28(2):241–7.
65. Papaemmanuil E, Gerstung M, Malcovati L, Tauro S, Gundem G, Van Loo P, et al. Clinical and biological implications of driver mutations in myelodysplastic syndromes. Blood. 2013;122(22):3616–27.
66. Weinberg OK, Seetharam M, Ren L, Seo K, Ma L, Merker JD, et al. Clinical characterization of acute myeloid leukemia with myelodysplasia-related changes as defined by the 2008 WHO classification system. Blood. 2009;113(9):1906–8.
67. Arber DA, Stein AS, Carter NH, Ikle D, Forman SJ, Slovak ML. Prognostic impact of acute myeloid leukemia classification. Importance of detection of recurring cytogenetic abnormalities and multilineage dysplasia on survival. Am J Clin Pathol. 2003;119(5):672–80.
68. Hasserjian RP, Campigotto F, Klepeis V, Fu B, Wang SA, Bueso-Ramos C, et al. De novo acute myeloid leukemia with 20–29% blasts is less aggressive than acute myeloid leukemia with ≥30% blasts in older adults: a Bone Marrow Pathology Group study. Am J Hematol. 2014;89(11):E193–9.
69. Lindsley RC, Mar BG, Mazzola E, Grauman PV, Shareef S, Allen SL, et al. Acute myeloid leukemia ontogeny is defined by distinct somatic mutations. Blood. 2015;125(9):1367–76.
70. Papaemmanuil E, Gerstung M, Bullinger L, Gaidzik VI, Paschka P, Roberts ND, et al. Genomic classification and prognosis in acute myeloid leukemia. N Engl J Med. 2016;374(23):2209–21.
71. Devillier R, Mansat-De Mas V, Gelsi-Boyer V, Demur C, Murati A, Corre J, et al. Role of ASXL1 and TP53 mutations in the molecular classification and prognosis of acute myeloid leukemias with myelodysplasia-related changes. Oncotarget. 2015;6(10):8388–96.
72. Ohgami RS, Ma L, Merker JD, Gotlib JR, Schrijver I, Zehnder JL, et al. Next-generation sequencing of acute myeloid leukemia identifies the significance of TP53, U2AF1, ASXL1, and TET2 mutations. Mod Pathol. 2015;28(5):706–14.
73. Morton LM, Dores GM, Tucker MA, Kim CJ, Onel K, Gilbert ES, et al. Evolving risk of therapy-related acute myeloid leukemia following cancer chemotherapy among adults in the United States, 1975–2008. Blood. 2013;121(15):2996–3004.
74. Radivoyevitch T, Sachs RK, Gale RP, Molenaar RJ, Brenner DJ, Hill BT, et al. Defining AML and MDS second cancer risk dynamics after diagnoses of first cancers treated or not with radiation. Leukemia. 2016;30(2):285–94.
75. Mauritzson N, Albin M, Rylander L, Billström R, Ahlgren T, Mikoczy Z, et al. Pooled analysis of clinical and cytogenetic features in treatment-related and de novo adult acute myeloid leukemia and myelodysplastic syndromes based on a consecutive series of 761 patients analyzed 1976–1993 and on 5098 unselected cases reported in the literature 1974–2001. Leukemia. 2002;16(12):2366–78.
76. Rowley JD, Olney HJ. International workshop on the relationship of prior therapy to balanced chromosome aberrations in therapy-related myelodysplastic syndromes and acute leukemia: overview report. Genes Chromosomes Cancer. 2002;33(4):331–45.
77. Kayser S, Döhner K, Krauter J, Köhne CH, Horst HA, Held G, et al. The impact of therapy-related acute myeloid leukemia (AML) on outcome in 2853 adult patients with newly diagnosed AML. Blood. 2011;117(7):2137–45.

78. Nardi V, Winkfield KM, Ok CY, Niemierko A, Kluk MJ, Attar EC, et al. Acute myeloid leukemia and myelodysplastic syndromes after radiation therapy are similar to de novo disease and differ from other therapy-related myeloid neoplasms. J Clin Oncol. 2012;30(19):2340–7.
79. Andersen MK, Larson RA, Mauritzson N, Schnittger S, Jhanwar SC, Pedersen-Bjergaard J. Balanced chromosome abnormalities inv(16) and t(15;17) in therapy-related myelodysplastic syndromes and acute leukemia: report from an international workshop. Genes Chromosomes Cancer. 2002;33(4):395–400.
80. Borthakur G, Lin E, Jain N, Estey EE, Cortes JE, O'Brien S, et al. Survival is poorer in patients with secondary core-binding factor acute myelogenous leukemia compared with de novo core-binding factor leukemia. Cancer. 2009;115(14):3217–21.
81. Ok CY, Patel KP, Garcia-Manero G, Routbort MJ, Fu B, Tang G, et al. Mutational profiling of therapy-related myelodysplastic syndromes and acute myeloid leukemia by next generation sequencing, a comparison with de novo diseases. Leuk Res. 2015;39(3):348–54.
82. Shih AH, Chung SS, Dolezal EK, Zhang SJ, Abdel-Wahab OI, Park CY, et al. Mutational analysis of therapy-related myelodysplastic syndromes and acute myelogenous leukemia. Haematologica. 2013;98(6):908–12.
83. Roy A, Cowan G, Mead AJ, Filippi S, Bohn G, Chaidos A, et al. Perturbation of fetal liver hematopoietic stem and progenitor cell development by trisomy 21. Proc Natl Acad Sci U S A. 2012;109(43):17579–84.
84. Tunstall-Pedoe O, Roy A, Karadimitris A, de la Fuente J, Fisk NM, Bennett P, et al. Abnormalities in the myeloid progenitor compartment in Down syndrome fetal liver precede acquisition of GATA1 mutations. Blood. 2008;112(12):4507–11.
85. Chou ST, Opalinska JB, Yao Y, Fernandes MA, Kalota A, Brooks JS, et al. Trisomy 21 enhances human fetal erythro-megakaryocytic development. Blood. 2008;112(12):4503–6.
86. Wechsler J, Greene M, McDevitt MA, Anastasi J, Karp JE, Le Beau MM, et al. Acquired mutations in GATA1 in the megakaryoblastic leukemia of Down syndrome. Nat Genet. 2002;32(1):148–52.
87. Alford KA, Reinhardt K, Garnett C, Norton A, Böhmer K, von Neuhoff C, et al. Analysis of GATA1 mutations in Down syndrome transient myeloproliferative disorder and myeloid leukemia. Blood. 2011;118(8):2222–38.
88. Roberts I, Alford K, Hall G, Juban G, Richmond H, Norton A, et al. GATA1-mutant clones are frequent and often unsuspected in babies with Down syndrome: identification of a population at risk of leukemia. Blood. 2013;122(24):3908–17.
89. Yoshida K, Toki T, Okuno Y, Kanezaki R, Shiraishi Y, Sato-Otsubo A, et al. The landscape of somatic mutations in Down syndrome-related myeloid disorders. Nat Genet. 2013;45(11):1293–9.
90. Nikolaev SI, Santoni F, Vannier A, Falconnet E, Giarin E, Basso G, et al. Exome sequencing identifies putative drivers of progression of transient myeloproliferative disorder to AMKL in infants with Down syndrome. Blood. 2013;122(4):554–61.
91. Hasle H, Niemeyer CM, Chessells JM, Baumann I, Bennett JM, Kerndrup G, et al. A pediatric approach to the WHO classification of myelodysplastic and myeloproliferative diseases. Leukemia. 2003;17(2):277–82.
92. Bolouri H, Farrar JE, Triche T Jr, Ries RE, Lim EL, Alonzo TA, et al. The molecular landscape of pediatric acute myeloid leukemia reveals recurrent structural alterations and age-specific mutational interactions. Nat Med. 2018;24(1):103–12.
93. Harrison CJ, Hills RK, Moorman AV, Grimwade DJ, Hann I, Webb DK, et al. Cytogenetics of childhood acute myeloid leukemia: United Kingdom Medical Research Council Treatment trials AML 10 and 12. J Clin Oncol. 2010;28(16):2674–81.
94. von Neuhoff C, Reinhardt D, Sander A, Zimmermann M, Bradtke J, Betts DR, et al. Prognostic impact of specific chromosomal aberrations in a large group of pediatric patients with acute myeloid leukemia treated uniformly according to trial AML-BFM 98. J Clin Oncol. 2010;28(16):2682–9.

95. Sandahl JD, Kjeldsen E, Abrahamsson J, Ha SY, Heldrup J, Jahnukainen K, et al. Ploidy and clinical characteristics of childhood acute myeloid leukemia: a NOPHO-AML study. Genes Chromosomes Cancer. 2014;53(8):667–75.
96. Rasche M, von Neuhoff C, Dworzak M, Bourquin JP, Bradtke J, Göhring G, et al. Genotype-outcome correlations in pediatric AML: the impact of a monosomal karyotype in trial AML-BFM 2004. Leukemia. 2017;31(12):2807–14.
97. Balgobind BV, Raimondi SC, Harbott J, Zimmermann M, Alonzo TA, Auvrignon A, et al. Novel prognostic subgroups in childhood 11q23/MLL-rearranged acute myeloid leukemia: results of an international retrospective study. Blood. 2009;114(12):2489–96.
98. Huret JL, Brizard A, Slater R, Charrin C, Bertheas MF, Guilgot F, et al. Cytogenetic heterogeneity in t(11;19) acute leukemia: clinical, hematological and cytogenetic analyses of 48 patients—updated published cases and 16 new observations. Leukemia. 1993;7(2):152–60.

Chapter 15
Chronic Myeloid Neoplasms

Maria E. Arcila and Caleb Ho

Key Points

- The detection of relevant gene mutations can aid in the diagnosis and classification of chronic myeloid neoplasm, but the finding alone is insufficient for definitive diagnosis, and peripheral blood counts and marrow morphologic findings remain crucial.
- With the appropriate clinical context and peripheral blood findings, certain gene rearrangements/translocations (e.g., *BCR-ABL1*, *PDGFRA/B* rearrangements) and chromosomal level losses or gains are diagnostic of myeloid neoplasms.
- While mutations in certain genes (e.g., *DNMT3A*, *TET2*, *ASXL1*) can be found in a variety of chronic myeloid neoplasms, others (e.g., *JAK2*, *CALR*, *SF3B1*) are more associated with particular types of myeloid neoplasms.

Key Online Resources

- US National Library of Medicine Genetics Home Reference: https://ghr.nlm.nih.gov/condition
- Leukemia and Lymphoma Society Free Publications: https://www.lls.org/resource-center/download-or-order-free-publications
- National Comprehensive Cancer Network Clinical Guidelines: https://www.nccn.org/professionals/physician_gls/default.aspx

M. E. Arcila (✉) · C. Ho
Department of Pathology, Memorial Sloan Kettering Cancer Center, New York, NY, USA
e-mail: arcilam@mskcc.org; hoc@mskcc.org

L. J. Tafe, M. E. Arcila (eds.), *Genomic Medicine*,
https://doi.org/10.1007/978-3-030-22922-1_15

Introduction

Chronic myeloid neoplasms are a heterogenous group of disorders encompassing several disease subgroups. The discovery of genetic alterations affecting a core set of genes has revolutionized our overall understanding and diagnostic approach of this group of diseases. However, significant overlap exists among subgroups, such that the ultimate diagnosis and subclassification rely on an integrated multimodality approach that carefully incorporates the clinical, morphologic, and genetic features of each case. Based on the revised World Health Organization classification of tumors of hematopoietic and lymphoid tissues (WHO 2016) [1], chronic myeloid neoplasms can be broadly classified into five major categories:

myelodysplastic syndromes (MDS), myeloproliferative neoplasms (MPN), overlap syndromes (MDS/MPN), mastocytosis, and myeloid neoplasms associated with eosinophilia and abnormalities of PDGFR (A or B) or FGFR1. Each of the major categories is further subdivided into subcategories as summarized in Table 15.1.

Table 15.1 General categorization of chronic myeloid neoplasms

Category	Subcategory
Myeloproliferative neoplasms (MPN)	Chronic myeloid leukemia (CML), BCR-ABL1 positive Chronic neutrophilic leukemia (CNL) Polycythemia vera (PV) Primary myelofibrosis (PMF) Essential thrombocythemia (ET) Chronic eosinophilic leukemia, not otherwise specified (CEL, NOS) Myeloproliferative neoplasm, unclassifiable (MPN-U)
Mastocytosis	Cutaneous mastocytosis (CM) Systemic mastocytosis (SM) Systemic mastocytosis with associated hematologic neoplasm (SM-AHN) Mast cell leukemia
Myeloid/lymphoid neoplasms with eosinophilia and gene rearrangement	Myeloid/lymphoid neoplasms with PDGFRA rearrangement Myeloid/lymphoid neoplasms with PDGFRB rearrangement Myeloid/lymphoid neoplasms with FGFR1 rearrangement Provisional entity: myeloid/lymphoid neoplasms with PCM1-JAK2
Myelodysplastic/myeloproliferative neoplasms (MDS/MPN)	Chronic myelomonocytic leukemia(CMML) Atypical chronic myeloid leukemia (aCML), BCR-ABL1-negative Juvenile myelomonocytic leukemia (JMML) Myelodysplastic/myeloproliferative neoplasm with ring sideroblasts and thrombocytosis (MDS/MPN-RS-T) Myelodysplastic/myeloproliferative neoplasm, unclassifiable (MDS/MPN-U)

Table 15.1 (continued)

Category	Subcategory
Myelodysplastic syndromes (MDS)	Myelodysplastic syndrome with single lineage dysplasia Myelodysplastic syndrome with ring sideroblasts Myelodysplastic syndrome with multilineage dysplasia Myelodysplastic syndrome with excess blasts Myelodysplastic syndrome with excess blasts and erythroid predominance Myelodysplastic syndrome with excess blasts and fibrosis Myelodysplastic syndrome with isolated del(5q) Myelodysplastic syndrome, unclassifiable Childhood myelodysplastic syndrome Refractory cytopenia of childhood

Myeloproliferative Neoplasms (MPNs)

Myeloproliferative neoplasms are clonal hematopoietic disorders characterized by the proliferation of cells in one or more of the myeloid lineages. Patients most often present with variable age-matched bone marrow hypercellularity, with proliferation of one or more marrow hematopoietic lineages characterized and effective maturation, leading to increased number of myeloid elements, red blood cells, and/or platelets in the peripheral blood (cytosis). All MPNs, although insidious in the mode of onset, have the potential to progress to bone marrow failure related to myelofibrosis or to transform to acute leukemia.

Most MPNs are associated with genetic abnormalities affecting protein tyrosine kinases. Activating genetic abnormalities include translocations, insertions, deletions, and point mutations in several genes (summarized in Table 15.2). *BCR-ABL1* fusions are identified in most patients with chronic myeloid leukemia (CML). At diagnosis, 90–95% of cases have the characteristic t(9;22)(q34;q11) translocation [2] which results in the formation of the Philadelphia chromosome (Ph) and gives rise to the *BCR-ABL1* fusion gene [2–5]. The alteration can be detected by routine cytogenetics, FISH, or RT-PCR [6]. In a small proportion of cases, more complex chromosomal abnormalities or cryptic translocations may be involved, which mask translocation detection by routine cytogenetic assessment, but the fusion is detectable by FISH or RT-PCR (depending on assay design) [6]. The breakpoint region within the *BCR* gene can vary, generating proteins of different sizes which influence the phenotype of the disease. The most common protein is the p210 (210 kDa). Rarely, a p230 kDa fusion protein is encoded and is often associated with prominent neutrophilic maturation and/or thrombocytosis [6, 7]. The p190 (190 kDa) protein is seen in a small proportion of cases as the predominant fusion and is associated with an increased number of monocytes [8]. All fusions lead to constitutive activation of the kinase and confer sensitivity to imatinib and other specific kinase inhibitors

Table 15.2 Common molecular and cytogenetic alterations associated with myeloproliferative neoplasms

Myeloproliferative neoplasms	Common molecular alterations	Common cytogenetic abnormalities
Chronic myeloid leukemia (CML)	BCR-ABL1 fusions	t(9, 22)(q34;q11)
Chronic neutrophilic leukemia (CNL)	CSF3R alone or together with SETBP or ASXL1	
Polycythemia vera (PV)	JAK2 p.V617F or JAK2 exon 12[a]	+8,+9,9p−,13q−,20q−
Primary myelofibrosis (PMF)	Major clonal mutations: JAK2 (50–60%), CALR (30%), or MPL (8%)[a]	20q−, 1q+, +8, +9, 13q−, and der(6) t(1;6) strongly suggestive of PMF
Essential thrombocythemia (ET)	Major clonal mutations: JAK2 (50–60%), CALR (30%), or MPL (3%)[a]	+8, +9, 20q−
Chronic eosinophilic leukemia (CEL), NOS	No disease-specific mutation, but demonstration of somatic mutation associated with myeloid neoplasms provides evidence of clonality[a]	+8, 7−, Iso17q,
Myeloproliferative neoplasm, unclassifiable (MPN-U)	No disease-specific mutation, but demonstration of somatic mutation associated with myeloid neoplasms provides evidence of clonality[a]	

[a]Examples of other mutations associated with myeloid neoplasms: *ASXL1*, *EZH2*, *TET2*, *IDH1*, *IDH2*, *SRSF2*, and *SF3B1*

[9–11]. Following treatment, some patients may acquire point mutations in *ABL1* which confer resistance to ABL kinase inhibitors [12]. Disease progression is associated with clonal evolution. At the time of transformation to accelerated or blast phase, approximately 80% of patients show additional cytogenetic changes, including isochromosome 17q, gains of chromosomes 8 and/ or 19, and extra copies of the Ph chromosome. Other alterations are reported in the transformed stages of CML, affecting *TP53*, *RB1*, *MYC*, *CDKN2A*, *NRAS*, *KRAS*, *RUNX1*, *EVI1*, *TET2*, *CBL*, *ASXL1*, *IDH1*, and *IDH2* genes. Their role in transformation is not well defined [13, 14].

Among MPNs that are *BCR-ABL1* negative, mutations affecting one of four genes – *JAK2*, *MPL*, *CALR*, and *CSF3R* – have been shown to induce the MPN phenotype [15]. Mutations in any of these genes are associated with constitutive activation of common downstream signaling pathways – STAT, PI3K, and MAPK – as outlined in Fig. 15.1. *JAK2* mutations are the most important and most frequently occurring [16]. Although present in virtually all cases of polycythemia vera (PV), *JAK2* mutations are not unique to this entity and are found in 50–60% of cases of primary myelofibrosis (PMF) and essential thrombocythemia (ET) [17]. They may also be present in small subsets of acute myeloid leukemia (AML), MDS, MDS/MPN such as chronic myelomonocytic leukemia (CMML), other myeloid

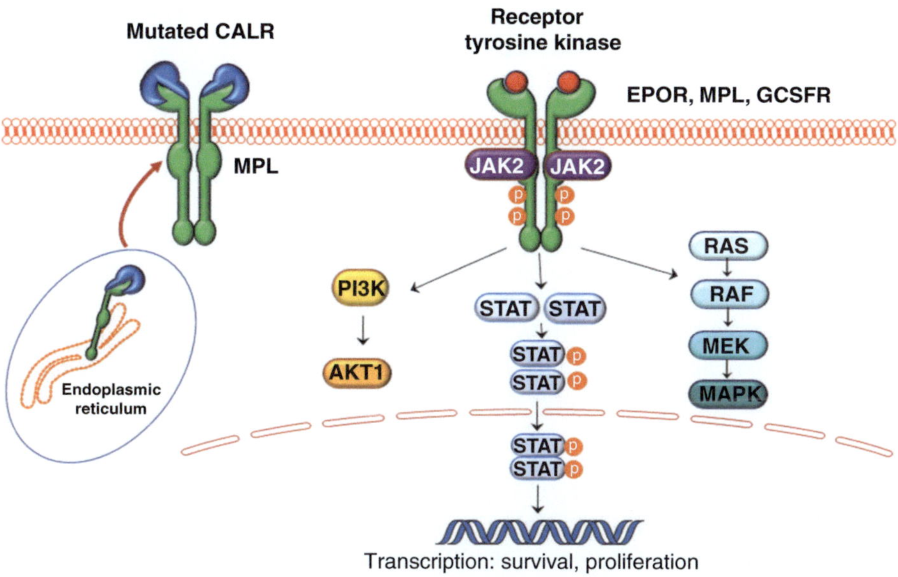

Fig. 15.1 Mutations in JAK2, CALR, MPL, and CSF3R are associated with constitutive activation of common downstream signaling pathways – STAT, PI3K, and MAPK. JAK2 is a kinase protein that associates with the cytoplasmic portions of various membrane-bound receptors including EPOR (receptor for erythropoietin), MPL (receptor for thrombopoietin), and G-CSFR (receptor for granulocyte/macrophage colony-stimulating factor). Mutated JAK2 renders the protein constitutively active with subsequent downstream activation of intracellular signaling. Mutations in CALR lead to formation of MPL-CALR complexes in the endoplasmic reticulum which then travel to the cell surface. Complexing of MPL with mutated CALR or mutations in the MPL receptor itself lead to constitutive activation of MPL and deregulated downstream signaling

neoplasms, clonal hematopoiesis of indeterminate potential (CHIP), and even B-lymphoblastic leukemia (B-ALL) [18]. Of the pathogenic *JAK2* mutations, the p.V617F mutation is by far the most common, constituting over 95% of cases. Variants involving other locations of *JAK2* have been reported in small proportion of PV (*JAK2* exon 12) and in B-ALL (*JAK2* exon 14) [15].

Mutations in *CALR* occur in 20–35% of patients with ET and PMF and are generally mutually exclusive with *JAK2* mutations, although rare exceptions do occur [19–21]. Known pathogenic *CALR* mutations are mostly insertions/deletions located within exon 9, giving rise to frameshifts that alter the reading frame of the protein and primarily affect the C-terminal sequence. The most common *CALR* exon 9 alterations include a 52bp deletion (known in the literature as Type 1 mutation) and a 5bp insertion (Type 2 mutation) [22]. Alterations in *MPL* are less frequent and identified in less than 10% of ET and PMF. The most common pathogenic mutations affect the W515 position and lead to constitutive activation of MPL [23–26].

In addition to the major phenotypic driver mutations (*CALR*, *JAK2*, and *MPL*), there is emerging evidence of several other somatic alterations which may coexist and enhance the effect of the driver mutations [27]. Affected genes function as epigenetic regulators, transcription factors, or signaling molecules (including *ASXL1*, *EZH2*, *TET2*, *IDH1/2*, *SRSF2*, *SF3B1*, and others) which alone are not defining of any particular subtype of MPN and are common to other myeloid neoplasms, such as MDS and acute leukemias. Poor survival and increased risk of leukemic transformation correlate with increasing number of somatic alterations in these patient [21, 28]. Similar mutations may also be present in the absence of the major driver mutations, in approximately 10–20% of PMF and ET (so-called triple negative MPNs). Detection of these genetic alterations may help establish the clonal nature of the process and would facilitate the diagnosis of MPN, provided that other clinical and pathologic criteria are met.

Activating mutations in the gene encoding a granulocyte colony-stimulating factor (G-CSF) receptor, *CSF3R*, which also signals through JAK2, are strongly associated with chronic neutrophilic leukemia (CNL). Mutations cluster in the extracellular domain of the gene [29, 30] and are often identified in conjunction with alterations in *SETBP1* or *ASXL1* [29, 31]. The coexistence of *ASXL1* mutations is associated with worse prognosis [32].

In addition to the mutations and fusions described, cytogenetic abnormalities are also common in MPNs. They are identified in approximately 20% of cases at the time of diagnosis and increase in later stages of each disease, in association with myelofibrosis leukemic transformation [33]. Common abnormalities are summarized in Table 15.2.

Mastocytosis

Mastocytosis is a distinct subset of hematopoietic disorders characterized by the abnormal growth and accumulation of mast cells (MC) in one or more organ system. Some major subtypes include cutaneous mastocytosis (with only skin involvement), systemic mastocytosis (almost always with bone marrow involvement), and mast cell leukemia. Clinical symptoms of the disease usually occur as a result of the pathologic infiltration and the release of chemical mediators in the various tissues affected. Acquired alterations in the *KIT* gene are described in a large proportion of patients [34, 35]. The most common mutation is the p.D816V, but other mutations have also been reported. Patients with aggressive systemic mastocytosis and systemic mastocytosis with an associated hematologic neoplasm (SM-AHN) may have additional mutations in other genes commonly associated with myeloid neoplasms, such as *TET2*, *SRSF2*, *ASXL1*, *CBL*, *RUNX1*, and *RAS* [36–39]. Similar to other myeloid neoplasms, the accumulation of other mutations appears to be of prognostic significance [40].

Myeloid/Lymphoid Neoplasms with Eosinophilia and Gene Rearrangements

This subcategory includes three specific disease subgroups and a provisional entity as outlined in Table 15.1. Eosinophilia, while proclaimed a characteristic feature of all entities in this category, is not necessarily invariable, and classification relies heavily on the presence of a fusion involving *PDGFRA*, *PDGFRB*, *FGFR1*, or *JAK2*. Importantly, however, while classification increasingly relies on molecular markers, the diagnosis must still be made in conjunction with the histomorphology and clinical and laboratory criteria, as similar fusions can be found in other entities as well. Clinicopathologic presentation may also vary widely. In addition to myeloproliferative neoplasms (MPN), patients can present with myelodysplastic syndrome/MPN, as well as de novo or secondary mixed-phenotype leukemias, making the diagnosis of these entities highly complex.

In addition to the diagnostic value, the accurate detection of fusions in this category is important for treatment and prognostic assessment. Neoplasms with *PDGFRA*- and *PDGFRB*-rearrangements are sensitive to the tyrosine kinase inhibitor imatinib and have better prognosis. In contrast, patients with *FGFR1* and *JAK2* fusion TK genes exhibit a more aggressive course and variable sensitivity to current TK inhibitors. Multiple fusions involving PDGFRA, PDGFRB, and FGFR1 have been described in the literature. The *FIP1L1-PDGFRA* fusion gene was the first fusion described for PDGFRA [41]. Seven additional fusion partners have also been reported, including *BCR*, *ETV6*, *KIF5B*, *CDK5RAP2*, *STRN*, *TNKS2*, and *FOXP1* [42]. For PDGFRB, more than 30 partners have been reported, with ETV6 as the first described and most common partner [43]. At least 14 fusion partners have been reported for FGRF1, *ZMYM2*, *CNTRL*, and *FGFR1OP* are the most common [44].

Myeloid and lymphoid neoplasms associated with fusions of *JAK2* partnering with *PCM1* share characteristic features that have justified their recent recognition as a provisional entity under the last update of the WHO classification. More recently, other *JAK2* fusion variants involving *ETV6* and *BCR* as partners have also been reported and may be considered variants of this provisional entity [45].

Myelodysplastic/Myeloproliferative Neoplasms (MDS/MPN)

This subcategory includes five disease entities with overlapping clinical and pathologic features of myelodysplastic and myeloproliferative neoplasms [46]. The marrow findings are characterized by effective proliferation of at least one hematopoietic lineage, as well as an ineffective proliferation of another lineage, leading to the presence of both cytosis and cytopenia in different lineages in the peripheral blood. Most mutations reported in this category are not disease specific. To further complicate the interpretation, many of these mutations may also be found in patients with CHIP and who do not meet criteria for a myeloid neoplasm. Genetic changes must be interpreted with caution and in the context for the clinical, laboratory findings, such as peripheral blood counts, and marrow and peripheral blood morphologic findings.

Chronic myelomonocytic leukemia (CMML) is characterized by a proliferation of monocytic lineage precursors, resulting in relative and absolute monocytosis in the peripheral blood, usually in combination with anemia and/or thrombocytopenia. The most common somatic mutations found in CMML include *ASXL1*, *TET2*, and *SRSF2* [46–50]. *Other less frequent mutations include those in NRAS*, *KRAS*, *CBL*, *RUNX1*, and *SETBP1*. Although none is specific to CMML, the detection of these mutations in a patient may aid in the separation of CMML from other myeloid neoplasms with reactive monocytosis.

Atypical chronic myeloid leukemia (aCML) is characterized by proliferation of myeloid precursors, leading to leukocytosis with left-shifted granulocytes in the peripheral blood, without significant relative monocytosis, and usually in combination with anemia and/or thrombocytopenia. Mutations in *ETNK1* are found in a significant subset of aCML cases [51] and can aid in separation from CNL, a MPN that is a major differential diagnosis from aCML. *Mutations in SETBP1* are also common in aCML and are associated with an increase in white blood cell count and with poor prognosis [52]. The most common alterations for the MDS/MPN entities are summarized in Table 15.3.

Table 15.3 Common molecular alterations associated with myelodysplastic/myeloproliferative neoplasms

Myelodysplastic/myeloproliferative neoplasms	Common alterations
Chronic myelomonocytic leukemia (CMML)	ASXL1, TET2, SRSF2, RUNX1, NRAS, KRAS, CBL, SETBP1
Atypical chronic myeloid leukemia (aCML) (BCR-ABL1 negative)	SETBP1, ETNK1
Juvenile myelomonocytic leukemia (JMML)	PTPN11, KRAS, NRAS, CBL, NF1
Myelodysplastic/myeloproliferative neoplasms with ring sideroblasts and thrombocytosis (MDS/MPN-RS-T)	SF3B1 with or without JAK2 p.V617F, less commonly with MPL p.W515K/L
Myelodysplastic/myeloproliferative neoplasm, unclassifiable (MDS/MPN-U)	No disease-specific mutation, but demonstration of somatic mutation associated with myeloid neoplasms provides evidence of clonality[a]

[a]Examples of mutations associated with myeloid neoplasms: *JAK2*, *CALR*, *MPL*, *ASXL1*, *EZH2*, *TET2*, *IDH1*, *IDH2*, *SRSF2*, and *SF3B1*

Myelodysplastic Syndrome (MDS)

Myelodysplastic syndrome is a group of myeloid neoplasms characterized by dysplasia in one or more of the major myeloid lineages, leading to ineffective hematopoiesis in corresponding marrow hematopoietic lineages, and peripheral cytopenias. In a significant portion of the patients, MDS is associated with recurrent genetic abnormalities. Genetic alterations play a critical role in the risk stratification of patients, together with the blast count and the degree of cytopenias. Both somatic mutations and cytogenetic abnormalities are common in MDS and, when combined, are present in over 90% of the cases. Although somatic mutations are not formally incorporated into the diagnostic criteria for MDS in the revised WHO classification (Ref: WHO, 2016), they serve as supportive evidence in the proper clinical context and marrow morphologic findings [1]. Despite the high prevalence of genetic alterations in these diseases, the diagnosis and subclassification of MDS remain challenging, due to the high clinical and genetic heterogeneity that is typical of this myeloid disease category. None of the mutations involved are pathognomonic for MDS, nor present in more than 25% of patients. Importantly, a subset of the mutations can also be detected in a large proportion of healthy older individuals, a phenomenon known as CHIP [53, 54].

The most common somatic mutations and recurrent cytogenetics abnormalities associated with MDS are summarized in Table 15.4 [55–57].

At present, a definitive diagnosis of MDS in a patient with clinical cytopenia requires the demonstration of significant morphologic features of dysplasia in one or more hematopoietic cell lineage or MDS-defining cytogenetic abnormalities. Since morphologic dysplasia can also be seen in a variety of nonneoplastic conditions, such as chemotherapy for solid malignancies, medication use, nutritional deficiency, chronic inflammatory/autoimmune conditions, and certain infectious processes, those processes must be excluded before a confident diagnosis of MDS can be rendered. Cytogenetic abnormalities have been fully integrated as part of the prognostic scoring of patients with MDS. The current comprehensive cytogenetic scoring system (CCSS) contains five prognostic subgroups which are summarized in Fig. 15.2[58]. These are further incorporated into the revised International Prognosis Scoring System (IPSS-R) which factors in the percent of bone marrow blasts and the degree of cytopenia to predict survival risk of evolution to AML (Table 15.5) [59]. For patients with normal cytogenetics and lacking distinctive features of dysplasia, ring sideroblasts, or increased blasts, the diagnosis of MDS cannot be rendered with the current diagnostic criteria, despite the presence of cytopenias.

Mutations in MDS are identified in numerous genes which can be divided into several categories based on their general function (summarized in

Table 15.4 Common molecular and cytogenetic alterations associated with myelodysplastic syndromes

Myelodysplastic syndromes	Most common mutated genes	Recurrent unbalanced cytogenetic abnormalities
Myelodysplastic syndrome (MDS) –general	ASXL1, CBL, DNMT3A, EZH2, IDH1, IDH2, KRAS, NRAS, RUNX1, SETBP1, STAG2, SRSF2, TET2, TP53, U2AF1, ZRSR2	Monosomy 5/deletion 5q Monosomy 7/deletion 7q Deletion 11q Deletion 12p/translocation 12p Monosomy 13/deletion 13q Iso (17q)/translocation 17p Idic(X)(q13) Trisomy 8[a] Deletion 20q[a] Loss of Chr. Y[a] Complex karyotype (≥3 abnormalities)
Myelodysplastic syndrome with ring sideroblasts and single lineage dysplasia or multilineage dysplasia (MDS-RS-SLD or MDS-RS-MLD)	SF3B1	See MDS – general above
Myelodysplastic syndrome with isolated del (5q)	See MDS – general above	Isolated deletion 5q or deletion 5q in combination with only one other chromosomal abnormality not involving chr. 7

[a]These cytogenetics abnormalities alone are insufficient for a diagnosis of MDS in the absence of significant morphologic dysplasia

Fig. 15.3). Mutations affect genes in a defined hierarchical fashion [55–57, 60]. Mutations in genes that encode epigenetic modifiers (*DNMT3A*, *TET2*, *ASXL1*, *EZH2*, etc.) or RNA splicing factors (*SF3B1*, *U2AF1*, and *SRSF2*), for example, tend to arise during the early phase of disease. Acquisition of additional mutations in genes that drive growth factor signaling pathways (*NRAS*, *KRAS*, *PTPN11*, *FLT3*, etc.) occurs during later stages. The accumulation of more somatic mutations generally correlates with worse prognosis [60–63]. There is also mutual exclusivity of alterations affecting genes in the same category. Point mutations in genes coding splicing factors, for instance, rarely co-occur in the same patient, and similar findings have been described for the cohesion genes [64, 65]. Conversely, mutations in *TP53* and *PPM1D*, which are frequently associated with therapy-related myeloid neoplasms, are known to co-occur [66].

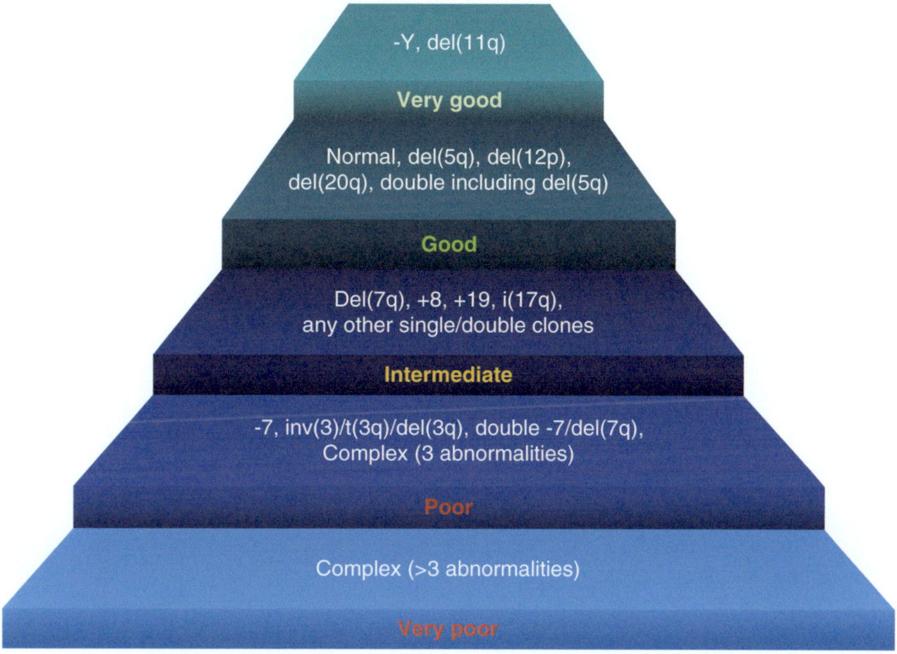

Fig. 15.2 Comprehensive cytogenetic scoring system for myelodysplastic syndromes. Each patient is stratified into one of the five prognostic groups based on cytogenetics abnormalities. Complex cytogenetics findings (three or more distinct abnormalities) are associated with poor or very poor prognoses [58]

Table 15.5 International prognostic scoring system revised (IPSS-R) [59,67,68]

Risk category	**Risk score**			**Median survival (years)**			
Very low	≤1.5			8.8			
Low	>1.5 but ≤3.0			5.8			
Intermediate	>3.0 but ≤4.5			3.0			
High	>4.5 but ≤6.0			1.6			
Very high	>6.0			0.8			
Variable	**Score**						
	0	0.5	1.0	1.5	2	3	4
Cytogenetics Category	Very good		Good		Intermediate	Poor	Very poor
Bone marrow blasts (%)	≤2		>2 but <5		5–10	>10	
Absolute neutrophil count (10^9/L)	≥0.8	<0.8					
Hemoglobin (g/dL)	≥10		≥8 but <10	<8			
Platelets (10^9/L)	≥100	≥50 but <100	<50				

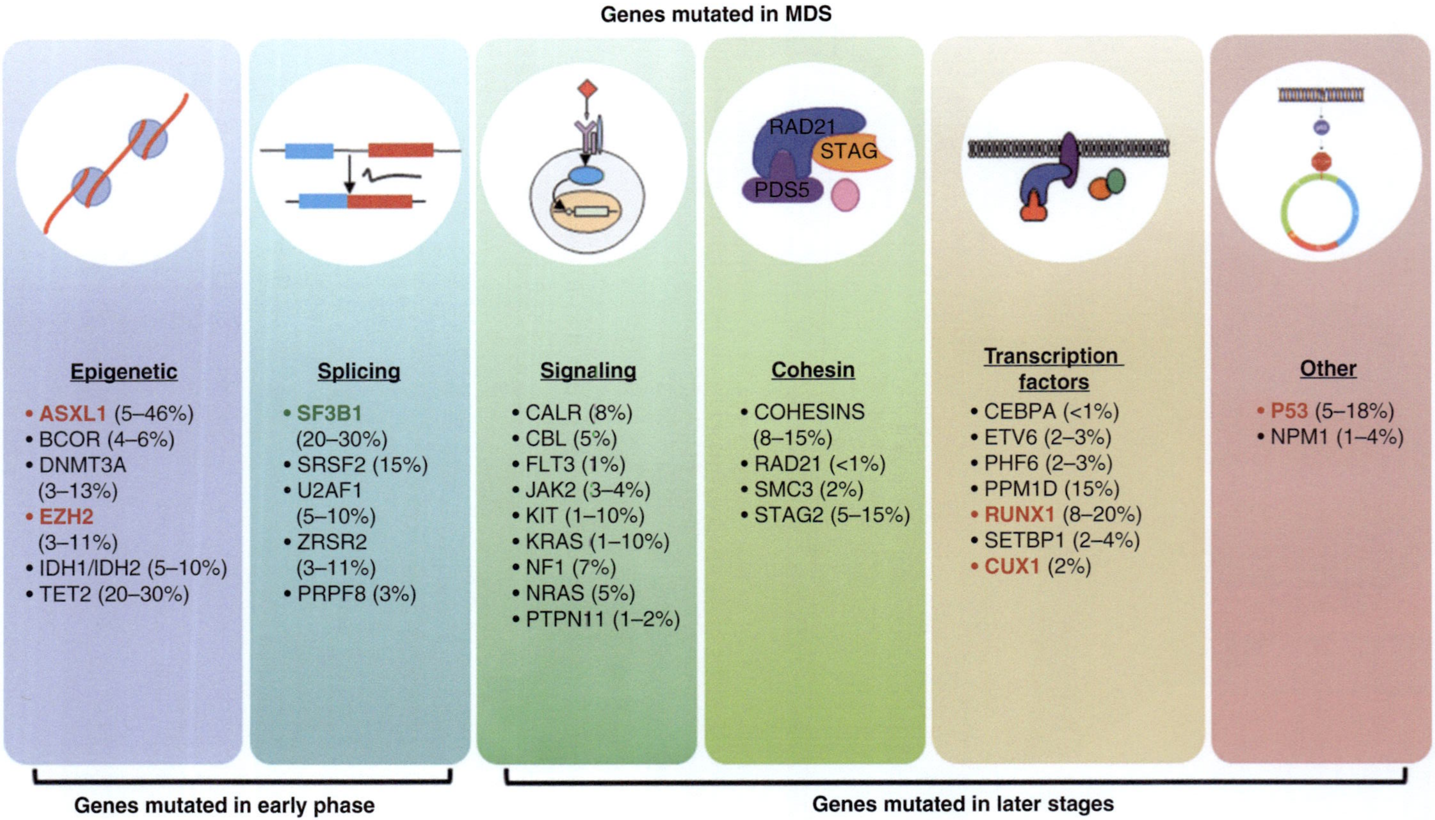

Fig. 15.3 Genes commonly mutated in myelodysplastic syndromes stratified by their general function including epigenetic regulation, RNA splicing, signaling pathways, cohesin complex, and transcription factors. Genes bolded in green are categorized as IPSS-independent good prognostic indicator, and those bolded in red are IPSS-independent poor prognostic indicator. Other genes have no clear role as independent prognosticator

References

1. Arber DA, Orazi A, Hasserjian R, Thiele J, Borowitz MJ, Le Beau MM, Bloomfield CD, Cazzola M, Vardiman JW. The 2016 revision to the World Health Organization classification of myeloid neoplasms and acute leukemia. Blood. 2016;127:2391–405.
2. Rowley JD. Letter: a new consistent chromosomal abnormality in chronic myelogenous leukaemia identified by quinacrine fluorescence and Giemsa staining. Nature. 1973;243:290–3.
3. Bartram CR, de Klein A, Hagemeijer A, van Agthoven T, Geurts van Kessel A, Bootsma D, Grosveld G, Ferguson-Smith MA, Davies T, Stone M, et al. Translocation of c-ab1 oncogene correlates with the presence of a Philadelphia chromosome in chronic myelocytic leukaemia. Nature. 1983;306:277–80.
4. Melo JV, Barnes DJ. Chronic myeloid leukaemia as a model of disease evolution in human cancer. Nat Rev Cancer. 2007;7:441–53.
5. Nowell PC, Hungerford DA. Chromosome studies on normal and leukemic human leukocytes. J Natl Cancer Inst. 1960;25:85–109.
6. Melo JV. The diversity of BCR-ABL fusion proteins and their relationship to leukemia phenotype. Blood. 1996;88:2375–84.
7. Pane F, Frigeri F, Sindona M, Luciano L, Ferrara F, Cimino R, Meloni G, Saglio G, Salvatore F, Rotoli B. Neutrophilic-chronic myeloid leukemia: a distinct disease with a specific molecular marker (BCR/ABL with C3/A2 junction). Blood. 1996;88:2410–4.
8. Melo JV, Myint H, Galton DA, Goldman JM. P190BCR-ABL chronic myeloid leukaemia: the missing link with chronic myelomonocytic leukaemia. Leukemia. 1994;8:208–11.
9. Druker BJ, Talpaz M, Resta DJ, Peng B, Buchdunger E, Ford JM, Lydon NB, Kantarjian H, Capdeville R, Ohno-Jones S, Sawyers CL. Efficacy and safety of a specific inhibitor of the BCR-ABL tyrosine kinase in chronic myeloid leukemia. N Engl J Med. 2001;344:1031–7.
10. Druker BJ, Tamura S, Buchdunger E, Ohno S, Segal GM, Fanning S, Zimmermann J, Lydon NB. Effects of a selective inhibitor of the Abl tyrosine kinase on the growth of Bcr-Abl positive cells. Nat Med. 1996;2:561–6.
11. Weisberg E, Manley PW, Cowan-Jacob SW, Hochhaus A, Griffin JD. Second generation inhibitors of BCR-ABL for the treatment of imatinib-resistant chronic myeloid leukaemia. Nat Rev Cancer. 2007;7:345–56.
12. Apperley JF. Part I: mechanisms of resistance to imatinib in chronic myeloid leukaemia. Lancet Oncol. 2007;8:1018–29.
13. Makishima H, Jankowska AM, McDevitt MA, O'Keefe C, Dujardin S, Cazzolli H, Przychodzen B, Prince C, Nicoll J, Siddaiah H, Shaik M, Szpurka H, Hsi E, Advani A, Paquette R, Maciejewski JP. CBL, CBLB, TET2, ASXL1, and IDH1/2 mutations and additional chromosomal aberrations constitute molecular events in chronic myelogenous leukemia. Blood. 2011;117:e198–206.
14. Soverini S, de Benedittis C, Mancini M, Martinelli G. Mutations in the BCR-ABL1 kinase domain and elsewhere in chronic myeloid leukemia. Clin Lymphoma Myeloma Leuk. 2015;15 Suppl:S120–8.
15. Skoda RC, Duek A, Grisouard J. Pathogenesis of myeloproliferative neoplasms. Exp Hematol. 2015;43:599–608.
16. Kralovics R, Passamonti F, Buser AS, Teo SS, Tiedt R, Passweg JR, Tichelli A, Cazzola M, Skoda RC. A gain-of-function mutation of JAK2 in myeloproliferative disorders. N Engl J Med. 2005;352:1779–90.
17. Tefferi A, Guglielmelli P, Larson DR, Finke C, Wassie EA, Pieri L, Gangat N, Fjerza R, Belachew AA, Lasho TL, Ketterling RP, Hanson CA, Rambaldi A, Finazzi G, Thiele J, Barbui T, Pardanani A, Vannucchi AM. Long-term survival and blast transformation in molecularly annotated essential thrombocythemia, polycythemia vera, and myelofibrosis. Blood. 2014;124:2507–13; quiz 2615.

18. Steensma DP, Dewald GW, Lasho TL, Powell HL, McClure RF, Levine RL, Gilliland DG, Tefferi A. The JAK2 V617F activating tyrosine kinase mutation is an infrequent event in both "atypical" myeloproliferative disorders and myelodysplastic syndromes. Blood. 2005;106:1207–9.
19. Klampfl T, Gisslinger H, Harutyunyan AS, Nivarthi H, Rumi E, Milosevic JD, Them NC, Berg T, Gisslinger B, Pietra D, Chen D, Vladimer GI, Bagienski K, Milanesi C, Casetti IC, Sant'Antonio E, Ferretti V, Elena C, Schischlik F, Cleary C, Six M, Schalling M, Schonegger A, Bock C, Malcovati L, Pascutto C, Superti-Furga G, Cazzola M, Kralovics R. Somatic mutations of calreticulin in myeloproliferative neoplasms. N Engl J Med. 2013;369:2379–90.
20. Nangalia J, Massie CE, Baxter EJ, Nice FL, Gundem G, Wedge DC, Avezov E, Li J, Kollmann K, Kent DG, Aziz A, Godfrey AL, Hinton J, Martincorena I, Van Loo P, Jones AV, Guglielmelli P, Tarpey P, Harding HP, Fitzpatrick JD, Goudie CT, Ortmann CA, Loughran SJ, Raine K, Jones DR, Butler AP, Teague JW, O'Meara S, McLaren S, Bianchi M, Silber Y, Dimitropoulou D, Bloxham D, Mudie L, Maddison M, Robinson B, Keohane C, Maclean C, Hill K, Orchard K, Tauro S, Du MQ, Greaves M, Bowen D, Huntly BJP, Harrison CN, Cross NCP, Ron D, Vannucchi AM, Papaemmanuil E, Campbell PJ, Green AR. Somatic CALR mutations in myeloproliferative neoplasms with nonmutated JAK2. N Engl J Med. 2013;369:2391–405.
21. Lundberg P, Karow A, Nienhold R, Looser R, Hao-Shen H, Nissen I, Girsberger S, Lehmann T, Passweg J, Stern M, Beisel C, Kralovics R, Skoda RC. Clonal evolution and clinical correlates of somatic mutations in myeloproliferative neoplasms. Blood. 2014;123:2220–8.
22. Pietra D, Rumi E, Ferretti VV, Di Buduo CA, Milanesi C, Cavalloni C, Sant'Antonio E, Abbonante V, Moccia F, Casetti IC, Bellini M, Renna MC, Roncoroni E, Fugazza E, Astori C, Boveri E, Rosti V, Barosi G, Balduini A, Cazzola M. Differential clinical effects of different mutation subtypes in CALR-mutant myeloproliferative neoplasms. Leukemia. 2016;30:431–8.
23. Pardanani AD, Levine RL, Lasho T, Pikman Y, Mesa RA, Wadleigh M, Steensma DP, Elliott MA, Wolanskyj AP, Hogan WJ, McClure RF, Litzow MR, Gilliland DG, Tefferi A. MPL515 mutations in myeloproliferative and other myeloid disorders: a study of 1182 patients. Blood. 2006;108:3472–6.
24. Schnittger S, Haferlach C, Beelen DW, Bojko P, Dengler R, Diestelrath A, Eckart MJ, Eckert R, Fries S, Kochling G, Laubenstein HP, Planker M, Pihusch R, Kern W, Haferlach T. Detection of three different MPLW515 in 10.1% of All JAK2 V617 unmutated ET and 9.3% of All JAK2 V617F unmutated OMF: a study of 387 patients. Blood. 2007;110:2546.
25. Beer P, Campbell P, Erber WN, Scott L, Bench AJ, Bareford D, Bridget W, Wheatley K, Buck G, Harrison CN, Green A. Clinical significance of MPL mutations in essential thrombocythemia: analysis of PT-1 cohort. Blood. 2007;110:677.
26. Vannucchi AM, Antonioli E, Pancrazzi A, Guglielmelli P, Di Lollo S, Alterini R, Guerini V, Baroni G, Rambaldi A, Bosi A, Barbui T. The clinical phenotype of patients with essential thrombocythemia harboring *MPL 515W>L/K* mutation. Blood. 2007;110:678.
27. Vainchenker W, Delhommeau F, Constantinescu SN, Bernard OA. New mutations and pathogenesis of myeloproliferative neoplasms. Blood. 2011;118:1723–35.
28. Guglielmelli P, Lasho TL, Rotunno G, Score J, Mannarelli C, Pancrazzi A, Biamonte F, Pardanani A, Zoi K, Reiter A, Duncombe A, Fanelli T, Pietra D, Rumi E, Finke C, Gangat N, Ketterling RP, Knudson RA, Hanson CA, Bosi A, Pereira A, Manfredini R, Cervantes F, Barosi G, Cazzola M, Cross NC, Vannucchi AM, Tefferi A. The number of prognostically detrimental mutations and prognosis in primary myelofibrosis: an international study of 797 patients. Leukemia. 2014;28:1804–10.
29. Maxson JE, Gotlib J, Pollyea DA, Fleischman AG, Agarwal A, Eide CA, Bottomly D, Wilmot B, McWeeney SK, Tognon CE, Pond JB, Collins RH, Goueli B, Oh ST, Deininger MW, Chang BH, Loriaux MM, Druker BJ, Tyner JW. Oncogenic CSF3R mutations in chronic neutrophilic leukemia and atypical CML. N Engl J Med. 2013;368:1781–90.
30. Pardanani A, Lasho TL, Laborde RR, Elliott M, Hanson CA, Knudson RA, Ketterling RP, Maxson JE, Tyner JW, Tefferi A. CSF3R T618I is a highly prevalent and specific mutation in chronic neutrophilic leukemia. Leukemia. 2013;27:1870–3.

31. Menezes J, Makishima H, Gomez I, Acquadro F, Gomez-Lopez G, Grana O, Dopazo A, Alvarez S, Trujillo M, Pisano DG, Maciejewski JP, Cigudosa JC. CSF3R T618I co-occurs with mutations of splicing and epigenetic genes and with a new PIM3 truncated fusion gene in chronic neutrophilic leukemia. Blood Cancer J. 2013;3:e158.
32. Elliott MA, Pardanani A, Hanson CA, Lasho TL, Finke CM, Belachew AA, Tefferi A. ASXL1 mutations are frequent and prognostically detrimental in CSF3R-mutated chronic neutrophilic leukemia. Am J Hematol. 2015;90:653–6.
33. Andrieux JL, Demory JL. Karyotype and molecular cytogenetic studies in polycythemia vera. Curr Hematol Rep. 2005;4:224–9.
34. Jara-Acevedo M, Teodosio C, Sanchez-Munoz L, Alvarez-Twose I, Mayado A, Caldas C, Matito A, Morgado JM, Munoz-Gonzalez JI, Escribano L, Garcia-Montero AC, Orfao A. Detection of the KIT D816V mutation in peripheral blood of systemic mastocytosis: diagnostic implications. Mod Pathol. 2015;28:1138–49.
35. Theoharides TC, Valent P, Akin C. Mast cells, mastocytosis, and related disorders. N Engl J Med. 2015;373:1885–6.
36. Tefferi A, Levine RL, Lim KH, Abdel-Wahab O, Lasho TL, Patel J, Finke CM, Mullally A, Li CY, Pardanani A, Gilliland DG. Frequent TET2 mutations in systemic mastocytosis: clinical, KITD816V and FIP1L1-PDGFRA correlates. Leukemia. 2009;23:900–4.
37. Traina F, Visconte V, Jankowska AM, Makishima H, O'Keefe CL, Elson P, Han Y, Hsieh FH, Sekeres MA, Mali RS, Kalaycio M, Lichtin AE, Advani AS, Duong HK, Copelan E, Kapur R, Olalla Saad ST, Maciejewski JP, Tiu RV. Single nucleotide polymorphism array lesions, TET2, DNMT3A, ASXL1 and CBL mutations are present in systemic mastocytosis. PLoS One. 2012;7:e43090.
38. Wilson TM, Maric I, Simakova O, Bai Y, Chan EC, Olivares N, Carter M, Maric D, Robyn J, Metcalfe DD. Clonal analysis of NRAS activating mutations in KIT-D816V systemic mastocytosis. Haematologica. 2011;96:459–63.
39. Schwaab J, Schnittger S, Sotlar K, Walz C, Fabarius A, Pfirrmann M, Kohlmann A, Grossmann V, Meggendorfer M, Horny HP, Valent P, Jawhar M, Teichmann M, Metzgeroth G, Erben P, Ernst T, Hochhaus A, Haferlach T, Hofmann WK, Cross NC, Reiter A. Comprehensive mutational profiling in advanced systemic mastocytosis. Blood. 2013;122:2460–6.
40. Jawhar M, Schwaab J, Schnittger S, Meggendorfer M, Pfirrmann M, Sotlar K, Horny HP, Metzgeroth G, Kluger S, Naumann N, Haferlach C, Haferlach T, Valent P, Hofmann WK, Fabarius A, Cross NC, Reiter A. Additional mutations in SRSF2, ASXL1 and/or RUNX1 identify a high-risk group of patients with KIT D816V(+) advanced systemic mastocytosis. Leukemia. 2016;30:136–43.
41. Cools J, DeAngelo DJ, Gotlib J, Stover EH, Legare RD, Cortes J, Kutok J, Clark J, Galinsky I, Griffin JD, Cross NC, Tefferi A, Malone J, Alam R, Schrier SL, Schmid J, Rose M, Vandenberghe P, Verhoef G, Boogaerts M, Wlodarska I, Kantarjian H, Marynen P, Coutre SE, Stone R, Gilliland DG. A tyrosine kinase created by fusion of the PDGFRA and FIP1L1 genes as a therapeutic target of imatinib in idiopathic hypereosinophilic syndrome. N Engl J Med. 2003;348:1201–14.
42. Elling C, Erben P, Walz C, Frickenhaus M, Schemionek M, Stehling M, Serve H, Cross NC, Hochhaus A, Hofmann WK, Berdel WE, Muller-Tidow C, Reiter A, Koschmieder S. Novel imatinib-sensitive PDGFRA-activating point mutations in hypereosinophilic syndrome induce growth factor independence and leukemia-like disease. Blood. 2011;117:2935–43.
43. Golub TR, Barker GF, Lovett M, Gilliland DG. Fusion of PDGF receptor beta to a novel ets-like gene, tel, in chronic myelomonocytic leukemia with t(5;12) chromosomal translocation. Cell. 1994;77:307–16.
44. Savage N, George TI, Gotlib J. Myeloid neoplasms associated with eosinophilia and rearrangement of PDGFRA, PDGFRB, and FGFR1: a review. Int J Lab Hematol. 2013;35:491–500.
45. Bain BJ, Ahmad S. Should myeloid and lymphoid neoplasms with PCM1-JAK2 and other rearrangements of JAK2 be recognized as specific entities? Br J Haematol. 2014;166: 809–17.

46. Mughal TI, Cross NC, Padron E, Tiu RV, Savona M, Malcovati L, Tibes R, Komrokji RS, Kiladjian JJ, Garcia-Manero G, Orazi A, Mesa R, Maciejewski JP, Fenaux P, Itzykson R, Mufti G, Solary E, List AF. An International MDS/MPN Working Group's perspective and recommendations on molecular pathogenesis, diagnosis and clinical characterization of myelodysplastic/myeloproliferative neoplasms. Haematologica. 2015;100:1117–30.
47. DiNardo CD, Daver N, Jain N, Pemmaraju N, Bueso-Ramos C, Yin CC, Pierce S, Jabbour E, Cortes JE, Kantarjian HM, Garcia-Manero G, Verstovsek S. Myelodysplastic/myeloproliferative neoplasms, unclassifiable (MDS/MPN, U): natural history and clinical outcome by treatment strategy. Leukemia. 2014;28:958–61.
48. Foucar K. Myelodysplastic/myeloproliferative neoplasms. Am J Clin Pathol. 2009;132:281–9.
49. Orazi A, Germing U. The myelodysplastic/myeloproliferative neoplasms: myeloproliferative diseases with dysplastic features. Leukemia. 2008;22:1308–19.
50. Geyer JT, Orazi A. Myeloproliferative neoplasms (BCR-ABL1 negative) and myelodysplastic/myeloproliferative neoplasms: current diagnostic principles and upcoming updates. Int J Lab Hematol. 2016;38 Suppl 1:12–9.
51. Gambacorti-Passerini CB, Donadoni C, Parmiani A, Pirola A, Redaelli S, Signore G, Piazza V, Malcovati L, Fontana D, Spinelli R, Magistroni V, Gaipa G, Peronaci M, Morotti A, Panuzzo C, Saglio G, Usala E, Kim DW, Rea D, Zervakis K, Viniou N, Symeonidis A, Becker H, Boultwood J, Campiotti L, Carrabba M, Elli E, Bignell GR, Papaemmanuil E, Campbell PJ, Cazzola M, Piazza R. Recurrent ETNK1 mutations in atypical chronic myeloid leukemia. Blood. 2015;125:499–503.
52. Meggendorfer M, Bacher U, Alpermann T, Haferlach C, Kern W, Gambacorti-Passerini C, Haferlach T, Schnittger S. SETBP1 mutations occur in 9% of MDS/MPN and in 4% of MPN cases and are strongly associated with atypical CML, monosomy 7, isochromosome i(17)(q10), ASXL1 and CBL mutations. Leukemia. 2013;27:1852–60.
53. Jaiswal S, Fontanillas P, Flannick J, Manning A, Grauman PV, Mar BG, Lindsley RC, Mermel CH, Burtt N, Chavez A, Higgins JM, Moltchanov V, Kuo FC, Kluk MJ, Henderson B, Kinnunen L, Koistinen HA, Ladenvall C, Getz G, Correa A, Banahan BF, Gabriel S, Kathiresan S, Stringham HM, McCarthy MI, Boehnke M, Tuomilehto J, Haiman C, Groop L, Atzmon G, Wilson JG, Neuberg D, Altshuler D, Ebert BL. Age-related clonal hematopoiesis associated with adverse outcomes. N Engl J Med. 2014;371:2488–98.
54. Genovese G, Kahler AK, Handsaker RE, Lindberg J, Rose SA, Bakhoum SF, Chambert K, Mick E, Neale BM, Fromer M, Purcell SM, Svantesson O, Landen M, Hoglund M, Lehmann S, Gabriel SB, Moran JL, Lander ES, Sullivan PF, Sklar P, Gronberg H, Hultman CM, McCarroll SA. Clonal hematopoiesis and blood-cancer risk inferred from blood DNA sequence. N Engl J Med. 2014;371:2477–87.
55. Papaemmanuil E, Gerstung M, Malcovati L, Tauro S, Gundem G, Van Loo P, Yoon CJ, Ellis P, Wedge DC, Pellagatti A, Shlien A, Groves MJ, Forbes SA, Raine K, Hinton J, Mudie LJ, McLaren S, Hardy C, Latimer C, Della Porta MG, O'Meara S, Ambaglio I, Galli A, Butler AP, Walldin G, Teague JW, Quek L, Sternberg A, Gambacorti-Passerini C, Cross NC, Green AR, Boultwood J, Vyas P, Hellstrom-Lindberg E, Bowen D, Cazzola M, Stratton MR, Campbell PJ. Chronic Myeloid Disorders Working Group of the International Cancer Genome C: clinical and biological implications of driver mutations in myelodysplastic syndromes. Blood. 2013;122:3616–27; quiz 3699.
56. Haferlach T, Nagata Y, Grossmann V, Okuno Y, Bacher U, Nagae G, Schnittger S, Sanada M, Kon A, Alpermann T, Yoshida K, Roller A, Nadarajah N, Shiraishi Y, Shiozawa Y, Chiba K, Tanaka H, Koeffler HP, Klein HU, Dugas M, Aburatani H, Kohlmann A, Miyano S, Haferlach C, Kern W, Ogawa S. Landscape of genetic lesions in 944 patients with myelodysplastic syndromes. Leukemia. 2014;28:241–7.
57. Makishima H, Yoshizato T, Yoshida K, Sekeres MA, Radivoyevitch T, Suzuki H, Przychodzen B, Nagata Y, Meggendorfer M, Sanada M, Okuno Y, Hirsch C, Kuzmanovic T, Sato Y, Sato-Otsubo A, LaFramboise T, Hosono N, Shiraishi Y, Chiba K, Haferlach C, Kern W, Tanaka H, Shiozawa Y, Gomez-Segui I, Husseinzadeh HD, Thota S, Guinta KM, Dienes B, Nakamaki

T, Miyawaki S, Sauntharajah Y, Chiba S, Miyano S, Shih LY, Haferlach T, Ogawa S, Maciejewski JP. Dynamics of clonal evolution in myelodysplastic syndromes. Nat Genet. 2017;49:204–12.
58. Schanz J, Tuchler H, Sole F, Mallo M, Luno E, Cervera J, Granada I, Hildebrandt B, Slovak ML, Ohyashiki K, Steidl C, Fonatsch C, Pfeilstocker M, Nosslinger T, Valent P, Giagounidis A, Aul C, Lubbert M, Stauder R, Krieger O, Garcia-Manero G, Faderl S, Pierce S, Le Beau MM, Bennett JM, Greenberg P, Germing U, Haase D. New comprehensive cytogenetic scoring system for primary myelodysplastic syndromes (MDS) and oligoblastic acute myeloid leukemia after MDS derived from an international database merge. J Clin Oncol. 2012;30:820–9.
59. Greenberg PL, Tuechler H, Schanz J, Sanz G, Garcia-Manero G, Sole F, Bennett JM, Bowen D, Fenaux P, Dreyfus F, Kantarjian H, Kuendgen A, Levis A, Malcovati L, Cazzola M, Cermak J, Fonatsch C, Le Beau MM, Slovak ML, Krieger O, Luebbert M, Maciejewski J, Magalhaes SM, Miyazaki Y, Pfeilstocker M, Sekeres M, Sperr WR, Stauder R, Tauro S, Valent P, Vallespi T, van de Loosdrecht AA, Germing U, Haase D. Revised international prognostic scoring system for myelodysplastic syndromes. Blood. 2012;120:2454–65.
60. Lindsley RC, Mar BG, Mazzola E, Grauman PV, Shareef S, Allen SL, Pigneux A, Wetzler M, Stuart RK, Erba HP, Damon LE, Powell BL, Lindeman N, Steensma DP, Wadleigh M, DeAngelo DJ, Neuberg D, Stone RM, Ebert BL. Acute myeloid leukemia ontogeny is defined by distinct somatic mutations. Blood. 2015;125:1367–76.
61. Corces-Zimmerman MR, Hong WJ, Weissman IL, Medeiros BC, Majeti R. Preleukemic mutations in human acute myeloid leukemia affect epigenetic regulators and persist in remission. Proc Natl Acad Sci U S A. 2014;111:2548–53.
62. Badar T, Patel KP, Thompson PA, DiNardo C, Takahashi K, Cabrero M, Borthakur G, Cortes J, Konopleva M, Kadia T, Bohannan Z, Pierce S, Jabbour EJ, Ravandi F, Daver N, Luthra R, Kantarjian H, Garcia-Manero G. Detectable FLT3-ITD or RAS mutation at the time of transformation from MDS to AML predicts for very poor outcomes. Leuk Res. 2015;39:1367–74.
63. Kim T, Tyndel MS, Kim HJ, Ahn JS, Choi SH, Park HJ, Kim YK, Yang DH, Lee JJ, Jung SH, Kim SY, Min YH, Cheong JW, Sohn SK, Moon JH, Choi M, Lee M, Zhang Z, Kim DDH. The clonal origins of leukemic progression of myelodysplasia. Leukemia. 2017;31:1928–35.
64. Yoshida K, Sanada M, Shiraishi Y, Nowak D, Nagata Y, Yamamoto R, Sato Y, Sato-Otsubo A, Kon A, Nagasaki M, Chalkidis G, Suzuki Y, Shiosaka M, Kawahata R, Yamaguchi T, Otsu M, Obara N, Sakata-Yanagimoto M, Ishiyama K, Mori H, Nolte F, Hofmann WK, Miyawaki S, Sugano S, Haferlach C, Koeffler HP, Shih LY, Haferlach T, Chiba S, Nakauchi H, Miyano S, Ogawa S. Frequent pathway mutations of splicing machinery in myelodysplasia. Nature. 2011;478:64–9.
65. Lee SC, Dvinge H, Kim E, Cho H, Micol JB, Chung YR, Durham BH, Yoshimi A, Kim YJ, Thomas M, Lobry C, Chen CW, Pastore A, Taylor J, Wang X, Krivtsov A, Armstrong SA, Palacino J, Buonamici S, Smith PG, Bradley RK, Abdel-Wahab O. Modulation of splicing catalysis for therapeutic targeting of leukemia with mutations in genes encoding spliceosomal proteins. Nat Med. 2016;22:672–8.
66. Shih AH, Chung SS, Dolezal EK, Zhang SJ, Abdel-Wahab OI, Park CY, Nimer SD, Levine RL, Klimek VM. Mutational analysis of therapy-related myelodysplastic syndromes and acute myelogenous leukemia. Haematologica. 2013;98:908–12.
67. Jaffe ES, Arber DA, Campo E, Harris NL, Quintanilla-Martinez L. Hematopathology. In: Hasserjian R, Head D, editors. Myelodysplastic syndromes. 2nd ed. Philadelphia: Elsevier; 2017. p. 793–815.
68. Greenberg PL, Stone RM, Bejar R, Bennett JM, Bloomfield CD, Borate U, De Castro CM, Deeg HJ, DeZern AE, Fathi AT, Frankfurt O, Gaensler K, Garcia-Manero G, Griffiths EA, Head D, Klimek V, Komrokji R, Kujawski LA, Maness LJ, O'Donnell MR, Pollyea DA, Scott B, Shami PJ, Stein BL, Westervelt P, Wheeler B, Shead DA, Smith C. National comprehensive cancer: myelodysplastic syndromes, version 2. J Natl Compr Canc Netw. 2015;13:261–72.

Chapter 16
Lymphomas

Vignesh Shanmugam and Annette S. Kim

Key Points

- Recurrent structural rearrangements, copy number changes, and somatic mutations are frequent in essentially all lymphoma subtypes.
- Many diagnoses display complex molecular genetic aberrations beyond the single -hallmark reciprocal translocations that formerly were thought to characterize particular diagnostic lymphoma entities.
- Individual molecular genetic lesions are seldom pathognomonic for any individual diagnosis, but key lesions in conjunction with mutational patterns can be diagnostically, prognostically, and therapeutically informative.
- Mutations patterns may subdivide individual morphologic diagnostic categories, but may also show molecular genetic relatedness between morphologically distinct diagnoses.

Key Online Resources

- http://atlasgeneticsoncology.org/Anomalies/Anomliste.html#NHL
- http://www.cbioportal.org/
- NCCN Guidelines for B-cell lymphomas, T-cell lymphomas, Hodgkin lymphoma, Chronic lymphocytic leukemia/small lymphocytic lymphoma, and hairy cell leukemia:https://www.nccn.org/professionals/physician_gls/default.aspx

V. Shanmugam · A. S. Kim (✉)
Department of Pathology, Brigham and Women's Hospital/Harvard Medical School, Boston, MA, USA
e-mail: vshanmugam@bwh.harvard.edu; askim@bwh.harvard.edu

L. J. Tafe, M. E. Arcila (eds.), *Genomic Medicine*,
https://doi.org/10.1007/978-3-030-22922-1_16

Atlas of Genetics and Cytogenetics has a non-Hodgkin lymphoma page that is focused on larger structural aberrations. cBioPortal.org can be searched for lymphoma somatic mutations. The NCCN guidelines have a very limited view on molecular genetic testing, but what little there is, is incorporated into clinical therapy decision-making.

Introduction

Lymphomas encompass a diverse group of mature lymphoid neoplasms with a wide range of histologic and clinical presentations, etiologies, and responses to therapy [1]. Historically, lymphomas have been challenging to categorize. Originally, classification schema relied upon morphology, followed by immunophenotypic markers of cell of origin and stage of maturation categories that predominate even today [2–4]. Yet the first genetic lesion discovered to cause tumorigenesis was in the field of lymphomas, the reciprocal translocation involving *MYC*, identified in 1958 as the underlying cause of Burkitt's lymphoma [5]. Subsequently, several other reciprocal translocations were identified in other non-Hodgkin lymphomas (NHL), such as t(14;18) and t(11;14). Today, molecular genetic aberrations play a key role in diagnosis, prognosis, and therapy selection in NHL and are increasingly informing our understanding of the underlying biology that differentiates the many diagnostic entities within the lymphomas.

Recurrent Molecular Aberrancies in B-Cell Neoplasms

Hodgkin Lymphoma (HL)

Hodgkin lymphoma is a B-cell-derived malignancy that bimodally affects young adults and the elderly. These tumors can be broadly divided into classic Hodgkin lymphoma (CHL) and nodular lymphocyte predominant Hodgkin lymphoma (NLPHL), each with distinct clinical and morphologic features [6]. The former accounts for 95% of cases of HL. Both subtypes are histologically characterized by the presence of only a small number of neoplastic large atypical mononucleated and multinucleated (designated Hodgkin and Reed–Sternberg cells or lymphocyte predominant cells) of germinal center B-cell origin embedded in an abundant and heterogeneous mixture of nonneoplastic inflammatory cells. Recurrent genetic alterations involving the NF-kB and JAK-STAT signaling pathways are common to both subtypes of HL, and diverse genetic mechanisms of immune evasion typify the genomes of the malignant HRS cells (Tables 16.1, 16.2, and 16.3; Fig. 16.1). By

Table 16.1 Frequent structural variants in HL

Rearrangement/gene partners	Description	Frequency	Clinical utility	Refs
CIITA rearrangements	Leads to downregulation of MHC class II expression	15%		[48]
IGH rearrangements	Rearrangements involve diverse proto-oncogenes (BCL6, BCL3, BCL2, REL, MYC) likely leading to overexpression	10%		[49]
t(4;9)(q21;p24)/*SEC31A-JAK2*	Leads to constitutive JAK-STAT pathway activation	1%	Sensitive to JAK inhibitors in vitro	[50]

Table 16.2 Frequent copy number alterations in HL

Copy number change	Gene(s) involved	Frequency	Clinical utility	Refs
2p gain	*REL*	28–54%		[51–53]
4q loss		7–25%		[51–53]
6q loss		5–30%		[51–53]
9p gain	*PD-L1/2, JAK2*	24–40%	Response to PD-L1 inhibitor therapy is largely independent of PD-L1 expression or amplification	[51–53]
11q loss		3–25%		[51–53]
12q gain	*MDM2*	37–40%		[51–53]
13q loss		22–35%		[51–53]
14q gain		7–30%		[51–53]
16p gain	*ABCC1*	24–30%	Increased ABCC1 expression associated with risk of refractory disease or early relapse	[51–53]
17p gain		25–40%		[51–53]
17q gain	*MAP3K14*	20–70%		[51–53]
20q gain	*CD40*	15–23%		[51–53]

contrast, NLPHL does not show inactivating *TNFAIP3* or *NFKBIA* mutations, instead harboring frequent BCL6 gene rearrangements (35%) [6].

Chronic Lymphocytic Leukemia/Small Lymphocytic Lymphoma (CLL/SLL)

CLL/SLL is the most common adult chronic leukemia in Western countries. The majority of patients present with leukemic disease (CLL), and isolated lymphomatous involvement is uncommon (SLL). Although this is generally considered to be

Table 16.3 Frequent somatic variants in HL

Pathway	Gene	Description	Most common mutations reported	Frequency	Clinical utility (diagnostic/ prognostic)	Refs
NF-κB signaling	*TNFAIP3*	Negative regulator of NF-κB signaling	Loss of function mutations	22–40%		[54–56]
	NFKBIA	Negative regulator of NF-κB signaling	Loss of function mutations	15%		[57]
	NFKBIE	Negative regulator of NF-kB signaling	Loss of function mutations	15%		[58]
Cell cycle regulation/ DNA repair	*TP53*	Tumor suppressor	Loss of function mutations	10%		[59]
Apoptosis	*CD95*	Death receptor	Loss of function mutations	10%		[60, 61]
JAK/STAT	*SOCS1*	Negative regulator of JAK-STAT signaling; mutations likely lead to loss of function	Missense mutations involving the SH3 domain and truncating mutations involving the JAK kinase domain	40–60%	Also identified in NLPHL, poor prognosis	[56, 62, 63]
	STAT6	STAT family transcription factor	Activating missense mutations within DNA-binding domain	30%		[64]
	PTPN1	Negative regulator of JAK-STAT signaling; mutations lead to loss of function and activation of JAK-STAT signaling	Missense and truncating mutations	20%		[65]
Nuclear export	*XPO1*	Importin-beta-superfamily of nuclear export proteins	Hotspot missense mutation (p.E571K)	25%	Can be detected in plasma, potential role in minimal residual disease monitoring	[66]
Immune evasion	*B2M*	Component of MHC class I	Loss of function mutations	70%		[56]

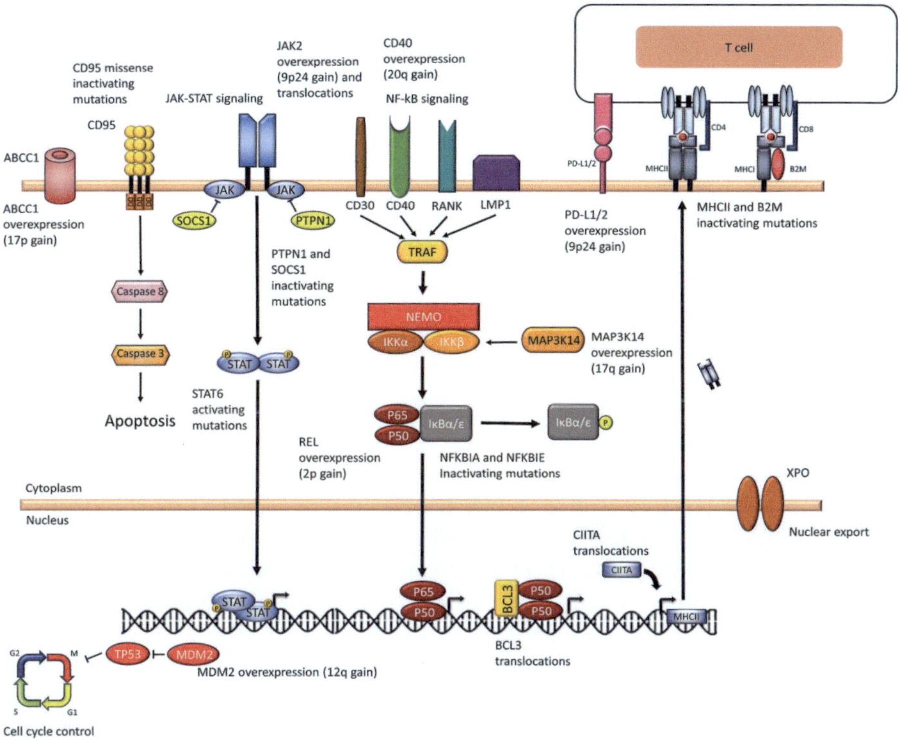

Fig. 16.1 Overview of molecular alterations in classic Hodgkin lymphoma. Pathways implicated in Hodgkin lymphoma include the STAT6 pathways and NF-κB pathway

an indolent disease, this is significant heterogeneity in clinical outcomes [6]. A small subset of tumors can progress into more aggressive disease, such as diffuse large B-cell lymphoma or Hodgkin lymphoma (less common). A large proportion of cases show recurrent genetic alterations that have powerful prognostic and predictive value. While reciprocal translocations are not recurrent in CLL, there are frequent copy number alterations and somatic variants (Tables 16.4 and 16.5; Fig. 16.2) [1, 6].

Resistance Mutations to Ibrutinib Therapy Ibrutinib, a Bruton's tyrosine kinase (BTK) inhibitor, has transformed the treatment of relapsed/refractory CLL. As its use has become widespread in the community, resistance to this therapy is increasingly being appreciated in a subset of patients. Some of these patients have been found to carry mutations involving the B-cell receptor signaling pathway that confer resistance to ibrutinib therapy (Table 16.6).

Table 16.4 Frequent copy number alterations in CLL

Copy number change	Gene(s) involved	Frequency	Clinical utility	Refs
13q14 loss		50–60%	Good prognosis	[67]
11q22-23 loss	*ATM*	17%	Poor prognosis	[68–70]
17p13 loss	*TP53*	8%	Poor prognosis, predicts resistance to fludarabine therapy	[70]
Trisomy 12		20%	Intermediate prognosis, associated with atypical morphologic features and CD11c expression	[70, 71]

Mantle Cell Lymphoma (MCL)

MCL is a CD5-positive mature B-cell neoplasm characterized by the hallmark reciprocal translocation involving *IGH* and *CCND1* (t(11;14)), resulting in overexpression for cyclin D1 (Table 16.7). Rarely, in cases that are negative for t(11;14), variant translocations involving light chains or *CCND2* or *CCND3* may be observed (Table16.7). Among the small B-cell lymphomas, MCL has a relatively more aggressive disease course with shorter overall survival, and morphologic variants, such as the pleomorphic and blastoid variants, may predict an even poorer prognosis. Other molecular genetic changes affect a wide range of pathways (Tables 16.8 and 16.9; Fig. 16.2) [1, 6].

Extranodal Marginal Zone Lymphoma (Extranodal MZL, Mucosa-Associated Lymphoid Tissue Lymphoma, MALT)

MZLs can be divided into three distinct entities that show different clinical, pathologic, and molecular genetic features: extranodal MZL of mucosa-associated lymphoid tissue (MALT lymphomas), nodal MZL, and splenic MZL. MALT lymphomas are the most common among the MZLs. While the three entities show highly convergent genetic alterations involving similar pathways, there are also key differences (Table 16.10; Fig. 16.3). For example, MALT lymphomas are frequently driven by reciprocal translocations culminating in NF-κB pathway activation unlike nodal and splenic MZL, wherein such rearrangements are uncommon but where copy number alterations (especially in splenic MZL) are more frequent (Table 16.11). Several genes in the NF-κB pathway are also recurrently mutated in MZLs (Table 16.12; Fig. 16.2) [1, 6].

Table 16.5 Frequent somatic variants in CLL

Pathway	Gene	Description	Most common mutations reported	Frequency	Clinical utility (diagnostic/prognostic)	Refs
DNA damage/cell cycle regulation	*TP53*	Tumor suppressor	Loss of function mutations	15%	Poor prognosis	[72–75]
	ATM	Tumor suppressor gene involved in double-strand break repair	Loss of function mutations	9%	Biallelic inactivation associated with poor prognosis	[72–74, 76]
Notch signaling	*NOTCH1*	Notch family receptor; mutation results in loss of PEST domain and increased protein stability leading to gain of function	2bp deletion (c.7541_7542delCT) in PEST domain	4–12%	Predicts poor response to addition of rituximab to fludarabine + cyclophosphamide	[72–75, 77–79]
Inflammatory signaling	*MYD88*	Essential cytosolic adapter protein in Toll-like receptor and interleukin-1 signaling	Activating missense mutations (p.L265P)	10%	Younger, advanced stage disease	[72–74, 77]
Splicing	*SF3B1*	Spliceosome component	Missense mutational hot spots (most common p.K700E, also p.K662, p.K666, and other mutations in p.580-p.780 range) lead to altered splicing	5–20%	Poor prognosis	[72–75, 80–82]

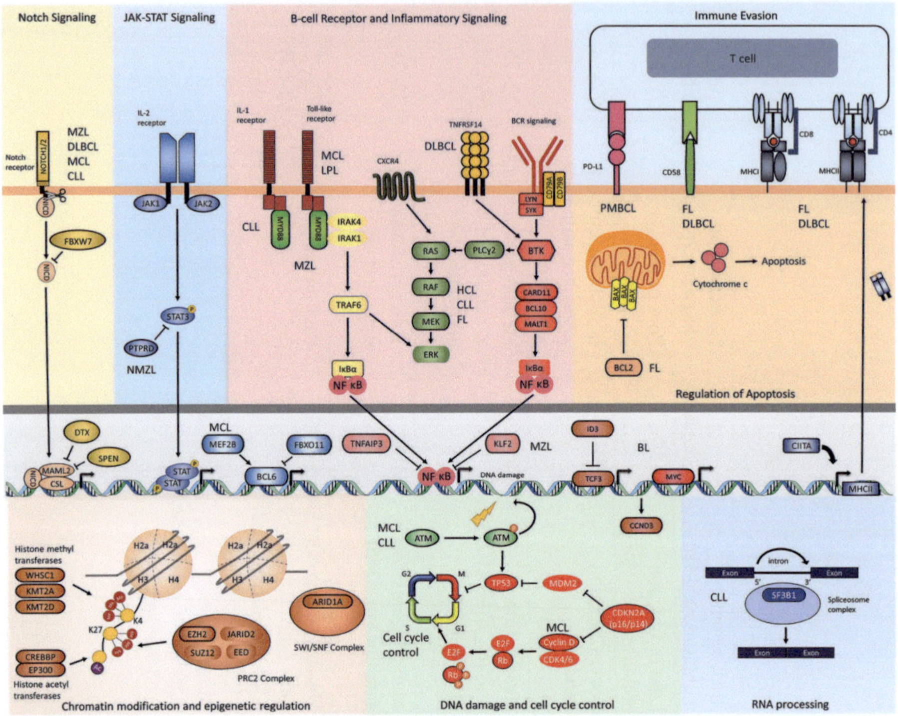

Fig. 16.2 Overview of molecular alterations in mature B-cell lymphomas with a focus on small B-cell lymphomas. Genes that are recurrently mutated are depicted with bold outlines. Key pathways are color coded and disease commonly associated with the pathways are noted. From left to right and top to bottom, the signaling pathways include Notch signaling, JAK-STAT signaling, B-cell receptor and inflammatory signaling, immune evasion signaling, chromatin modifiers, DNA damage and cell cycling, and RNA processing. Abbreviations: MZL marginal zone lymphoma, DLBCL diffuse large B-cell lymphoma, MCL mantle cell lymphoma, CLL chronic lymphocytic leukemia, LPL lymphoplasmacytic lymphoma, PMBCL primary mediastinal B-cell lymphoma, FL follicular lymphoma, HCL hairy cell lymphoma

Table 16.6 Frequent resistance mutations in CLL patients on ibrutinib

Pathway	Gene	Description	Most common mutations reported	Refs
BCR signaling	*BTK*	Mutations result in reversible inhibition by ibrutinib	Missense mutations at ibrutinib-binding site (p.C481S)	[83, 84]
	PLCG2	Activating mutations result in activation of BCR signaling in a BTK-independent manner	GOF	[84, 85]

Table 16.7 Frequent structural variants in MCL

Rearrangement/gene partners	Description	Frequency	Clinical utility	Refs
t(11;14)(q13;q32)/*CCND1-IGH*	Leads to overexpression of cyclin D proteins	90–99%	Diagnostic	[86, 87]
t(2;11)(p11;q13)/*CCND1-IGK*		<1%		[87]
t(11;22)(q13;q11)/*CCND1-IGL*		<1%		[87]
t(12;14)(p13;q32)/*CCND2-IGH*		<1%		[87]
t(2;12)(p11;p13)/*CCND2-IGK*		<1%		[87]
t(12;22)(p13;q21)/*CCND2-IGL*		<1%		[87]
t(6;14)(p21;q32)/*CCND3-IGH*		<1%		[87]

Table 16.8 Frequent copy number alterations in MCL

Copy number change	Gene(s) involved	Frequency	Clinical utility	Refs
9p21.3 loss	*CDKN2A/B*	20–30%	Associated with blastoid and pleomorphic morphology	[87–91]
3q gain		32–70%	Associated with blastoid and pleomorphic morphology	[87–91]
7p gain		5–27%	Associated with blastoid and pleomorphic morphology	[87–91]
8q gain	*MYC*	10–32%		[87–91]
12q gain	*CDK4*	5–30%	Associated with blastoid and pleomorphic morphology	[87–91]
15q gain		4–26%		[87–91]
18q gain	*BCL2*	7–26%		[87–91]
1p loss	*CDKN2C/FAF1*	24–52%		[87–91]
6q loss	*TNGAIP3/LATS1*	13–37%		[87–91]
8p loss	*MCPH1*	7–79%		[87–91]
9q loss		5–21%		[87–91]
10p loss		3–18%		[87–91]
11q loss	*ATM, BIRC3*	19–37%		[87–91]
13q loss	*RB1*	17–70%		[87–91]
17p loss	*TP53*	4–30%	Associated with blastoid and pleomorphic morphology	[87–91]

Table 16.9 Frequent somatic variants in MCL

Pathway	Gene	Description	Most common mutations reported	Frequency	Clinical utility (diagnostic/prognostic)	Refs
DNA damage/cell cycle regulation	*ATM*	Tumor suppressor	Loss of function mutations	40–50%		[25, 92–95]
	CCND1	D-type cyclin; mutations lead to increased protein stability	Missense mutation involving N-terminus (exon 1)	20–34%		[25, 92–95]
	TP53	Tumor suppressor	Loss of function mutations	7–31%	Poor prognosis (poor response to regimens including cytarabine, rituximab, and autologous stem cell transplant	[25, 92–96]
	UBR5	E3 ubiquitin-protein ligase; truncating mutations lead to loss of conserved cysteine residue on C-terminus likely resulting in loss of E3 ligase activity	Frameshift mutations involving C-terminus (exon 58)	7–18%		[25, 92–95]
Inflammatory signaling	*BIRC3*	Negative regulator of alternative NF-kB signaling; mutations likely lead to activation of alternate NF-kB signaling via NIK disinhibition	Missense and truncating mutations involving the C-terminus (CARD and RING E3 ligase domains	5–10%		[25, 92–95]
	TRAF2	Mediates signal transduction from TNF receptors; mutations likely lead to activation of alternate NF-kB signaling via NIK disinhibition	Missense and truncating mutations	7%		[25, 92–95]
Chromatin modifiers	*WHSC1*	Histone 3 methyltransferase of lysine-36	Missense mutations involving SET domain (E1099K, T1150A)	7–13%		[25, 92–95]
	KMT2D	Histone methyltransferase	Loss of function mutations	12–20%		[25, 92–95]
	KMT2C	Histone methyltransferase	Loss of function mutations	16%		[25, 92–95]
Notch signaling	*NOTCH1*	Notch family receptor; hyperactive Notch signaling due to increased stability of the cleaved intracellular domain (NICD)	Truncating mutations involving the PEST domain	6–14%	Poor prognosis	[25, 92–95]
	NOTCH2	Notch family receptor	Truncating PEST domain mutations, resulting in activation	5%	Poor prognosis	[25, 92–95]

Table 16.10 Frequent structural variants in MZL

Rearrangement/gene partners	Description	Frequency	Clinical utility	Refs
t(11;18)(q22;q21)/*BIRC3 (API2)-MALT1*	Leads to loss of RING domain of BIRC3 while keeping BIR domains intact leading to BCR-independent dimerization and loss of ubiquitination of BCL10 resulting in activation of NF-κB signaling	15–50%	More associated with GI and pulmonary MALT	[97, 98]
t(1;14)(p22;q32)/*BCL10-IGH*	Leads to overexpression of BCL10 under the control of the *IGH* enhancer resulting in NF-kB activation	1–2%	More associated with GI and pulmonary MALT	[97, 98]
t(14;18)(q32;q21)/*IGH-MALT1*	Leads to overexpression of MALT under the control of the *IGH* enhancer resulting in NF-κB activation	15–20%	More associated with ocular, salivary gland, thyroid, and cutaneous MALT	[99]
t(3;14)(p14.1;q32)/*FOXP1-IGH*	Leads to overexpression of FOXP1 under the control of the *IGH* enhancer	10%	More associated with ocular, salivary gland, thyroid, and cutaneous MALT	[100]

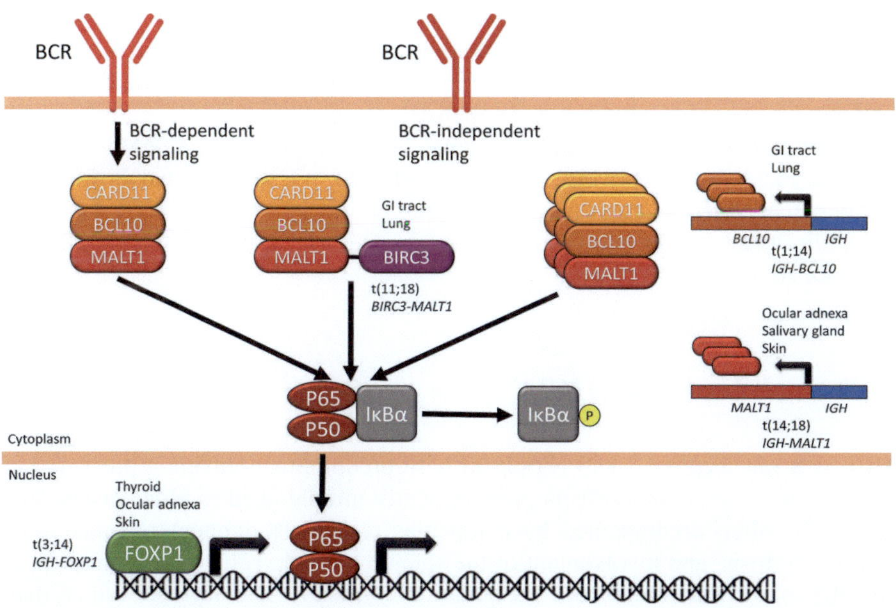

Fig. 16.3 Overview of molecular alterations in extranodal marginal zone lymphoma. Recurrent translocations, their protein consequences, and common sites of disease are shown

Table 16.11 Frequent copy number alterations in MZL

Copy number change	Gene(s) involved	Frequency			Clinical utility	Refs
		MALT	NMZL	SMZL		
Trisomy 3		25–30%	25%	20%		[101, 102]
Trisomy 18		20%	25%	15%		[101, 102]
Trisomy 12		10%	10%	10%		[101, 102]
7q deletion		Rare	Rare	25–30%		[101, 102]
6q23 deletion		15%	15%	Rare		[101–103]
17p deletion	*TP53*	Rare	Rare	17%		[101, 102]
8p deletion		Rare	Rare	13%	Combination of del 8p and 17p predicts poor prognosis	[101, 102]

Lymphoplasmacytic Lymphoma/Waldenström Macroglobulinemia (LPL/WM)

Lymphoplasmacytic lymphoma (LPL) is an uncommon B-cell neoplasm of mature adults with generally an indolent course (median survival 10 years), accounting for approximately 2% of NHLs [2, 7, 8]. LPL is associated with the clinical presentation of WM, defined as LPL with BM involvement and typically an IgM monoclonal gammopathy. Although 18% of patients with LPL have a first-degree relative with a B-cell lymphoproliferative disorder, no familial predisposition mutations have been identified at this time [9]. Copy number alterations and somatic variants are commonly used to distinguish LPL from other entities in the differential diagnosis, including marginal zone lymphoma and IgM myeloma (Tables 16.13 and 16.14; Fig. 16.2). The *MYD88* p.L265P variant is found in greater than 90% of cases of LPL and predicts response to the BTK inhibitor, ibrutinib, which can be mitigated by co-occurring mutations in *CXCR4* [10–14]. Translocations are rare in LPL.

Hairy Cell Leukemia (HCL)

HCL is a rare mature B-cell neoplasm with predominant leukemic presentation and indolent course that affects predominantly middle-aged to older males. The disease is often accompanied by cytopenias (especially monocytopenia), bone marrow fibrosis, and involvement of the splenic red pulp [2]. Up to 10% of cases of HCL show variant clinical presentation (typically leukocytosis rather than cytopenias), morphology, and immunophenotype. These cases do not respond well to traditional therapies for HCL (e.g., purine analogues such as cladribine

Table 16.12 Frequent somatic variants in MZL

Pathway	Gene	Description	Most common mutations reported	Frequency			Clinical utility (diagnostic/prognostic)	Refs
				MALT	NMZL	SMZL		
NF-κB signaling	*TNFAIP3*	Negative regulator of NF-κB signaling	Loss of function mutations	25%	25%	8%	Relatively specific to MZL among small B-cell lymphomas	[103]
	BIRC3	E3 ligase; mutations disrupt RING domain	Missense mutations	0%	5%	10%		[104–106]
	MYD88	Essential cytosolic adapter protein in Toll-like receptor and interleukin-1 signaling; mutations affect a conserved beta-beta loop of the TIR domain leading to spontaneous and uncontrolled MYD88/IRAK complex formation	Missense mutations (L265P)	10%	10%	15%		[104, 106–109]
	TRAF3	Mediates signal transduction from TNF receptors; mutations result in loss of the C-terminal MATH domain	Loss of function mutations	1%	5%	5%		[104–106]
	CARD11	NF-kB signaling	Missense mutations; mutations involve coiled coil domain leading to spontaneous protein multimerization, CBM complex formation, and NF-kB activation	2%	5–10%	5–10%		[104, 106, 109]

(continued)

Table 16.12 (continued)

Pathway	Gene	Description	Most common mutations reported	Frequency			Clinical utility (diagnostic/prognostic)	Refs
				MALT	NMZL	SMZL		
NOTCH signaling	*NOTCH1*	Notch family receptor; hyperactive Notch signaling due to increased stability of the cleaved intracellular domain (NICD)	Truncating mutations involving the PEST domain	0%	0%	5%		[104, 106, 109]
	NOTCH2	Notch family receptor	Truncating PEST domain mutations, resulting in activation	<5%	25%	10–25%	Specific to NMZL and SMZL, among small B-cell lymphoma; possibly poor prognosis	[104, 106, 109, 110]
	SPEN	Inhibitor of RBPJ	Loss of function mutations	0%	8%	5%		[104, 106, 109]
	DTX1	RING finger ubiquitin ligase	Missense mutations	3%	6%	2%		[104, 106, 109]
	MAML2	Part of Notch2 transcriptional complex	Missense mutations	0%	0%	2%		[104, 106, 109]
KLF2 pathway	*KLF2*	Transcription factor	Loss of function mutations	8%	10%	20%		[104, 111]
PTPRD pathway	*PTPRD*	Receptor-type protein tyrosine phosphatase; mutations involve tyrosine phosphatase domain leading to loss of function	Missense mutations	0%	20%	0%	Specific to NMZL	[104]

Epigenetic regulation	*KMT2D*	Histone methyltransferase	Loss of function mutations	15%	35%	15%		[104, 106, 109, 112, 113]
	SIN3A	Component of histone deacetylase complex		0%	0%	7.50%		[104, 106, 109, 112, 113]
	ARID1A	Component of SWI/SNF complex	Loss of function mutations	0%	6%	10%		[104, 106, 109, 112, 113]
	EP300	Histone acetyltransferase	Predominantly missense mutations in the HAT domain	0%	6%	5%		[104, 106, 109, 112, 113]
	CREBBP	Histone acetyltransferase	Truncating mutations	17%	9%	5%		[104, 106, 109, 110, 112, 113]
	TBL1XR1	Component of SMR T-CoR transcriptional co-repressor		19%	15%	10%		[104, 106, 109, 112, 113]
Cell cycle regulation /DNA damage	*TP53*	Tumor suppressor	Loss of function mutations	3%	3%	15%		[104, 106, 109, 110, 114]

Table 16.13 Frequent copy number alterations in LPL

Copy number change	Gene(s) involved	Frequency	Clinical Utility	Refs
del(6q)		50%	poor prognosis	[115–117]
Trisomy 4		20%		[118]
Gain 3q				[119, 120]
Gain 8q				[119, 120]
Gain 18				[119, 120]
Gain Xq				[119, 120]
Loss 11q23				[119, 120]
Loss 13q14				[119, 120]
Loss 17p	*TP53*			[119, 120]

and pentostatin), and are provisionally classified as "hairy cell leukemia variant" (HCLv) [2]. Although recurrent copy number alterations are identified (Table 16.15), the presence of a *BRAF* p.V600E mutation is 98–100% sensitive for classical HCL and is also highly specific since the mutation has not been identified in entities typically on the differential diagnosis of HCL, such as splenic marginal zone lymphoma, hairy cell leukemia variant, and splenic diffuse red pulp small B-cell lymphoma (Table 16.16; Fig. 16.2) [15–18]. BRAF inhibitors have been demonstrated to rapidly induce durable remission in relapsed/refractory HCL, with response rates of 96–100% in clinical trials [19]. In contrast to classical HCL, HCLv involves activating mutations of *MAP2K1* in 42% of cases, mutually exclusive of *BRAF* p.V600E [20].

Follicular Lymphoma (FL)

FL is the second most common B-cell lymphoma, found primarily in adults and accounting for approximately 20% of all lymphomas [2]. FL subtypes are broken out based upon clinical behavior, including primary cutaneous FL, pediatric-type FL, and FL of specific extranodal sites, such as the duodenum or testes. FL may transform to a more aggressive lymphoma in 25–35% of cases, typically a diffuse large B-cell lymphoma (DLBCL) [2]. The *IGH-BCL2* translocation, t(14;18)(q32,q21), is found in approximately 85–90% of cases of FL, but is not specific as it is also found in 20–25% of de novo DLBCLs (not transformed from a known prior FL), occasional cases of CLL, and rarely in other lymphomas (Table 16.17) [21–26]. Copy number alterations are also not specific (Table 16.18). Epigenetic genes, especially histone modifiers, are recurrently mutated in FL with inactivating mutations of *KMT2D* found in more than 80% of cases (Table 16.19, Fig. 16.2) [27–29]. An integrated clinicogenetic profile has been incorporated into the modified Follicular Lymphoma International Prognostic Index, including mutational status of seven key genes (m7-FLIPI) [30].

Table 16.14 Frequent somatic variants in LPL

Pathway	Gene	Description	Most common mutations reported	Frequency	Clinical utility	Refs
Signaling	*MYD88*	Essential cytosolic adapter protein in Toll-like receptor and interleukin-1 signaling; constitutive activation of NF-κB signaling	Predominantly p.L265P	>90%	diagnostic, sensitivity to ibrutinib	[121]
	CXCR4	Prolonged signaling through CXCR4	Nonsense mutation that truncates last 15–20 amino acids or frameshift mutations in the terminal 44 amino acids	27–36%	decreases sensitivity to ibrutinib	[13, 14]
	CD79B	B-cell receptor complex		<10%		[13]
	TRAF2	TNF receptor-associated factor (TRAF) protein family		<10%		[13]
	TRAF3			<10%		[13]
	NOTCH2	Notch family receptor	Truncating PEST domain mutations, resulting in activation	<10%		[13]
Chromatin modification	*ARID1A*	SWI/SWF family		17%		[13]
Cell cycling, DNA repair	*TP53*	Tumor suppressor	Loss of function mutations	<10%		[13]
Transcriptional regulator	*MYBBP1A*	Transcriptional regulator through interaction with MYB		<10%		[13]
Mucin	*MUC16*			<10%		[13]
Gene rearrangement	*RAG2*			<10%		[13]

Table 16.15 Frequent copy number alterations in HCL

Copy number change	Gene(s) involved	Frequency	Clinical Utility	Refs
Gains of 5		20%		[122–124]
Loss 7q		10%		[122–124]

Table 16.16 Frequent somatic variants in HCL

Pathway	Gene	Description	Most common mutations reported	Frequency	Clinical utility	Refs
Signaling	*BRAF*	RAS/RAF/ MAPK signaling	p.V600E	98–100%	diagnostic, targetable	[15]
	MAP2K1	MAPK signaling	Activating missense hot spots in the kinase domain (including p. C121S) and negative regulatory domain	rare	More common in HCLv (42%) associated with IGHV4-34 in HCLv and rarely in HCL	[20, 125]

Table 16.17 Frequent structural variants in FL

Rearrangement/ gene partners	Description	Frequency	Clinical utility	Refs
t(14;18) (*IGH-BCL2*)	Overexpression of BCL2;MBR (50–70%); mcr (5–15%); icr (~13%)	85–90%	Diagnosis	[21, 26, 126, 127]
BCL6 (3q27) rearrangements	overexpression of BCL6; numerous partners	Seen only in FL grade 3 lymphomas that are negative for t(14;18)	Prognosis	[128–131]

Legend: *MBR* major breakpoint region, *mcr* minor cluster region; *icr* intermediate cluster region

Table 16.18 Frequent copy number alterations in FL

Copy number change	Gene(s) involved	Frequency	Clinical utility	Refs
Loss 1p36	*TNFRSF14*			[132]
Loss 6q	*PRDM1, FOXO3, TNFAIP3, TMEM30A*		Poor prognosis	[132–134]
Gain 7				[132]
Gain 18				[132]
Gain X				[132]
Loss 17p13	*TP53*		Poor prognosis	[132–134]
Loss 9p21.3	*CDKN2A/B, MLLT3*		Poor prognosis	[132–134]
Loss of LOH 1p16			Associated with diffuse FL	[135, 136]

Table 16.19 Frequent somatic variants in FL

Pathway	Gene	Description	Most common mutations reported	Frequency	Clinical utility	Refs
Chromatin modification	*KMT2D*	Histone methyltransferase	Loss of function mutations	80%		[28]
	CREBBP	Histone acetyltransferase	Truncating mutations	33%	m7-FLIPI prognostic, progression	[27–30, 132, 137]
	EZH2	Polycomb group of transcriptional repressors	Truncating and missense mutations within SET domain	27%	m7-FLIPI prognostic, progression	[27–30, 132, 137]
	EP300	Histone acetyltransferase	Predominantly missense mutations in the HAT domain	9%	m7-FLIPI prognostic	[27–30]
	ARID1A	SWI/SWF family	Loss of function		m7-FLIPI prognostic	[30]
	BCL7A	Tumor suppressor	Loss of function			[30]
	TNFRSF14	TNF receptor superfamily member	Truncating mutations	19–46% (29% PTNFL)	Poor prognosis, pediatric FL diagnosis	[30, 138]
	CARD11	NF-κB signaling	Predominantly missense mutations throughout the gene		m7-FLIPI prognostic	[30]
Signaling	*MAP2K1*	MAPK signaling	Activating missense hot spots in the kinase domain (including p.C121S) and negative regulatory domain	10–40%	Pediatric FL diagnosis	[138]
	MAPK1	MAPK signaling	Activating mutations	<10%	pediatric FL diagnosis	[138]
	RRAS	RAS/RAF/MAPK pathway	Activating mutations	<5%	pediatric FL diagnosis	[138]

(continued)

Table 16.19 (continued)

Pathway	Gene	Description	Most common mutations reported	Frequency	Clinical utility	Refs
Transcription	*MEF2B*	Transcriptional activator	Predominantly N-terminal missense mutations	15%	m7-FLIPI prognostic, progression	[27–30, 132, 137]
	FOXP1	Forkhead transcription factor family	Predominantly missense mutations		m7-FLIPI prognostic	[30]
Cell cycling, DNA repair	*CDKN2A*	Inhibitor of CDK4 kinase, stabilizes p53	Deletion/loss of function mutations		Progression	[30, 139]
	CDKN2B	Inhibitor of CDK4 kinase	Deletion/loss of function mutations		Progression	[30, 139]
	MYC	Transcription factor regulating cell cycle progression, apoptosis, and cellular transformation	Gain of function, overexpression		Progression	[132]
	TP53	Tumor suppressor	Loss of function mutations		Progression	[30, 132]
Cell death	*BCL2*	Anti-apoptosis	Gain of function		Progression	[132, 137]
Immune modulators	*B2M*	Component of MHC class I	Loss of function mutations		Progression	[132]
	HLA	Regulation of immune response			Progression	[132]
	CD58	mediates complement effect on cells			Progression	[132]
	IRF8	Transcription factor in the interferon pathway	Missense mutations in the IRF domain and C-terminal truncating mutations	10–50%	Pediatric FL diagnosis	[138]

Legend: m7-FLIPI, Follicular Lymphoma International Prognostic Index, including seven mutated genes

Diffuse Large B-Cell Lymphoma (DLBCL) and Other High-Grade B-Cell Lymphomas (HGBCL)

DLBCL, NOS, is the most common adult lymphoma and accounts for 30–40% of cases of NHL [2]. Although there is marked heterogeneity in the clinical presentation and outcomes, recent molecular profiling efforts have identified new molecularly defined subdivisions [31, 32] that cross or refine many of the former immunophenotypic and transcriptional profiling-based cell-of-origin (COO) as well as genetic categories. COO categories were originally defined by gene expression profiling that identified (1) a germinal center B-cell-like subtype (GCB DLBCLs), (2) activated B-cell-like (ABC-like) subtype, and (3) a "type 3" category that does not cluster with either the GCB or ABC groups [33–36]. This distinction is of prognostic significance since GCB DLBCL has a five-year overall survival of 60%, while ABC DLBCL has only a 35% five-year overall survival [34, 37]. Two recent studies have identified several molecularly defined subgroups of DLBCL that further stratify prognosis, even within the ABC and GCB categories (Tables 16.20, 16.21, and 16.22; Figs. 16.2 and 16.4) [31, 32].

Table 16.20 Frequent structural variants in DLBCL

Rearrangement/ gene partners	Description	Frequency	Clinical utility	Refs
BCL6 (3q27) rearrangements	Overexpression of BCL6; 20 different partners (57% with Ig genes). MBR (region encompassing 5′ flanking region, first noncoding exon, and first intron)	19–45%	Most common in GCB lymphomas which carry a better prognosis, but can be seen in non-GCB DLBCL (Cluster 1)	[32, 140, 141]
t(14;18)	Overexpression of BCL2; MBR (50–70%); mcr (5–15%); icr (~13%), with IGH enhancer in 97% of cases	21%	Diagnosis, prognosis, EZB, Cluster 3 (FL-like, a/w worse prog within GCB)	[31, 32, 140, 141]
BCL10 rearrangements	Overexpression of BCL10 in the NFκB pathway	18%	Diagnosis, prognosis	[140, 141]
MYC rearrangements	Overexpression of MYC; multiple partners (58% with Ig genes)	8–16%	Diagnosis, poor prognosis with TP53 mutations, and as part of double- or triple-hit lymphomas	[32, 140, 141]
t(2;17)(p23;q23)	*CLTC-ALK* fusion		Diagnosis of ALK+ DLBCL	

(continued)

Table 16.20 (continued)

Rearrangement/ gene partners	Description	Frequency	Clinical utility	Refs
PDL1, PDL2 rearrangements	9p24.1	5%	ABC, Cluster 1 (MZL-like, better prognosis within ABC)	[32]
TBL1XR1 rearrangements	Component of SMR T-CoR transcriptional co-repressor	4%		[32]
TP63 rearrangements	p63 is a p53 tumor suppressor family member	3%		[32]
CIITA rearrangements	Transcriptional activator of MHC class II genes	3%		[32]
ETV6 rearrangements	ETS family transcription factor	2%		[32]

Table 16.21 Frequent copy number alterations in DLBCL

Copy number change	Gene(s) involved	Frequency	Clinical utility	Refs
17p13	Deletion (*TP53*)	24%	Cluster 2 (poor prog)	[32]
13q14.2	Deletion (*RB1*)	7%	Cluster 2 (poor prog)	[32]
9p21.13	Deletion (*CDKN2A/B*)	35–50%	Cluster 2 (poor prog)	[27, 142]
Numerous changes, often associated with loci where there are concomitant mutations or rearrangements			Cluster 2 (poor prog)	[32]
18q21.33	Gain (*BCL2*)	5%	Cluster 5 (a/w extranodal dz), independent poor prog in multivariante analysis	[32]
Loss 10q23.31	Loss *PTEN*	8%	GCB, Cluster 3 (FL-like, a/w worse prog within GCB)	[32]
2p16.1	Gain/amplification *REL*	15%	GCB, EZB	[31]
13q31.3	Gain/amplification (miR-17-92)	9%	Cluster 2, EZB, independent poor prog in multivariate analysis	[31, 32]
13q14.2	Loss miR-15/16, *RB1*	14%	Cluster 2	[32]
1q42.12	Loss	8%	Independent poor prog in multivariate analysis	[32]
18p	Gain	23%	Independent poor prog in multivariante analysis	[32]

Table 16.22 Frequent somatic variants in DLBCL

Pathway	Gene	Description	Most common mutations reported	Frequency	Clinical utility	Refs
	TP53	Tumor suppressor	Loss of function mutations	21–23%	Cluster 2 (poor prognosis, associated with CNAs)	[32, 143, 144]
Immune modulator	*CD58*	Immunoglobulin superfamily member; binds to CD2 on T-cells	Loss of function (truncating or missense mutations throughout the gene)	6–11%	GCB, Cluster 4: better prognosis within the GCB category	[32, 143, 145]
	CD83	Immunoglobulin superfamily member involved in B-cell activation	Predominantly missense mutations in the SET domain	3–6%		[32]
	CD70	TNF receptor superfamily member; binds to CD27 on T-cells	Missense mutations in the TNF domain or truncating mutations	9%		[32]
Signaling	*RHOA*	RHOA signaling	Missense mutations that disrupt ARHGEF binding, resulting in increased AKT signaling	4–5%		[32]
	GNA13		Truncating and missense mutations throughout the gene	8–11%		[132, 138, 140, 141, 146]
	SGK1		Predominantly missense mutations (fewer truncating) in the N-terminus and kinase domain	9%		[32]
	BRAF	RAS/RAF signaling	Activating mutations in the kinase domain	3–6%		[32]
	STAT3	JAK/STAT signaling	Activating missense mutations in src homology 2 (SH2) domain (exon 12; p.D566, p.D616, p.D661)	6–9%		[32]
	CARD11	NF-κB signaling	Predominantly missense mutations throughout the gene	11–14%		[32, 145]
	NFKBIE		Loss of function mutations	3–7%		[32]
	NFKBIA		Loss of function mutations	4–5%		[32]

(continued)

Table 16.22 (continued)

Pathway	Gene	Description	Most common mutations reported	Frequency	Clinical utility	Refs
Chromatin modification	*KMT2D*	Histone methyltransferase	Loss of function mutations; predominantly truncating throughout the gene	25–31%	GCB, Cluster 3: worse prognosis within the GCB category; associated with *BCL2-IGH* t(14;18) translocation; FL-like; can acquire additional structural rearrangements in *MYC* leading to double hit lymphoma	[132, 138, 140, 141, 145]
	TNFRSF14	TNF receptor superfamily member	Truncating and missense mutations	13–14%		[32]
	EZH2	Polycomb group of transcriptional repressors	Truncating and missense mutations within SET domain	7–8%		[132, 134, 138, 140, 141, 145]
	CREBBP	Histone acetyltransferase	Truncating mutations or missense mutations in the HAT domain	16–17%		[31, 32, 143, 145]
	EP300	Histone acetyltransferase	Predominantly missense mutations in the HAT domain	8%		[31, 143, 145]
Transcription factor	*MEF2B*	Transcriptional activator	Predominantly N-terminal missense mutations	7–11%		[31, 143]
Signaling	*PTEN*	AKT/MTOR pathway; associated with loss of the *PTEN* locus on 10q23 and the EZB subgroup with gain of the microRNA group, miR-17-92, on 13q31.3, both of which would contribute further to AKT/MTOR dysregulation	Loss of function mutations (predominantly truncating)	3–4%		[31, 32]
	MTOR		Activating mutations	3%		[31]
Immune modulators	*IRF8*	Transcription factor in the interferon pathway	Missense mutations in the IRF domain and C-terminal truncating mutations	8–11%		[32]
	CIITA	Transcriptional activator of MHC class II genes	Missense mutations in the NACHT domain	3–5%		[31, 145]
	HLA-DMA	MHC class II antigen	Predominantly missense mutations in the MHC domain	1–2%		[31]

Signaling	*CD79A*	B-cell receptor complex	Gain of function mutations	3–14%	ABC, Cluster5, MCD: worse prognosis within the ABC category; associated with extranodal disease	[31, 32, 143, 145]
	MYD88	Essential cytosolic adapter protein in Toll-like receptor and interleukin-1 signaling; constitutive activation of NF-κB signaling	Missense mutations, p.L265P most common	18–27%		[31, 32, 143, 145]
	PIM1	Kinase in multiple signaling pathways	Missense and truncating mutations clusters in the N-terminal half of the gene	22–28%		[32, 145]
Metabolism	*GRHPR*	Glyoxylate and hydroxypyruvate reductase		6%		[32]
Transcription regulation	*ETV6*	ETS family transcription factor	N terminal truncating mutations or ETS domain missense mutations	7–9%		[32]
	TBL1XR1	Component of SMR T-CoR transcriptional co-repressor	Predominantly missense or inframe mutations in the WD domains	7–13%		[32]
	PRDM1	Transcription activator in post germinal center B-cells	Loss of function missense or truncating mutations, especially in the SET domain	7–11%		[31, 145]
Cell cycle	*CDKN2A*	Inhibitor of CDK4 kinase, stabilizes p53	deletion/loss of function mutations	6%		[31]
	BTG1	Antiproliferative cell cycle regulator	Predominantly missense mutations in the BTG domain	14–15% (*BTG2* 18%)		[31, 32]
Apoptosis	*BCL2*	Antiapoptotic	Missense mutations throughout the gene	10–17%		[32]

(continued)

Table 16.22 (continued)

Pathway	Gene	Description	Most common mutations reported	Frequency	Clinical utility	Refs
Transcription factor	*BCL6*	Germinal center transcription factor	Predominantly missense mutations in the BTB domain and C-terminus	6–11%	ABC, BN2, Cluster 1: better prognosis within the ABC category; MZL-like	[31, 32]
Notch signaling pathway	*NOTCH2*	Notch family receptor	Truncating PEST domain mutations, resulting in activation	7–8%		[31, 32]
	SPEN	Negative regulator of NOTCH signaling	Truncating loss of function mutation throughout the gene	9–10%		[32]
	DTX1	NOTCH target	Missense mutations in the N-terminal WWE domain	12–15%		[31]
Immune modulator	*B2M*	Component of MHC class I	Loss of function mutations (truncating and missense)	9–16%		[32, 143, 145]
Signaling	*FAS*	NF-κB signaling	Truncating or missense mutations in the Death domain	8–9%		[32]
	TNFAIP3		Predominantly truncating mutations throughout the gene	9–17%		[31, 32, 143, 145]
	BCL10		Predominantly C-terminal truncating mutations	5–9%		[31, 32]
	PRKCB		Missense mutations	5%		[31]
Notch signaling pathway	*NOTCH1*	Notch family receptor	Truncating PEST domain mutations, resulting in activation	3%	ABC, N1: poor prognosis	[31]
Transcription factor	*IRF4*	Transcription factor	Activating missense mutations in the IRF domain	9%		[31]
	ID3	Negative transcriptional regulator of *TCF3*	Loss of function	4%		[31)
	BCOR	*BCL6* co-repressor	Loss of function mutations	5%		[31]

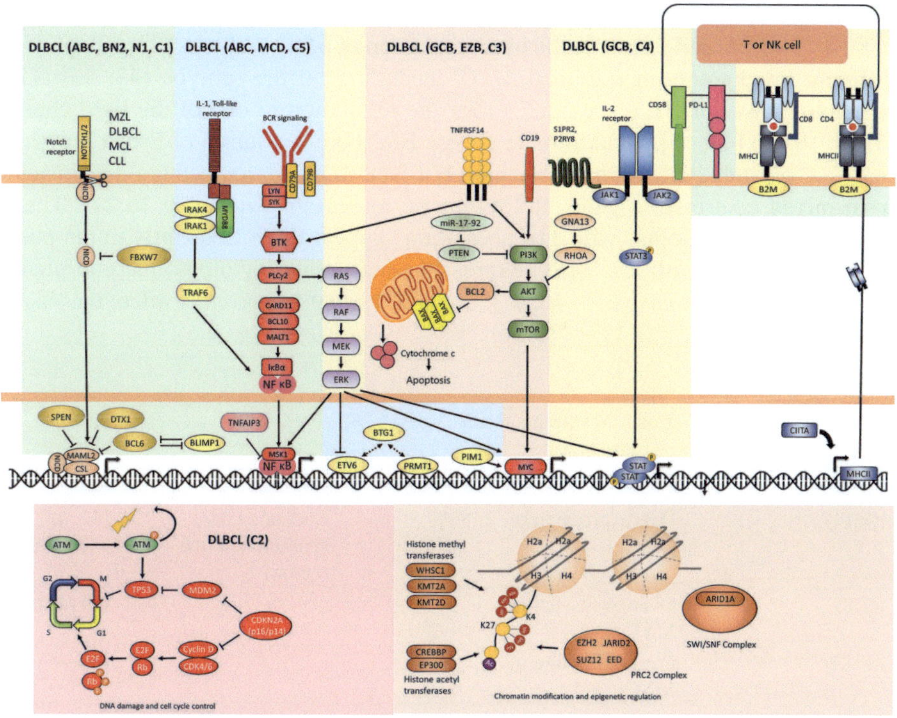

Fig. 16.4 Overview of molecular alterations in diffuse large B-cell lymphoma. Somatic mutations, rearrangements, and copy number alterations are categorized into color-coded groups by cell of origin and prognostic subgroups. Subgroups (left to right) include signaling through the Notch pathway, p53, MYD88, and CD79A and NF-κB pathway, PTEN/AKT pathways, chromatin modifiers, JAK-STAT pathway, and immune evasion pathway. Abbreviations: GCB germinal center B-cell, ABC activated B-cell, C1 cluster 1, C2 cluster 2, C3 cluster 3, C4 cluster 4, C5 cluster 5, BN2 group characterized by *BCL6* and *NOTCH2* mutations, N1 group characterized by *NOTCH1* mutations, MCD group characterized by *MYD88* and *CD79A* mutations, EZB group characterized by *EZH2* and *BCL2* mutations

Burkitt's Lymphoma (BL)

BL is a highly aggressive B-cell neoplasm that can manifest as one of the three subtypes that have different epidemiologic and molecular bases while related by their common dependence upon *MYC* dysregulation [2]. The endemic variant of BL is prevalent in young children of equatorial Africa, associated in approximately 95% of cases with Epstein-Barr virus (EBV) [5]. Sporadic BL is found predominantly in adolescents and young adults of Western countries, with less frequent association with EBV in 5–30% of cases [2, 38, 39]. Immunodeficiency-associated BL is the third biologic subtype, often associated with human immunodeficiency virus (HIV) and, in approximately 25–40% of cases, with clonal EBV as well [40,

41]. The t(8;14)(q24;q32), juxtaposing *MYC* with the *IGH* locus, can be identified in 80% of all BL and results in the overexpression of *MYC* (Table 16.23), albeit with different breakpoints in *IGH* and *MYC* depending on the subtype [42, 43]. The remaining cases of BL place *MYC* under the regulation of one of the light chains (Table 16.23) [44, 45]. In addition to classic BL, there is a subset of B-cell lymphomas that resemble BL morphologically, but lack *MYC* rearrangement and instead have mixed centromeric gains and telomeric losses on 11q (Table 16.24). These "Burkitt-like lymphomas with 11q aberration" appear more frequently in the post-transplant setting with less MYC expression and greater cytologic pleomorphism and karyotypic complexity [6, 46, 47]. Somatic variants recurrently affect the *TCF3* pathway (Table 16.25 and Fig. 16.2).

Table 16.23 Frequent structural variants in BL

Rearrangement/gene partners	Description	Frequency	Clinical utility	Refs
t(8;14)	Overexpression of MYC	80%	Endemic (JH), sporadic (switch region)	[42, 43, 147–150]
t(2;8)	Overexpression of MYC			[44, 45]
t(8;22)	Overexpression of MYC			[44, 45]

Table 16.24 Frequent copy number alterations in BL

Copy number change	Gene(s) involved	Frequency	Clinical utility	Refs
11q		centromeric gains, telomeric losses	Diagnostic for provisional Burkitt-like with 11q	[46, 47]

Table 16.25 Frequent somatic variants in BL

Pathway	Gene	Description	Most common mutations reported	Frequency	Clinical utility	Refs
TCF3 pathway	*TCF3*	Master B-cell transcriptional regulator	Gain of function	23%		[151–153]
	CCND3	Downstream target of *TCF3*, involved in cell cycling	Gain of function mutations (truncating or missense) in the C-terminus	38%		[151–153]
	ID3	Negative transcriptional regulator of *TCF3*	Loss of function	68%		[151–153]

Recurrent Molecular Aberrancies in T-Cell Neoplasms

Angioimmunoblastic T-Cell Lymphoma (AITL) and Other Nodal T-Cell Lymphomas with T-Follicular Helper (TFH) Phenotype

AITL is an EBV-associated peripheral T-cell lymphoma that usually affects older adults with nodal involvement, often presenting with prominent and protean systemic manifestations (e.g., cold agglutinin disease with hemolytic anemia, polyclonal hypergammaglobulinemia). The putative cell of origin of this neoplasm is a CD4+ T-follicular helper cell (TFH), based on the observation that the neoplastic T-cells uniformly show expression of markers of TFH differentiation (PD-1, CD10, BCL-6, CXCL13, ICOS). Recurrent cytogenetic and molecular findings target T-cell stimulatory pathways (Tables 16.26, 16.27, and 16.28, Fig. 16.5) [1, 6].

Anaplastic Large-Cell Lymphoma (ALCL)

ALCL is a predominantly nodal T-cell lymphoma that is histologically characterized by a proliferation of large anaplastic cells that show strong CD30 expression. These tumors can be classified into two distinct entities based on the presence of

Table 16.26 Frequent structural variants in AITL

Rearrangement/gene partners	Description	Frequency	Clinical utility	Refs
CTLA4-CD28	Likely the result of partial gene duplication; fusion protein consists of the extracellular domain of CTLA4 and the cytoplasmic region of CD28, likely capable of transforming inhibitory signals into stimulatory signals for T-cell activation	58%	Potential target for anti-CTLA4 Immunotherapy	[154]
t(5;9)(q33;q22) (*ITK-SYK*)	Both *ITK* and *SYK* are involved in normal antigen-induced lymphocyte activation. Fusion protein joins the Pleckstrin homology (PHD) and TEC homology domains (THD) of ITK with the SYK kinase domain leading to ligand-independent constitutive antigen receptor signaling	Rare	Confers sensitivity to SYK inhibitors	[155, 156]

Table 16.27 Frequent copy number alterations in AITL

Copy number change	Gene(s) involved	Frequency	Clinical utility	Refs
Trisomy 7		8%		[157]
Trisomy 5		15–41%	Poor prognosis	[157–159]
Trisomy 3		27%		[158]
Trisomy 21		41%		[158]
Trisomy 19		15%		[160]
9p23 amplification		60%		[159]
8q24.11 amplification		22%		[159]
6q loss		23%		[158]
5q gain		55%		[158]
3q loss		10%		[159]
3q gain		36%		[158]
22q gain		23%		[161]
19q13.43 amplification		32%		[159]
13q22.3 gain	*MYCBP2*	36%	Poor prognosis	[159]
13q loss		23%		[158]
11q13 gain	*CCND1, GSTP1*	13%		[158]

an ALK rearrangement (ALK+ ALCL and ALK− ALCL) (Table 16.29). These two entities have widely different clinical and prognostic features as well as molecular underpinnings, although both involve some level of signaling through the JAK-STAT pathway (Tables 16.30 and 16.31, Fig. 16.5) [1, 6]. ALK+ ALCL is more common in the young adult population, is highly chemosensitive, and has a relatively favorable prognosis (five-year survival, 80–90%). ALK-negative ALCL is more common in older adults and has a less favorable prognosis (five-year survival, 36%) [6].

Peripheral T-Cell Lymphoma, Not Otherwise Specified (PTCL, NOS)

The PTCL, NOS category includes a clinically and biologically heterogeneous group of T-cell neoplasms that do not meet diagnostic criteria for another WHO-defined category [6]. Therefore, the diagnosis is one of exclusion. The tumors that fall into this category do not appear to harbor specific cytogenetic or molecular genetic alterations, although there is some molecular overlap with AITL (Tables 16.32, 16.33, and 16.34, Fig. 16.5) [1, 6].

Table 16.28 Frequent somatic variants in AITL

Pathway	Gene	Description	Most common mutations reported	Frequency	Clinical utility (diagnostic/prognostic)	Refs
Signal transduction and actin nucleation	*RHOA*	GTPase molecular switch involved in signal transduction and regulating cell shape and motility; p.G17V mutations lead to loss of GTPase activity	Hot spot missense mutation (p.G17V)	53–68%	Driver mutation, relatively specific to AITL	[161, 162]
T-cell co-stimulation	*CD28*	T-cell-specific surface glycoprotein involved in proliferation, survival, cytokine production, and Th2 development; missense mutations are activating leading to constitutive T-cell stimulation and increased proliferation	Hot spot missense mutations (p.D124, p. T195)	10–11%		[163, 164]
Epigenetic regulation	*TET2*	Demethylates CpG sites by oxidation of 5-methyl group of 5-methyl cytosine	Loss of function mutations	76–83%	Coexist with *RHOA* and *DNMT3A* mutations	[162, 165–167]
	DNMT3A	DNA methyltransferase	Loss of function mutations	26–38%	Coexist with *TET2* mutations	[162, 165–167]
	IDH2	NADP(+)-dependent isocitrate dehydrogenase part of tricarboxylic acid cycle (citric acid cycle) cycle, mutation results in production of oncometabolite (*R*)-2-hydroxyglutarate which inhibits TET2 function	Hot spot missense mutations (predominantly p.R172 and less commonly p. R140)	45%	Relatively specific for AITL, possible role for MRD monitoring	[162, 165–168]

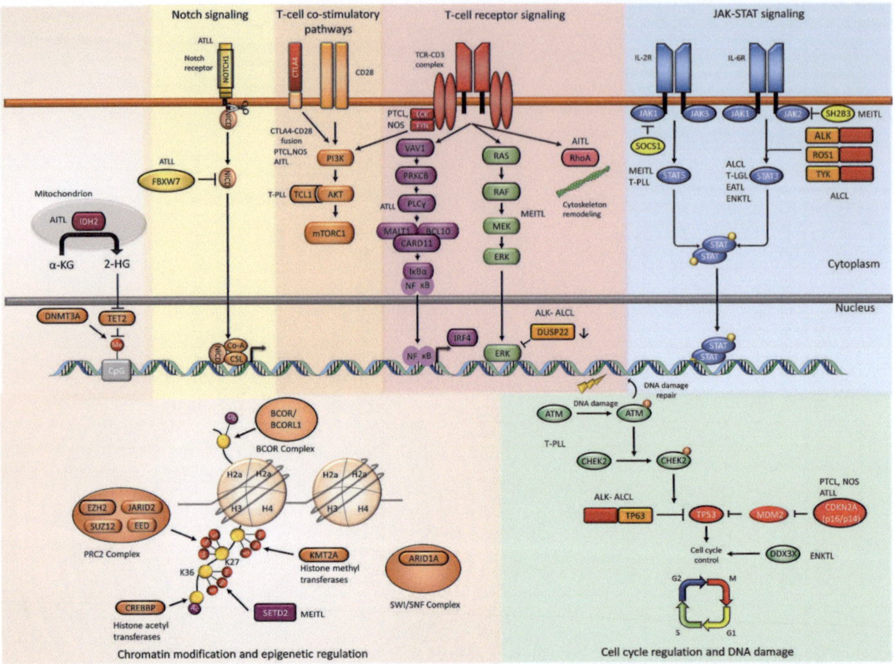

Fig. 16.5 Overview of recurrent molecular alterations in mature T-cell neoplasms. Somatic mutations, rearrangements, and copy number alterations across a wide variety of T-cell lymphomas converge on a limited set of pathways highlighted in this figure: T-cell receptor signaling, T-cell co-stimulatory signaling pathways, JAK-STAT signaling, DNA damage/cell cycle regulation, epigenetic regulation, and Notch signaling. Genes that are recurrently mutated in T-cell neoplasms are depicted with bold outlines. If a specific genetic alteration is relatively specific for a T-cell lymphoma entity, the respective T-cell lymphoma category is indicated next to the gene. Abbreviations: AITL angioimmunoblastic T-cell lymphoma, ATLL adult T-cell leukemia/lymphoma, PTCL, NOS peripheral T-cell lymphoma, not otherwise specified, MEITL monomorphic epitheliotropic intestinal T-cell lymphoma, T-PLL T-cell prolymphocytic leukemia, ALCL anaplastic large cell lymphoma, T-LGL T-cell large granular lymphocytic leukemia, EATL enteropathy-associated T-cell lymphoma

T-Cell Large Granular Lymphocytic (T-LGL) Leukemia

T-LGL leukemia is an indolent disorder of clonal circulating cytotoxic T-cells often associated with cytopenias (neutropenia or severe anemia, the latter a result of pure red cell aplasia). Associations with autoimmune diseases, such as rheumatoid arthritis, are well established. However, making a diagnosis of T-LGL leukemia is challenging because the differential diagnosis of an expanded population of LGLs is quite broad. Transient T-LGL expansions can be seen in the setting of allogeneic transplant setting, autoimmune disease, viral illness, and even as a response to an underlying B-cell neoplasm. Moreover, demonstration of clonality by TCR gene

Table 16.29 Frequent structural variants in ALCL

Rearrangement/gene partners	Description	Frequency	Clinical utility	Refs
ALK-positive anaplastic large-cell lymphoma				
t(2;5)(p23;q35.1)/*NPM1-ALK*	The fusion attaches the N-terminus of *NPM1* containing an oligomerization domain to the full tyrosine kinase domain of *ALK* resulting in constitutive kinase activity. Other fusion partners to *ALK* (*TPM3*, *ATIC*, etc.) also contain oligomerization domains, likely leading to constitutive ALK kinase activation by the same mechanism	84%	Diagnostic of ALK+ ALCL	[2]
t(1;2)(q25;p23)/*TPM3-ALK*		13%		[2]
inv(2)(p23;q35)/*ATIC-ALK*		1%		[2]
t(2;3)(p23;q21)/*TFG-ALK*		<1%		[2]
t(2;17)(p23;q23)/*CLTC-ALK*		<1%		[2]
t(2;X)(p23;q11-12)/*MSN-ALK*		<1%		[2]
t(2;22)(q23;p11.2)/*MYH9-ALK*		<1%		[2]
t(2;19)(p23;q13.1)/*TPM4-ALK*		<1%		[2]
t(2;17)(p23;q25)/*ALO17-ALK*		<1%		[2]
ALK-negative anaplastic large-cell lymphoma (including primary cutaneous ALCL)				
t(6;7)(p25.3;q32.2)/*DUSP22-FRA7H*	DUSP22 is a dual-specificity phosphatase that inhibits T-cell antigen receptor signaling by inactivating ERK2; translocation results in disruption of the *DUSP22* gene and decreased expression	20–45%	Favorable prognosis, relatively specific to ALK- ALCL, rarely reported in PTCLs but not other cutaneous T-cell lymphomas	[169, 170]
VAV1 rearrangements	VAV1 encodes a guanine exchange factor (GEF) critical in T-cell receptor signaling. The fusion results in loss of the C-terminal SH3 autoinhibitory domain leading to activating of VAV1 GEF activity culminating in RAC-dependent increase in growth and migration	16%		[171]
ROS1 rearrangements	Fusion partners (*NFKB2*, *NCOR2*) provide dimerization domains to the tyrosine kinase domains of *ROS1* and *TYK2* leading to constitutive kinase activity and JAK/STAT signaling	11%		[172]
TYK2 rearrangements		11%		[172]

(continued)

Table 16.29 (continued)

Rearrangement/gene partners	Description	Frequency	Clinical utility	Refs
inv(3)(q26q28)/*TP63-TBL1XR1*	p63 is a p53 family member; fusion results in loss of the N-terminal transactivation domain of TP63 leading to a dominant negative fusion product that inhibits the TP53 pathway	8%	Poor prognosis	[170, 173]
IRF4 rearrangements	Interferon regulatory factor (IRF) family transcription factor; IRF4 overexpression is oncogenic in vitro	57% (cALCL)		[174, 175]

Table 16.30 Frequent copy number alterations in ALCL

Copy number change	Gene(s) involved	Frequency		Clinical utility	Refs
		ALK+ ALCL	ALK– ALCL		
17p13.3-p12 loss	*TP53*	9%	42%	Poor prognosis	[181]
6q21 loss	*PRDM1, ATG5*	6%	56%	Poor prognosis	[181]
13q32.3-q33.3 loss		9%	23%		[181]
16q23.2 loss		3%	29%		[181]
1q gain		15%	32%		[181]
8q24.22 gain		12%	23%		[181]

Table 16.31 Frequent somatic variants in ALCL

Pathway	Gene	Description	Most common mutations reported	Frequency	Clinical utility (diagnostic/prognostic)	Refs
JAK-STAT signaling	*JAK1*	Protein-tyrosine kinase which regulates interferon signaling	Activating missense mutations in tyrosine kinase domain (p.G1097D/S)	7–15%	Not identified in histologic mimics, ALK+ ALCL or PTCL, NOS	[172, 176–180]
	STAT3	STAT family protein	Activating missense mutations in src homology 2 (SH2) domain (exon 12; p.Y640F, p.N647I, p.D661Y, p.A662V)	10–20%	Not identified in histologic mimics, ALK+ ALCL or PTCL, NOS	[172, 176–180]

Table 16.32 Frequent structural variants in PTCL

Rearrangement/ gene partners	Description	Frequency	Clinical utility	Refs
ITK-SYK	Both *ITK* and *SYK* are involved in normal antigen-induced lymphocytes activation. Fusion protein joins the Pleckstrin homology (PHD) and TEC homology domains (THD) of ITK with the SYK kinase domain leading to ligand-independent constitutive antigen receptor signaling	17%	Confers sensitivity to SYK inhibitors	[156, 182]
CTLA4-CD28	Likely the result of partial gene duplication; fusion protein consists of the extracellular domain of CTLA4 and the cytoplasmic region of CD28, likely capable of transforming inhibitory signals into stimulatory signals for T-cell activation	23%	Potential target for anti-CTLA4 immunotherapy	[154]
VAV1	*VAV1* encodes a guanine exchange factor (GEF) critical in T-cell receptor signaling. The fusion results in loss of the C-terminal SH3 autoinhibitory domain leading to activating of VAV1 GEF activity culminating in RAC1-dependent increase in growth and migration	11%	Sensitive to RAC1 inhibitors	[171]
t(6;14)(p25;q11.2)/*IRF4-TCRA*	Interferon regulatory factor (*IRF*) family transcription factor; rearrangement likely leads to overexpression of IRF4 which is oncogenic in vitro	Rare		[174, 175]

Table 16.33 Frequent copy number alterations in PTCL

Copy number change	Gene(s) involved	Frequency	Clinical utility	Refs
9p23 amplification		36%		[159]
8q24.11 amplification		33%		[159]
19q13.43 amplification		21%		[159]
3q loss		12%		[159]
9p21.3	*MTAP, CDKN2A, CDKN2B*	9–31%	Poor prognosis	[159, 183]
2p15-16 amplification	*REL*	10%		[184]
7p gain		20%	Poor prognosis	[183]
7q gain		31%	Poor prognosis	[183]
17q11-q25 gain		30%		[160]
8q24.21 gain		20%		[160]
22q12-qtel gain		20%		[160]
13q13-q33 loss		30%		[160]

Table 16.34 Frequent somatic variants in PTCL

Pathway	Gene	Description	Most common mutations reported	Frequency	Clinical utility (diagnostic/prognostic)	Refs
Epigenetic regulation	*DNMT3A*	DNA methyltransferase	Loss of function mutations	27–36%		[161, 166, 185]
	TET2	Demethylates CpG sites by oxidation of 5-methyl group of 5-methyl cytosine	Loss of function mutations	46–49%		[161, 166, 185]
Signal transduction and actin nucleation	*RHOA*	GTPase molecular switch involved in signal transduction and regulating cell shape and motility; G17V mutations lead to loss of GTPase activity	Hot spot missense mutation (p.G17V)	12–18%		[186, 187]
TCR signaling	*FYN*	Src family kinase involved T-cell receptor (TCR) signaling; missense mutations disrupt intramolecular inhibitory interaction of the SH2 domain with the C-terminal SRC-kinase-phosphorylated residue leading to FYN activation	Missense mutations (p.L174R, p.R176C, p.Y531H)	5%	Sensitive to TKIs	[186, 187]
	VAV1	Guanine exchange factor (GEF) critical in T-cell receptor signaling; focal deletion results in in-frame mis-splicing of exon 25 into a cryptic intraexonic splice acceptor motif in exon 26 resulting in expression of a VAV1 gain-of-function oncoprotein with an in-frame deletion	Focal in-frame deletion (Δ778-786)	5%		[187]
T-cell co-stimulation	*CD28*	Costimulatory molecule for T-cell activation	Hot spot missense mutations (p.D124, p.T195)	5%		[187]

Table 16.35 Frequent somatic variants in T-LGL

Pathway	Gene	Description	Most common mutations reported	Frequency	Clinical utility (diagnostic/ prognostic)	Refs
JAK-STAT signaling	*STAT3*	Mutations result in increased dimerization and STAT3 phosphorylation leading to increased JAK-STAT signaling	Hot spot missense mutations involving the SH2 domain involved in dimerization (exon 21; p.Y640, p.D661)	28–70%		[188–193]
	STAT5B	Mutations result in increased dimerization and STAT5b phosphorylation leading to increased JAK-STAT signaling	Missense mutations involving the SH2 domain (p.Y665H, p.N642H)	2%	p.N642H mutation associated with more aggressive disease and CD3+ CD56+ phenotype	[188–193]

rearrangement studies does not equate with neoplasia. In this context, the demonstration of a pathogenic somatic mutation in *STAT3* (or rarely *STAT5B*) would be supportive evidence of neoplasia (Table 16.35) [1, 6].

T-Cell Prolymphocytic Leukemia (T-PLL)

T-PLL is a rare aggressive T-cell neoplasm that predominantly presents with peripheral blood and bone marrow involvement. This neoplasm is characterized by hallmark translocations involving the oncogene TCL1 (Table 16.36). Like T-LGL, T-PLL has recurrent activation of the IL2-JAK-STAT pathway, but shows dependence upon *STAT5B* as well as frequent mutations or deletions of *ATM* (Tables 16.37 and 16.38; Fig. 16.5) [1, 6].

Enteropathy-Associated T-Cell Lymphoma (EATL) and Monomorphic Epitheliotropic Intestinal T-Cell Lymphoma (MEITL)

EATL is a rare intestinal T-cell lymphoma seen in association with Celiac disease most frequent in patients with Northern European ancestry. This is distinct from

Table 16.36 Frequent structural variants in T-PLL

Rearrangement/gene partners	Description	Frequency	Clinical utility	Refs
inv(14)(q11;q32.1)/ t(14;14)(q11;q32.1)/*TCL1A/B-TRA/D*	Leads to translocation of the *TCRA/D* locus next to the *TCL1* proto-oncogene resulting in overexpression and activation of AKT	73%	Relatively specific to T-PLL	[194]
t(X;14)(q28;q11)/*MTCP1-TRA/D*	*MTCP1* is a *TCL1* family member; translocation results in overexpression of *MTCP1*	7%	Relatively specific to T-PLL	[194, 195]
t(7;14)(q35;q32.1)/*TCL1-TRB*	Translocation of the *TCRB* locus next to the *TCL1* proto-oncogene resulting in overexpression and activation of AKT	Rare		[196]
t(9;17)(q34.12;q25.3)/*SEPT9-ABL1*		Rare	Resistant to ABL1 tyrosine kinase inhibitors	[197]

Table 16.37 Frequent copy number alterations in T-PLL

Copy number change	Gene(s) involved	Frequency	Clinical utility	Refs
8q gain [including i(8)(q10)]		61–77%	Associated with TCL1-TCRA/D translocations	[194, 198, 199]
14q32 gain	*TRA, TRD*	30%		[194]
6q loss		25%		[194, 198]
7q36 loss	*EZH2, GIMAP*	41–53%		[194, 199]
8p loss		61%		[194]
11q loss	*ATM*	69%	Associated with concurrent ATM mutations and TCRA/D translocations	[194, 199]
17p loss	*TP53*	31%	Associated with concurrent TP53 deletions and lack of TCRA/D rearrangements	[194]
22q loss	*SMARCB1*	33–37%		[194, 200]
10p loss		20%		[194]

Table 16.38 Frequent somatic variants in T-PLL

Pathway	Gene	Description	Most common mutations reported	Frequency	Clinical utility (diagnostic/ prognostic)	Refs
DNA damage/cell cycle regulation	*ATM*	Tumor suppressor gene involved in double-strand break repair; mutations lead to loss of protein function	Missense (C-terminal half) and truncating mutations	70–73%	Younger age and associated with TCL1 translocations, often with biallelic inactivation of ATM; no clear prognostic significance	[194, 199]
	TP53	Tumor suppressor gene; mutations lead to loss of protein function	Missense mutations (including p.R175)	14%	Older age and lack of TCL1 translocation; often with biallelic inactivation of TP53; no clear prognostic significance	[194, 199]
	CHEK2	Protein kinase involved in DNA damage response	Frameshift and missense mutations (loss of function)	5%		[194, 199]
JAK-STAT signaling	*STAT5B*	Mutations result in increased dimerization and STAT5b phosphorylation leading to increased JAK-STAT signaling	Missense mutations within SH2 domain (p.N642H)	36%		[194, 199]
	JAK3	Activating mutations leads to increased JAK-STAT signaling	Missense mutations (p.M511I between JH3 and pseudokinase JH2 domain)	21–34%	Associated with poor overall survival in univariate analysis	[194, 199]
	JAK1	Activating mutations leads to increased JAK-STAT signaling	Missense mutations in pseudokinase domain (p.V658F, p.S703I)	6–8%		[194, 199]
	IL2RG	Interleukin-2 receptor; activating mutations involving transmembrane domain result increased JAK-STAT signaling	Missense mutations/ in-frame deletions involving transmembrane domain	2%		[194, 199]

(continued)

Table 16.38 (continued)

Pathway	Gene	Description	Most common mutations reported	Frequency	Clinical utility (diagnostic/prognostic)	Refs
Epigenetic regulation	*EZH2*	Polycomb group of transcriptional repressors	Truncating and missense mutations within SET domain	13%		[194, 199]
	BCOR	BCL6 co-repressor	Missense mutations	8%		[194, 199]
Ubiquitination and proteasome degradation	*FBXW10*	member of F-box protein family of ubiquitin ligases	Truncating and missense mutations (loss of function)	8%		[194, 199]

MEITL, which occurs in Asian and Hispanic patients and which has no association with Celiac disease (formerly known as EATL type II). Taken together, these two entities account for a quarter of all primary small intestinal lymphomas. Both these entities show overlapping but somewhat distinct genetic profiles with frequent mutations involving epigenetic modifiers and JAK-STAT signaling (EATL resembling T-LGL and MEITL resembling T-PLL) and recurrent gain of *MYC* in MEITL (Tables 16.39 and 16.40; Fig. 16.5) [1, 6].

Adult T-Cell Leukemia/Lymphoma (ATLL)

ATLL is a distinct mature T-cell neoplasm that is driven by the human T-cell leukemia virus type 1 (HTLV-1). Accordingly, this disease is more common in regions with a higher prevalence of HTLV-1 infection, such as southwest Japan and the Caribbean basin. The clinical presentation and course of ATLL is highly variable with four distinct subtypes: acute, lymphomatous, chronic, and smoldering. The acute and lymphomatous subtypes are highly aggressive diseases with very poor prognosis, while the chronic and smoldering subtypes show an indolent clinical course. These clinical subtypes exhibit distinct molecular genetic differences that dictate prognosis (Tables 16.41, 16.42, and 16.43, Fig. 16.5) [1, 6].

Extranodal Natural Killer/T-Cell Lymphoma (ENKTL)

ENKTL is a rare aggressive EBV-driven neoplasm that usually presents in older adults at extranodal sites (e.g., upper aerodigestive tract, skin) characterized by prominent necrosis and angiocentricity [6]. Most cases show an NK-cell phenotype; rare cases can show a cytotoxic T-cell phenotype. This disease is far more prevalent in Asia and South America. As with several other T-cell neoplasms, epigenetic and JAK-STAT pathway mutations are recurrent as well as copy number loss on 6q (Tables 16.44, 16.45, and 16.46; Fig. 16.5).

Table 16.39 Frequent copy number alterations in EATL and MEITL

Copy number change	Gene(s) involved	Frequency	Clinical utility	Refs
9q gain		70–75%		[201–203]
16q12.1 loss		23%		[204]
1q32.2--q41 gain		47%	More frequent in EATL	[201, 204]
5q34-q35.2 gain		50%	More frequent in EATL	[203, 204]
8q24 gain	*MYC*	43%	More frequent in MEITL	[201–203]
7q gain		30%		[201, 205]

Table 16.40 Frequent somatic variants in EATL and MEITL

Pathway	Gene	Description	Most common mutations reported	Frequency	Clinical utility (diagnostic/prognostic)	Refs
Epigenetic regulation	*SETD2*	Tumor suppressor and H3K36-specific trimethyltransferase	Loss of function mutations	32–93%	Associated with copy number loss involving SETD2 (3p21.31); more frequent in MEITL	[205]
	CREBBP	Histone acetyltransferase	Truncating mutations	26%		[205]
JAK-STAT signaling	*STAT5B*	Mutations result in increased dimerization and STAT5b phosphorylation leading to increased JAK-STAT signaling	Hot spot missense mutations involving SH2 domain (N642H)	29–60%	More frequent in MEITL	[201, 205]
	JAK3	Activating mutations lead to increased JAK-STAT signaling	Missense mutations involving pseudokinase domain	23–46%	More frequent in MEITL	[201, 205]
	JAK1	Activating mutations lead to increased JAK-STAT signaling	Missense mutations (p.G1097)	23–50%	More frequent in EATL	[201, 205]
	STAT3	Hot spot activating mutations	Missense mutations (p.N647I, p.K658N)	16–25%	More frequent in EATL	[201, 205]
	SH2B3	Negative regulator of JAK-STAT signaling	Loss-of-function mutations	20%		[205]
	SOCS1	Negative regulator of JAK-STAT signaling	Loss-of-function mutations	7%	More frequent in EATL	[201, 205]

RAS/MAPK signaling	*BRAF*	RAF family serine/threonine protein kinase; reported variants are weakly activating/kinase impaired	Missense mutations	27%	More frequent in MEITL	[205]
	KRAS	Small GTPase involved in MAPK signaling; hotspot activating mutations involving codon 12/13	Missense mutations (codon 12/13)	7–20%	More frequent in MEITL	[201, 205]
	NRAS	Small GTPase involved in MAPK signaling; hot spot activating mutations involving codon 12/13	Missense mutations (codon 12/13)	10%		[201, 205]
DNA damage	*TP53*	Tumor suppressor	Loss–of-function mutations	10–33%		[201, 205]

Table 16.41 Frequent structural variants in ATLL

Rearrangement/gene partners	Description	Frequency	Clinical utility	Refs
CD28-CTLA4 fusion	Extracellular domain of CTLA4/ICOS fused to cytoplasmic region of CD28; chimeric protein is also under transcriptional control of *CTLA4* and *ICOS* leading to overexpression leading to excess co-stimulatory signaling	5%	Potential target for anti-CTLA4 immunotherapy	[206]
CD28-ICOS fusion		2%		[206]

Table 16.42 Frequent copy number alterations in ATLL

Copy number change	Gene(s) involved	Frequency	Clinical utility	Refs
9p24 amplification	*PD-L1*	10–20%	More common in aggressive subtype; poor prognosis independent of subtype	[206, 207]
6p22 deletion	*ATXN1*	10–20%		[206, 207]
6q21 deletion	*PRDM1*	10–20%		[206, 207]
9p21 deletion	*CDKN2A*	20–30%	More common in aggressive subtype; shorter OS in indolent subtype	[206, 207]
13q32 deletion	*GPR183*	20–30%		[206, 207]

Table 16.43 Frequent somatic variants in ATLL

Pathway	Gene	Description	Most common mutations reported	Frequency	Clinical utility (diagnostic/ prognostic)	Refs
Notch pathway	*NOTCH1*	Notch family receptor; likely gain of function	Missense mutations involving C-terminus	30%		[206–208]
	FBXW7	Part of E3 protein ligase complex; loss-of-function mutations	Missense mutations involving the substrate-binding domain	25%		[206, 207, 209]

Table 16.43 (continued)

Pathway	Gene	Description	Most common mutations reported	Frequency	Clinical utility (diagnostic/ prognostic)	Refs
Signal transduction and actin nucleation	*RHOA*	GTPase molecular switch involved in signal transduction and regulating cell shape and motility; mutations can lead to gain or loss of function	Missense mutations involving GTP-binding domains (codons 16, 17, 161)	15%		[206, 207, 210]
TCR and NF-kB signaling	*PLCG1*	Regulator of proximal TCR signaling; likely gain of function	Hot spot missense mutations (codons 48, 345, 520, 1163, 1165)	36%		[206, 207]
	PRKCB	PKC family protein; likely gain of function	Hot spot missense mutations (codon 427)	33%	Shorter OS in aggressive subtype	[206, 207]
	CARD11	Scaffold protein involved in NF-kB signaling; likely gain of function	Missense mutations involving coiled coil and autoinhibitory domains	24%		[206, 207]
	VAV1	Guanine exchange factor (GEF) critical in T-cell receptor signaling; likely gain of function	Missense mutations	18%		[206, 207]
	IRF4	Downstream target of NF-kB signaling	Hot spot missense mutations involving DNA-binding domain	14%	More common in aggressive subtype; shorter OS in indolent subtype	[206, 207]

(continued)

Table 16.43 (continued)

Pathway	Gene	Description	Most common mutations reported	Frequency	Clinical utility (diagnostic/ prognostic)	Refs
Chemokine receptor	*CCR4*	G-protein coupled receptor; likely gain of function	Truncating mutations involving C-terminal cytoplasmic domain	29%		[206, 207]
JAK-STAT signaling	*STAT3*	Gain of function mutations	Hot spot missense mutations involving the SH2 domain (Y640, D661)	22%	More common in indolent subtype	[206, 207]
Cell cycle regulation	*TP53*	Tumor suppressor	Loss of function mutations	16%	More common in aggressive subtype	[206, 207]

Table 16.44 Frequent structural variants in ENKTL

Rearrangement/gene partners	Description	Frequency	Clinical utility	Refs
CTLA4-CD28	Likely the result of partial gene duplication; fusion protein consists of the extracellular domain of CTLA4 and the cytoplasmic region of CD28, likely capable of transforming inhibitory signals into stimulatory signals for T-cell activation	29%	Potential target for anti-CTLA4 immunotherapy	[154]

Table 16.45 Frequent copy number alterations in ENKTL

Copy number change	Gene(s) involved	Frequency	Clinical utility	Refs
6q21-26 loss	*PRDM1*, *ATG5*, *HACE1*	44%		[170]

Table 16.46 Frequent somatic variants in ENKTL

Pathway	Gene	Description	Most common mutations reported	Frequency	Clinical utility (diagnostic/prognostic)	Refs
JAK-STAT signaling	*JAK3*	Activating mutations lead to increased JAK-STAT signaling	Missense mutations involving JH2 pseudokinase domain (p.A572V, p.A573V)	5–35%	Sensitive to JAK inhibitors in vitro	[211, 212]
	STAT3	Activating mutations lead to increased JAK-STAT signaling	Missense mutations involving SH2 domain (p.D661Y)	6–27%	Sensitive to JAK inhibitors in vitro	[212–214]
	STAT5B	Activating mutations lead to increased JAK-STAT signaling	Missense mutations involving SH2domain (p.N642H)	2–6%	Sensitive to JAK inhibitors in vitro	[213, 214]
Translation and ribosome assembly	*DDX3X*	RNA helicase; mutation results in decreased RNA unwinding, loss of cell cycle suppression and transcriptional activation of NF-kB and MAPK pathways	Truncating and missense mutations involving the ATP-binding helicase (residues 211-403) domain and the C-terminal helicase domain (residues 414-575)	20%	Poor prognosis	[214, 215]
Epigenetic regulation	*BCOR*	BCL6 co-repressor	Loss–of-function mutations	21%		[212, 215]
	KMT2D	Histone methyltransferase	Loss-of-function mutations	7–18%		[212, 214]
	ARID1A	SWI/SNF family component	Loss-of-function mutations	6%		[212, 214]
DNA damage	*TP53*	Tumor suppressor	Loss-of-function mutations	12–13%	Poor prognosis	[214]

References

1. Kim A, Wu C, Lovitch S. Molecular genetic aspects of non-hodgkin lymphomas. In: Greer JP, Appelbaum F, Arber DA, Dispenzieri A, Fehniger T, Glader B, et al., editors. Wintrobe's clinical hematology. 14th ed. Wolters Kluwer Health, Lippincott Williams & Wilkins; Philadelphia, PA: 2018.
2. Swerdlow SH, International Agency for Research on Cancer, World Health Organization. WHO classification of tumours of haematopoietic and lymphoid tissues. In: World Health Organization classification of tumours. 4th ed. Lyon: International Agency for Research on Cancer; 2008. p. 439.
3. Klein U, Dalla-Favera R. Germinal centres: role in B-cell physiology and malignancy. Nat Rev Immunol [Internet]. 2008;8(1):22–33. Available from: http://www.ncbi.nlm.nih.gov/entrez/query.fcgi?cmd=Retrieve&db=PubMed&dopt=Citation&list_uids=18097447
4. Shaffer AL, Rosenwald A, Staudt LM. Lymphoid malignancies: the dark side of B-cell differentiation. Nat Rev Immunol [Internet]. 2002;2(12):920–32. Available from: http://www.ncbi.nlm.nih.gov/entrez/query.fcgi?cmd=Retrieve&db=PubMed&dopt=Citation&list_uids=12461565
5. Burkitt DP. A sarcoma involving the jaws in African children. Br J Surg. 1958;46(197):218–23.
6. Swerdlow SH, Campo E, Pileri SA, Harris NL, Stein H, Siebert R, et al. The 2016 revision of the World Health Organization (WHO) classification of lymphoid neoplasms. Blood [Internet]. 2016;127(20):blood-2016-01-643569. Available from: http://www.ncbi.nlm.nih.gov/pubmed/26980727
7. Vijay A, Gertz MA. Waldenstrom macroglobulinemia. Blood [Internet]. 2007;109(12):5096–103. Available from: http://www.ncbi.nlm.nih.gov/entrez/query.fcgi?cmd=Retrieve&db=PubMed&dopt=Citation&list_uids=17303694%5Cnfile://c/CloudStation/Pictures/Literature PDFs/Vijay - Blood 2007-3735109633/Vijay - Blood 2007.pdf
8. Dimopoulos MA, Kyle RA, Anagnostopoulos A, Treon SP. Diagnosis and management of Waldenstrom's macroglobulinemia. J Clin Oncol [Internet]. 2005;23(7):1564–77. Available from: http://www.ncbi.nlm.nih.gov/pubmed/15735132
9. Treon SP, Hunter ZR, Aggarwal A, Ewen EP, Masota S, Lee C, et al. Characterization of familial Waldenstrom's macroglobulinemia. Ann Oncol [Internet]. 2006;17:488–94. Available from: http://www.ncbi.nlm.nih.gov/pubmed/16357024
10. Treon SP, Xu L, Hunter Z. MYD88 mutations and response to ibrutinib in Waldenström's macroglobulinemia. N Engl J Med [Internet]. 2015;373(6):584–6. Available from: http://www.nejm.org/doi/abs/10.1056/NEJMc1506192
11. Castillo JJ, Palomba ML, Advani RTS. Ibrutinib in Waldenström macroglobulinemia: latest evidence and clinical experience. Ther Adv Hematol. 2016;7(4):179–86.
12. Treon SP, Xu L, Yang G, Zhou Y, Liu X, Cao Y, et al. MYD88 L265P somatic mutation in Waldenström's macroglobulinemia. N Engl J Med. 2012;367:826–33.
13. Hunter ZR, Xu L, Yang G, Zhou Y, Liu X, Cao Y, et al. The genomic landscape of Waldenström macroglobulinemia is characterized by highly recurring MYD88 and WHIM-like CXCR4 mutations, and small somatic deletions associated with B-cell lymphomagenesis. Blood. 2014;123(11):1637–46.
14. Schmidt J, Federmann B, Schindler N, Steinhilber J, Bonzheim I, Fend F, et al. *MYD88* L265P and *CXCR4* mutations in lymphoplasmacytic lymphoma identify cases with high disease activity. Br J Haematol [Internet]. 2015. Available from: http://doi.wiley.com/10.1111/bjh.13361
15. Kreitman RJ. Hairy cell leukemia-new genes, new targets. Curr Hematol Malig Rep [Internet]. 2013;8(3):184–95. Available from: http://www.ncbi.nlm.nih.gov/pubmed/23892906
16. Davies H, Bignell GR, Cox C, Stephens P, Edkins S, Clegg S, et al. Mutations of the BRAF gene in human cancer. Nature [Internet]. 2002;417(6892):949–54. Available from: http://www.nature.com/doifinder/10.1038/nature00766
17. Blombery PA, Wong SQ, Hewitt CA, Dobrovic A, Maxwell EL, Juneja S, et al. Detection of BRAF mutations in patients with hairy cell leukemia and related lymphoproliferative disor-

ders. Haematologica [Internet]. 2012;97(5):780–3. Available from: http://www.ncbi.nlm.nih.gov/entrez/query.fcgi?cmd=Retrieve&db=PubMed&dopt=Citation&list_uids=22133769
18. Tiacci E, Trifonov V, Schiavoni G, Holmes A, Kern W, Martelli MP, et al. BRAF mutations in hairy-cell leukemia. N Engl J Med [Internet]. 2011;364(24):2305–15. Available from: http://www.ncbi.nlm.nih.gov/entrez/query.fcgi?cmd=Retrieve&db=PubMed&dopt=Citation&list_uids=21663470
19. Tiacci E, Park JH, De Carolis L, Chung SS, Broccoli A, Scott S, et al. Targeting mutant BRAF in relapsed or refractory hairy-cell leukemia. N Engl J Med [Internet]. 2015:150909140059008. Available from: http://www.nejm.org/doi/abs/10.1056/NEJMoa1506583
20. Waterfall JJ, Arons E, Walker RL, Pineda M, Roth L, Killian JK, et al. High prevalence of MAP2K1 mutations in variant and IGHV4-34-expressing hairy-cell leukemias. Nat Genet [Internet]. 2014;46(1):8–10. Available from: http://www.ncbi.nlm.nih.gov/pubmed/24241536%5Cn; http://www.pubmedcentral.nih.gov/articlerender.fcgi?artid=PMC3905739
21. Aster JC, Longtine JA. Detection of BCL2 rearrangements in follicular lymphoma. Am J Pathol [Internet]. 2002;160(3):759–63. Available from: http://www.ncbi.nlm.nih.gov/entrez/query.fcgi?cmd=Retrieve&db=PubMed&dopt=Citation&list_uids=11891173
22. Baseggio L, Geay MO, Gazzo S, Berger F, Traverse-Glehen A, Ffrench M, et al. In non-follicular lymphoproliferative disorders, IGH/BCL2-fusion is not restricted to chronic lymphocytic leukaemia. Br J Haematol [Internet]. 2012. Available from: http://www.ncbi.nlm.nih.gov/entrez/query.fcgi?cmd=Retrieve&db=PubMed&dopt=Citation&list_uids=22686190
23. Weiss LM, Warnke RA, Sklar J, Cleary ML. Molecular analysis of the t(14;18) chromosomal translocation in malignant lymphomas. N Engl J Med [Internet]. 1987;317(19):1185–9. Available from: http://www.ncbi.nlm.nih.gov/entrez/query.fcgi?cmd=Retrieve&db=PubMed&dopt=Citation&list_uids=3657890
24. Huang JZ, Sanger WG, Greiner TC, Staudt LM, Weisenburger DD, Pickering DL, et al. The t(14;18) defines a unique subset of diffuse large B-cell lymphoma with a germinal center B-cell gene expression profile. Blood [Internet]. 2002;99(7):2285–90. Available from: http://www.ncbi.nlm.nih.gov/entrez/query.fcgi?cmd=Retrieve&db=PubMed&dopt=Citation&list_uids=11895757
25. Kridel R, Meissner B, Rogic S, Boyle M, Telenius A, Woolcock B, et al. Whole transcriptome sequencing reveals recurrent NOTCH1 mutations in mantle cell lymphoma. Blood [Internet]. 2012;119(9):1963–71. Available from: http://www.ncbi.nlm.nih.gov/entrez/query.fcgi?cmd=Retrieve&db=PubMed&dopt=Citation&list_uids=22210878
26. Kridel R, Sehn LH, Gascoyne RD. Review series pathogenesis of follicular lymphoma. J Clin Invest. 2012;122(10):3424–31.
27. Pasqualucci L, Khiabanian H, Fangazio M, Vasishtha M, Messina M, Holmes A, et al. Genetics of follicular lymphoma transformation. Cell Rep. 2014;6(1):130–40.
28. Morin RD, Mendez-Lago M, Mungall AJ, Goya R, Mungall KL, Corbett RD, et al. Frequent mutation of histone-modifying genes in non-Hodgkin lymphoma. Nature [Internet]. 2011;476(7360):298–303. Available from: http://www.ncbi.nlm.nih.gov/entrez/query.fcgi?cmd=Retrieve&db=PubMed&dopt=Citation&list_uids=21796119
29. Okosun J, Bodor C, Wang J, Araf S, Yang CY, Pan C, et al. Integrated genomic analysis identifies recurrent mutations and evolution patterns driving the initiation and progression of follicular lymphoma. Nat Genet [Internet]. 2014;46(2):176–81. Available from: http://www.ncbi.nlm.nih.gov/pubmed/24362818
30. Pastore A, Jurinovic V, Kridel R, Hoster E, Staiger AM, Szczepanowski M, et al. Integration of gene mutations in risk prognostication for patients receiving first-line immunochemotherapy for follicular lymphoma: a retrospective analysis of a prospective clinical trial and validation in a population-based registry. Lancet Oncol. 2015;16(9):1111–22.
31. Schmitz R, Wright G, Huang D, Johnson C, Phelan J, Wang J, et al. Genetics and pathogenesis of diffuse large B-cell lymphoma. N Engl J Med. 2018;378(15):1396–407.
32. Chapuy B, Stewart C, Dunford A, Kim J, Kamburov A, Redd R, et al. Molecular subtypes of diffuse large B cell lymphoma are associated with distinct pathogenic mechanisms and outcomes. Nat Med. 2018;24(5):679–90.

33. Shipp MA, Ross KN, Tamayo P, Weng AP, Kutok JL, Aguiar RC, et al. Diffuse large B-cell lymphoma outcome prediction by gene-expression profiling and supervised machine learning. Nat Med [Internet]. 2002;8(1):68–74. Available from: http://www.ncbi.nlm.nih.gov/entrez/query.fcgi?cmd=Retrieve&db=PubMed&dopt=Citation&list_uids=11786909
34. Alizadeh AA, Eisen MB, Davis RE, Ma C, Lossos IS, Rosenwald A, et al. Distinct types of diffuse large B-cell lymphoma identified by gene expression profiling. Nature [Internet]. 2000;403(6769):503–11. Available from: http://www.ncbi.nlm.nih.gov/entrez/query.fcgi?cmd=Retrieve&db=PubMed&dopt=Citation&list_uids=10676951
35. Davis RE, Ngo VN, Lenz G, Tolar P, Young RM, Romesser PB, et al. Chronic active B-cell-receptor signalling in diffuse large B-cell lymphoma. Nature [Internet]. 2010;463(7277):88–92. Available from: http://www.pubmedcentral.nih.gov/articlerender.fcgi?artid=2845535&tool=pmcentrez&rendertype=abstract
36. Young RM, Wu T, Schmitz R, Dawood M, Xiao W, Phelan JD, et al. Survival of human lymphoma cells requires B-cell receptor engagement by self-antigens. Proc Natl Acad Sci U S A [Internet]. 2015;112(44):13447–54. Available from: http://www.pnas.org/content/112/44/13447.abstract
37. Rosenwald A, Wright G, Chan WC, Connors JM, Campo E, Fisher RI, et al. The use of molecular profiling to predict survival after chemotherapy for diffuse large-B-cell lymphoma. N Engl J Med [Internet]. 2002;346(25):1937–47. Available from: http://www.ncbi.nlm.nih.gov/entrez/query.fcgi?cmd=Retrieve&db=PubMed&dopt=Citation&list_uids=12075054
38. Roullet M, Bagg A. The basis and rational use of molecular genetic testing in mature B-cell lymphomas. Adv Anat Pathol [Internet]. 2010;17(5):333–58. Available from: http://www.ncbi.nlm.nih.gov/entrez/query.fcgi?cmd=Retrieve&db=PubMed&dopt=Citation&list_uids=20733353
39. Jarrett RF. Viruses and lymphoma/leukaemia. J Pathol [Internet]. 2006;208(2):176–86. Available from: http://www.ncbi.nlm.nih.gov/entrez/query.fcgi?cmd=Retrieve&db=PubMed&dopt=Citation&list_uids=16362996
40. Hamilton-Dutoit SJ, Raphael M, Audouin J, Diebold J, Lisse I, Pedersen C, et al. In situ demonstration of Epstein-Barr virus small RNAs (EBER 1) in acquired immunodeficiency syndrome-related lymphomas: correlation with tumor morphology and primary site. Blood [Internet]. 1993;82(2):619–24. Available from: http://www.ncbi.nlm.nih.gov/entrez/query.fcgi?cmd=Retrieve&db=PubMed&dopt=Citation&list_uids=8392401
41. Raphael M, Gentilhomme O, Tulliez M, Byron PA, Diebold J. Histopathologic features of high-grade non-Hodgkin's lymphomas in acquired immunodeficiency syndrome. The French Study Group of Pathology for human immunodeficiency virus-associated tumors. Arch Pathol Lab Med [Internet]. 1991;115(1):15–20. Available from: http://www.ncbi.nlm.nih.gov/entrez/query.fcgi?cmd=Retrieve&db=PubMed&dopt=Citation&list_uids=1987908
42. Dalla-Favera R, Bregni M, Erikson J, Patterson D, Gallo RC, Croce CM. Human c-myc onc gene is located on the region of chromosome 8 that is translocated in Burkitt lymphoma cells. Proc Natl Acad Sci U S A [Internet]. 1982;79(24):7824–7. Available from: http://www.ncbi.nlm.nih.gov/entrez/query.fcgi?cmd=Retrieve&db=PubMed&dopt=Citation&list_uids=6961453
43. Taub R, Kirsch I, Morton C, Lenoir G, Swan D, Tronick S, et al. Translocation of the c-myc gene into the immunoglobulin heavy chain locus in human Burkitt lymphoma and murine plasmacytoma cells. Proc Natl Acad Sci U S A [Internet]. 1982;79(24):7837–41. Available from: http://www.ncbi.nlm.nih.gov/entrez/query.fcgi?cmd=Retrieve&db=PubMed&dopt=Citation&list_uids=6818551
44. Hollis G, Mitchell K, Battey J, Potter H, Taub R, Lenoir G, et al. A variant translocation places the lambda immunoglobulin genes 3′ to the c-myc oncogene in Burkitt's lymphoma. Nature [Internet]. 1984;307(5953):752–5. Available from: http://www.scholaruniverse.com/ncbi-linkout?id=6422306%5Cn/Users/Suprawee/Desktop/Thesis/Background reading for thesis/Hollis - IgL-Myc translocation in Burkitt's lymphoma.pdf
45. Erikson J, Nishikura K, ar-Rushdi A, Finan J, Emanuel B, Lenoir G, et al. Translocation of an immunoglobulin kappa locus to a region 3' of an unrearranged c-myc oncogene enhances c-myc transcription. Proc Natl Acad Sci U S A [Internet]. 1983;80(24):7581–5. Available

from: http://www.ncbi.nlm.nih.gov/entrez/query.fcgi?cmd=Retrieve&db=PubMed&dopt=Citation&list_uids=6424112
46. Salaverria I, Martin-Guerrero I, Wagener R, Kreuz M, Kohler CW, Richter J, et al. A recurrent 11q aberration pattern characterizes a subset of MYC-negative high-grade B-cell lymphomas resembling Burkitt lymphoma. Blood. 2014;123(8):1187–98.
47. Ferreiro JF, Morscio J, Dierickx D, Marcelis L, Verhoef G, Vandenberghe P, Tousseyn T, Wlodarska I. Post-transplant molecularly defined Burkitt lymphomas are frequently MYC-negative and characterized by the 11q-gain/loss pattern. Haematologica. 2015;100:e275–9.
48. Steidl C, Shah SP, Woolcock BW, Rui L, Kawahara M, Farinha P, et al. MHC class II transactivator CIITA is a recurrent gene fusion partner in lymphoid cancers. Nature [Internet]. 2011 [cited 2018 Nov 12];471(7338):377–81. Available from: http://www.nature.com/doifinder/10.1038/nature09754
49. Martín-Subero JI, Klapper W, Sotnikova A, Callet-Bauchu E, Harder L, Bastard C, et al. Chromosomal breakpoints affecting immunoglobulin loci are recurrent in Hodgkin and reed-sternberg cells of classical hodgkin lymphoma. Cancer Res [Internet]. 2006 [cited 2018 Nov 12];66(21):10332–8. Available from: http://www.ncbi.nlm.nih.gov/pubmed/17079453
50. Van Roosbroeck K, Cox L, Tousseyn T, Lahortiga I, Gielen O, Cauwelier B, et al. JAK2 rearrangements, including the novel SEC31A-JAK2 fusion, are recurrent in classical Hodgkin lymphoma. Blood [Internet]. 2011 [cited 2018 Nov 12];117(15):4056–64. Available from: http://www.ncbi.nlm.nih.gov/pubmed/21325169
51. Chui DTY, Hammond D, Baird M, Shield L, Jackson R, Jarrett RF. Classical Hodgkin lymphoma is associated with frequent gains of 17q. Genes Chromosomes Cancer [Internet]. 2003 [cited 2018 Nov 12];38(2):126–36. Available from: http://www.ncbi.nlm.nih.gov/pubmed/12939740
52. Joos S, Menz CK, Wrobel G, Siebert R, Gesk S, Ohl S, et al. Classical Hodgkin lymphoma is characterized by recurrent copy number gains of the short arm of chromosome 2. Blood [Internet]. 2002 [cited 2018 Nov 12];99(4):1381–7. Available from: http://www.ncbi.nlm.nih.gov/pubmed/11830490
53. Steidl C, Telenius A, Shah SP, Farinha P, Barclay L, Boyle M, et al. Genome-wide copy number analysis of Hodgkin Reed-Sternberg cells identifies recurrent imbalances with correlations to treatment outcome. Blood [Internet]. 2010 [cited 2018 Nov 12];116(3):418–27. Available from: http://www.ncbi.nlm.nih.gov/pubmed/20339089
54. Schmitz R, Hansmann M-L, Bohle V, Martin-Subero JI, Hartmann S, Mechtersheimer G, et al. *TNFAIP3* (A20) is a tumor suppressor gene in Hodgkin lymphoma and primary mediastinal B cell lymphoma. J Exp Med [Internet]. 2009 [cited 2018 Nov 12];206(5):981–9. Available from: http://www.ncbi.nlm.nih.gov/pubmed/19380639
55. Etzel B-M, Gerth M, Chen Y, Wünsche E, Facklam T, Beck JF, et al. Mutation analysis of tumor necrosis factor alpha-induced protein 3 gene in Hodgkin lymphoma. Pathol Res Pract [Internet]. 2017 [cited 2018 Nov 12];213(3):256–60. Available from: http://www.ncbi.nlm.nih.gov/pubmed/28189285
56. Reichel J, Chadburn A, Rubinstein PG, Giulino-Roth L, Tam W, Liu Y, et al. Flow sorting and exome sequencing reveal the oncogenome of primary Hodgkin and Reed-Sternberg cells. Blood [Internet]. 2015 [cited 2018 Nov 12];125(7):1061–72. Available from: http://www.bloodjournal.org/cgi/doi/10.1182/blood-2014-11-610436
57. Lake A, Shield LA, Cordano P, Chui DTY, Osborne J, Crae S, et al. Mutations of NFKBIA, encoding IkappaB alpha, are a recurrent finding in classical Hodgkin lymphoma but are not a unifying feature of non-EBV-associated cases. Int J cancer [Internet]. 2009 [cited 2018 Nov 12];125(6):1334–42. Available from: http://doi.wiley.com/10.1002/ijc.24502
58. Emmerich F, Theurich S, Hummel M, Haeffker A, Vry MS, Döhner K, et al. Inactivating I kappa B epsilon mutations in Hodgkin/Reed-Sternberg cells. J Pathol [Internet]. 2003 [cited 2018 Nov 12];201(3):413–20. Available from: http://doi.wiley.com/10.1002/path.1454
59. Maggio EM, Stekelenburg E, Van den Berg A, Poppema S. TP53 gene mutations in Hodgkin lymphoma are infrequent and not associated with absence of Epstein-Barr virus. Int J Cancer [Internet]. 2001 [cited 2018 Nov 12];94(1):60–6. Available from: http://www.ncbi.nlm.nih.gov/pubmed/11668479

60. Maggio EM, Van Den Berg A, de Jong D, Diepstra A, Poppema S. Low frequency of FAS mutations in Reed-Sternberg cells of Hodgkin's lymphoma. Am J Pathol [Internet]. 2003 [cited 2018 Nov 12];162(1):29–35. Available from: http://linkinghub.elsevier.com/retrieve/pii/S0002944010637959
61. Müschen M, Re D, Bräuninger A, Wolf J, Hansmann ML, Diehl V, et al. Somatic mutations of the CD95 gene in Hodgkin and Reed-Sternberg cells. Cancer Res [Internet]. 2000 [cited 2018 Nov 12];60(20):5640–3. Available from: http://www.ncbi.nlm.nih.gov/pubmed/11059754
62. Lennerz JK, Hoffmann K, Bubolz A-M, Lessel D, Welke C, Rüther N, et al. Suppressor of cytokine signaling 1 gene mutation status as a prognostic biomarker in classical Hodgkin lymphoma. Oncotarget [Internet]. 2015 [cited 2018 Nov 12];6(30):29097–110. Available from: http://www.ncbi.nlm.nih.gov/pubmed/26336985
63. Weniger MA, Melzner I, Menz CK, Wegener S, Bucur AJ, Dorsch K, et al. Mutations of the tumor suppressor gene SOCS-1 in classical Hodgkin lymphoma are frequent and associated with nuclear phospho-STAT5 accumulation. Oncogene [Internet]. 2006 [cited 2018 Nov 12];25(18):2679–84. Available from: http://www.nature.com/articles/1209151
64. Tiacci E, Penson A, Schiavoni G, Ladewig E, Fortini E, Wang Y, et al. New recurrently mutated genes in classical Hodgkin lymphoma revealed by whole-exome sequencing of microdissected tumor cells. Blood [Internet]. 2016 [cited 2018 Nov 12];128(22). Available from: http://www.bloodjournal.org/content/128/22/1088
65. Gunawardana J, Chan FC, Telenius A, Woolcock B, Kridel R, Tan KL, et al. Recurrent somatic mutations of PTPN1 in primary mediastinal B cell lymphoma and Hodgkin lymphoma. Nat Genet [Internet]. 2014 [cited 2018 Nov 12];46(4):329–35. Available from: http://www.nature.com/articles/ng.2900
66. Camus V, Stamatoullas A, Mareschal S, Viailly P-J, Sarafan-Vasseur N, Bohers E, et al. Detection and prognostic value of recurrent exportin 1 mutations in tumor and cell-free circulating DNA of patients with classical Hodgkin lymphoma. Haematologica [Internet]. 2016 [cited 2018 Nov 12];101(9):1094–101. Available from: http://www.haematologica.org/cgi/doi/10.3324/haematol.2016.145102
67. Dohner H, Stilgenbauer S, Benner A, Leupolt E, Krober A, Bullinger L, et al. Genomic aberrations and survival in chronic lymphocytic leukemia. N Engl J Med [Internet]. 2000;343(26):1910–6. Available from: http://www.ncbi.nlm.nih.gov/entrez/query.fcgi?cmd=Retrieve&db=PubMed&dopt=Citation&list_uids=11136261
68. Crespo M, Bosch F, Villamor N, Bellosillo B, Colomer D, Rozman M, et al. ZAP-70 expression as a surrogate for immunoglobulin-variable-region mutations in chronic lymphocytic leukemia. N Engl J Med [Internet]. 2003;348(18):1764–75. Available from: http://www.ncbi.nlm.nih.gov/entrez/query.fcgi?cmd=Retrieve&db=PubMed&dopt=Citation&list_uids=12724482
69. Fabbri M, Bottoni A, Shimizu M, Spizzo R, Nicoloso MS, Rossi S, et al. Association of a microRNA/TP53 feedback circuitry with pathogenesis and outcome of B-cell chronic lymphocytic leukemia. JAMA [Internet]. 2011;305(1):59–67. Available from: http://www.ncbi.nlm.nih.gov/entrez/query.fcgi?cmd=Retrieve&db=PubMed&dopt=Citation&list_uids=21205967
70. Grever MR, Lucas DM, Dewald GW, Neuberg DS, Reed JC, Kitada S, et al. Comprehensive assessment of genetic and molecular features predicting outcome in patients with chronic lymphocytic leukemia: results from the US Intergroup Phase III Trial E2997. J Clin Oncol [Internet]. 2007;25(7):799–804. Available from: http://www.ncbi.nlm.nih.gov/entrez/query.fcgi?cmd=Retrieve&db=PubMed&dopt=Citation&list_uids=17283363
71. Matutes E, Oscier D, Garcia-Marco J, Ellis J, Copplestone A, Gillingham R, et al. Trisomy 12 defines a group of CLL with atypical morphology: correlation between cytogenetic, clinical and laboratory features in 544 patients. Br J Haematol [Internet]. 1996;92(2):382–8. Available from: http://www.ncbi.nlm.nih.gov/entrez/query.fcgi?cmd=Retrieve&db=PubMed&dopt=Citation&list_uids=8603004
72. Landau DA, Carter SL, Stojanov P, McKenna A, Stevenson K, Lawrence MS, et al. Evolution and impact of subclonal mutations in chronic lymphocytic leukemia. Cell. 2013;152(4):714–26.
73. Puente XS, Beà S, Valdés-Mas R, Villamor N, Gutiérrez-Abril J, Martín-Subero JI, et al. Non-coding recurrent mutations in chronic lymphocytic leukaemia. Nature

[Internet]. 2015;526(7574):519–24. Available from: http://www.ncbi.nlm.nih.gov/pubmed/26200345%5Cn; http://www.nature.com/doifinder/10.1038/nature14666
74. Puente XS, Pinyol M, Quesada V, Conde L, Ordonez GR, Villamor N, et al. Whole-genome sequencing identifies recurrent mutations in chronic lymphocytic leukaemia. Nature [Internet]. 2011;475(7354):101–5. Available from: http://www.ncbi.nlm.nih.gov/entrez/query.fcgi?cmd=Retrieve&db=PubMed&dopt=Citation&list_uids=21642962
75. Stilgenbauer S, Schnaiter A, Paschka P, Zenz T, Rossi M, Dohner K, et al. Gene mutations and treatment outcome in chronic lymphocytic leukemia: results from the CLL8 trial. Blood [Internet]. 2014 [cited 2018 Nov 12];123(21):3247–54. Available from: http://www.ncbi.nlm.nih.gov/pubmed/24652989
76. Austen B, Skowronska A, Baker C, Powell JE, Gardiner A, Oscier D, et al. Mutation status of the residual *ATM* allele is an important determinant of the cellular response to chemotherapy and survival in patients with chronic lymphocytic leukemia containing an 11q deletion. J Clin Oncol [Internet]. 2007 [cited 2018 Nov 12];25(34):5448–57. Available from: http://www.ncbi.nlm.nih.gov/pubmed/17968022
77. Wang L, Lawrence MS, Wan Y, Stojanov P, Sougnez C, Stevenson K, et al. SF3B1 and other novel cancer genes in chronic lymphocytic leukemia. N Engl J Med [Internet]. 2011;365(26):2497–506. Available from: http://www.ncbi.nlm.nih.gov/entrez/query.fcgi?cmd=Retrieve&db=PubMed&dopt=Citation&list_uids=22150006
78. Fabbri G, Rasi S, Rossi D, Trifonov V, Khiabanian H, Ma J, et al. Analysis of the chronic lymphocytic leukemia coding genome: role of NOTCH1 mutational activation. J Exp Med [Internet]. 2011;208(7):1389–401. Available from: http://www.ncbi.nlm.nih.gov/entrez/query.fcgi?cmd=Retrieve&db=PubMed&dopt=Citation&list_uids=21670202
79. Balatti V, Bottoni A, Palamarchuk A, Alder H, Rassenti LZ, Kipps TJ, et al. NOTCH1 mutations in CLL associated with trisomy 12. Blood [Internet]. 2012;119(2):329–31. Available from: http://www.ncbi.nlm.nih.gov/entrez/query.fcgi?cmd=Retrieve&db=PubMed&dopt=Citation&list_uids=22086416
80. Rossi D, Bruscaggin A, Spina V, Rasi S, Khiabanian H, Messina M, et al. Mutations of the SF3B1 splicing factor in chronic lymphocytic leukemia: association with progression and fludarabine-refractoriness. Blood [Internet]. 2011;118(26):6904–8. Available from: http://www.ncbi.nlm.nih.gov/entrez/query.fcgi?cmd=Retrieve&db=PubMed&dopt=Citation&list_uids=22039264
81. Landau DAA, Tausch E, Taylor-Weiner ANN, Stewart C, Reiter JGG, Bahlo J, et al. Mutations driving CLL and their evolution in progression and relapse. Nature. 2015;526(7574):525–30.
82. Guièze R, Wu CJ. Genomic and epigenomic heterogeneity in chronic lymphocytic leukemia. Blood. 2015;126(4):445–53.
83. Woyach JA, Furman RR, Liu T-M, Ozer HG, Zapatka M, Ruppert AS, et al. Resistance mechanisms for the Bruton's tyrosine kinase inhibitor ibrutinib. N Engl J Med. 2014;370(24):2286–94.
84. Ahn IE, Underbayev C, Albitar A, Herman SEM, Tian X, Maric I, et al. Clonal evolution leading to ibrutinib resistance in chronic lymphocytic leukemia. Blood [Internet]. 2017 [cited 2018 Nov 12];129(11):1469–79. Available from: http://www.ncbi.nlm.nih.gov/pubmed/28049639
85. Cheng S, Guo A, Lu P, Ma J, Coleman M, Wang YL. Functional characterization of BTK(C481S) mutation that confers ibrutinib resistance: exploration of alternative kinase inhibitors. Leukemia. 2015;29(4):895–900.
86. Fu K, Weisenburger DD, Greiner TC, Dave S, Wright G, Rosenwald A, et al. Cyclin D1-negative mantle cell lymphoma: a clinicopathologic study based on gene expression profiling. Blood [Internet]. 2005;106(13):4315–21. Available from: http://www.ncbi.nlm.nih.gov/entrez/query.fcgi?cmd=Retrieve&db=PubMed&dopt=Citation&list_uids=16123218
87. Royo C, Salaverria I, Hartmann EM, Rosenwald A, Campo E, Bea S. The complex landscape of genetic alterations in mantle cell lymphoma. Semin Cancer Biol [Internet]. 2011;21(5):322–34. Available from: http://www.ncbi.nlm.nih.gov/entrez/query.fcgi?cmd=Retrieve&db=PubMed&dopt=Citation&list_uids=21945515
88. Dreyling MH, Bullinger L, Ott G, Stilgenbauer S, Muller-Hermelink HK, Bentz M, et al. Alterations of the cyclin D1/p16-pRB pathway in mantle cell lymphoma. Cancer Res

[Internet]. 1997;57(20):4608–14. Available from: http://www.ncbi.nlm.nih.gov/entrez/query.fcgi?cmd=Retrieve&db=PubMed&dopt=Citation&list_uids=9377576
89. Pinyol M, Hernandez L, Cazorla M, Balbin M, Jares P, Fernandez PL, et al. Deletions and loss of expression of p16INK4a and p21Waf1 genes are associated with aggressive variants of mantle cell lymphomas. Blood [Internet]. 1997;89(1):272–80. Available from: http://www.ncbi.nlm.nih.gov/entrez/query.fcgi?cmd=Retrieve&db=PubMed&dopt=Citation&list_uids=8978301
90. Pinyol M, Cobo F, Bea S, Jares P, Nayach I, Fernandez PL, et al. p16(INK4a) gene inactivation by deletions, mutations, and hypermethylation is associated with transformed and aggressive variants of non-Hodgkin's lymphomas. Blood [Internet]. 1998;91(8):2977–84. Available from: http://www.ncbi.nlm.nih.gov/entrez/query.fcgi?cmd=Retrieve&db=PubMed&dopt=Citation&list_uids=9531609
91. Rosenwald A, Wright G, Wiestner A, Chan WC, Connors JM, Campo E, et al. The proliferation gene expression signature is a quantitative integrator of oncogenic events that predicts survival in mantle cell lymphoma. Cancer Cell [Internet]. 2003;3(2):185–97. Available from: http://www.ncbi.nlm.nih.gov/entrez/query.fcgi?cmd=Retrieve&db=PubMed&dopt=Citation&list_uids=12620412
92. Beà S, Valdés-Mas R, Navarro A, Salaverria I, Martín-Garcia D, Jares P, et al. Landscape of somatic mutations and clonal evolution in mantle cell lymphoma. Proc Natl Acad Sci U S A [Internet]. 2013;110(45):18250–5. Available from: http://www.pnas.org/content/110/45/18250
93. Zhang J, Jima D, Moffitt AB, Liu Q, Czader M, Hsi ED, et al. The genomic landscape of mantle cell lymphoma is related to the epigenetically determined chromatin state of normal B cells. Blood. 2014;123(19):2988–96.
94. Rahal R, Frick M, Romero R, Korn JM, Kridel R, Chun Chan F, et al. Pharmacological and genomic profiling identifies NF-κB–targeted treatment strategies for mantle cell lymphoma. Nat Med [Internet]. 2014 [cited 2018 Nov 12];20(1):87–92. Available from: http://www.ncbi.nlm.nih.gov/pubmed/24362935
95. Meissner B, Kridel R, Lim RS, Rogic S, Tse K, Scott DW, et al. The E3 ubiquitin ligase UBR5 is recurrently mutated in mantle cell lymphoma. Blood [Internet]. 2013 [cited 2018 Nov 12];121(16):3161–4. Available from: http://www.ncbi.nlm.nih.gov/pubmed/23407552
96. Eskelund CW, Dahl C, Hansen JW, Westman M, Kolstad A, Pedersen LB, et al. *TP53* mutations identify younger mantle cell lymphoma patients who do not benefit from intensive chemoimmunotherapy. Blood [Internet]. 2017 [cited 2018 Nov 12];130(17):1903–10. Available from: http://www.ncbi.nlm.nih.gov/pubmed/28819011
97. Auer IA, Gascoyne RD, Connors JM, Cotter FE, Greiner TC, Sanger WG, et al. t(11;18)(q21;q21) is the most common translocation in MALT lymphomas. Ann Oncol [Internet]. 1997;8(10):979–85. Available from: http://www.ncbi.nlm.nih.gov/entrez/query.fcgi?cmd=Retrieve&db=PubMed&dopt=Citation&list_uids=9402171
98. Ott G, Katzenberger T, Greiner A, Kalla J, Rosenwald A, Heinrich U, et al. The t(11;18)(q21;q21) chromosome translocation is a frequent and specific aberration in low-grade but not high-grade malignant non-Hodgkin's lymphomas of the mucosa-associated lymphoid tissue (MALT-) type. Cancer Res [Internet]. 1997;57(18):3944–8. Available from: http://www.ncbi.nlm.nih.gov/entrez/query.fcgi?cmd=Retrieve&db=PubMed&dopt=Citation&list_uids=9307277
99. Murga Penas EM, Callet-Bauchu E, Ye H, Gazzo S, Berger F, Schilling G, et al. The t(14;18)(q32;q21)/IGH-MALT1 translocation in MALT lymphomas contains templated nucleotide insertions and a major breakpoint region similar to follicular and mantle cell lymphoma. Blood [Internet]. 2010;115(11):2214–9. Available from: http://www.ncbi.nlm.nih.gov/entrez/query.fcgi?cmd=Retrieve&db=PubMed&dopt=Citation&list_uids=19965626
100. Streubel B, Vinatzer U, Lamprecht A, Raderer M, Chott A. T(3;14)(p14.1;q32) involving IGH and FOXP1 is a novel recurrent chromosomal aberration in MALT lymphoma. Leukemia

[Internet]. 2005;19(4):652–8. Available from: http://www.ncbi.nlm.nih.gov/entrez/query.fcgi?cmd=Retrieve&db=PubMed&dopt=Citation&list_uids=15703784
101. Kwee I, Rancoita PMV, Rinaldi A, Ferreri AJM, Bhagat G, Gascoyne RD, et al. Genomic profiles of MALT lymphomas: variability across anatomical sites. Haematologica [Internet]. 2011 [cited 2018 Nov 12];96(7):1064–6. Available from: http://www.haematologica.org/cgi/doi/10.3324/haematol.2011.040402
102. Rinaldi A, Mian M, Chigrinova E, Arcaini L, Bhagat G, Novak U, et al. Genome-wide DNA profiling of marginal zone lymphomas identifies subtype-specific lesions with an impact on the clinical outcome. Blood [Internet]. 2011 [cited 2018 Nov 12];117(5):1595–604. Available from: http://www.bloodjournal.org/cgi/doi/10.1182/blood-2010-01-264275
103. Novak U, Rinaldi A, Kwee I, Nandula S V., Rancoita PM V., Compagno M, et al. The NF- B negative regulator TNFAIP3 (A20) is inactivated by somatic mutations and genomic deletions in marginal zone lymphomas. Blood [Internet]. 2009 [cited 2018 Nov 12];113(20):4918–21. Available from: http://www.ncbi.nlm.nih.gov/pubmed/19258598
104. Spina V, Khiabanian H, Messina M, Monti S, Cascione L, Bruscaggin A, et al. The genetics of nodal marginal zone lymphoma. Blood [Internet]. 2016 [cited 2018 Nov 12];128(10):1362–73. Available from: http://www.ncbi.nlm.nih.gov/pubmed/27335277
105. Rossi D, Deaglio S, Dominguez-Sola D, Rasi S, Vaisitti T, Agostinelli C, et al. Alteration of BIRC3 and multiple other NF-κB pathway genes in splenic marginal zone lymphoma. Blood [Internet]. 2011 [cited 2018 Nov 12];118(18):4930–4. Available from: http://www.bloodjournal.org/cgi/doi/10.1182/blood-2011-06-359166
106. Rossi D, Trifonov V, Fangazio M, Bruscaggin A, Rasi S, Spina V, et al. The coding genome of splenic marginal zone lymphoma: activation of *NOTCH2* and other pathways regulating marginal zone development. J Exp Med [Internet]. 2012 [cited 2018 Nov 12];209(9):1537–51. Available from: http://www.ncbi.nlm.nih.gov/pubmed/22891273
107. Li Z-M, Rinaldi A, Cavalli A, Mensah AA, Ponzoni M, Gascoyne RD, et al. MYD88 somatic mutations in MALT lymphomas. Br J Haematol [Internet]. 2012 [cited 2018 Nov 12];158(5):662–4. Available from: http://www.ncbi.nlm.nih.gov/pubmed/22640364
108. Gachard N, Parrens M, Soubeyran I, Petit B, Marfak A, Rizzo D, et al. IGHV gene features and MYD88 L265P mutation separate the three marginal zone lymphoma entities and Waldenström macroglobulinemia/lymphoplasmacytic lymphomas. Leukemia [Internet]. 2013 [cited 2018 Nov 12];27(1):183–9. Available from: http://www.ncbi.nlm.nih.gov/pubmed/22944768
109. Kiel MJ, Velusamy T, Betz BL, Zhao L, Weigelin HG, Chiang MY, et al. Whole-genome sequencing identifies recurrent somatic NOTCH2 mutations in splenic marginal zone lymphoma. J Exp Med [Internet]. 2012 [cited 2018 Nov 12];209(9):1553–65. Available from: http://www.jem.org/lookup/doi/10.1084/jem.20120910
110. Parry M, Rose-Zerilli MJ, Ljungström V, Gibson J, Wang J, Walewska R, et al. Genetics and prognostication in splenic marginal zone lymphoma: revelations from deep sequencing. Clin Cancer Res [Internet]. 2015 [cited 2018 Nov 12];21(18):4174–83. Available from: http://clincancerres.aacrjournals.org/cgi/doi/10.1158/1078-0432.CCR-14-2759
111. Piva R, Deaglio S, Famà R, Buonincontri R, Scarfò I, Bruscaggin A, et al. The Krüppel-like factor 2 transcription factor gene is recurrently mutated in splenic marginal zone lymphoma. Leukemia [Internet]. 2015 [cited 2018 Nov 12];29(2):503–7. Available from: http://www.ncbi.nlm.nih.gov/pubmed/25283840
112. Johansson P, Klein-Hitpass L, Grabellus F, Arnold G, Klapper W, Pförtner R, et al. Recurrent mutations in NF-κB pathway components, KMT2D, and NOTCH1/2 in ocular adnexal MALT-type marginal zone lymphomas. Oncotarget [Internet]. 2016 [cited 2018 Nov 12];7(38):62627–39. Available from: http://www.ncbi.nlm.nih.gov/pubmed/27566587
113. Jung H, Yoo HY, Lee SH, Shin S, Kim SC, Lee S, et al. The mutational landscape of ocular marginal zone lymphoma identifies frequent alterations in TNFAIP3 followed by mutations in TBL1XR1 and CREBBP. Oncotarget [Internet]. 2017 [cited 2018 Nov 12];8(10):17038–49. Available from: http://www.ncbi.nlm.nih.gov/pubmed/28152507

114. Pillonel V, Juskevicius D, Ng CKY, Bodmer A, Zettl A, Jucker D, et al. High-throughput sequencing of nodal marginal zone lymphomas identifies recurrent BRAF mutations. Leukemia [Internet]. 2018 [cited 2018 Nov 12];32(11):2412–26. Available from: http://www.ncbi.nlm.nih.gov/pubmed/29556019
115. Mansoor A, Medeiros LJ, Weber DM, Alexanian R, Hayes K, Ones DJ, et al. Cytogenetic findings in lymphoplasmacytic lymphoma/Waldenström macroglobulinemia: chromosomal abnormalities are associated with the polymorphous subtype and an aggressive clinical course. Am J Clin Pathol. 2001;116(4):543–9.
116. Ocio EM, Schop RFJ, Gonzalez B, Van Wier SA, Hernandez-Rivas JM, Gutierrez NC, et al. 6q deletion in Waldenstrom macroglobulinemia is associated with features of adverse prognosis. Br J Haematol. 2007;136(1):80–6.
117. Schop RFJ, et al. 6q deletion discriminates Waldenstrom macroglobulinemia from IgM monoclonal gammopathy of undetermined significance. Cancer Genet Cytogenet. 2006;169(2):150–3.
118. Terré C, Nguyen-Khac F, Barin C, Mozziconacci MJ, Eclache V, Léonard C, Chapiro E, Farhat H, Bouyon A, Rousselot P, Choquet S, Spentchian M, Dubreuil P, Leblond VCS. Trisomy 4, a new chromosomal abnormality in Waldenström's macroglobulinemia: a study of 39 cases. Leukemia. 2006;20(9):1634–6.
119. Braggio E, Keats JJ, Leleu X, Wier SV, Jimenez-Zepeda VH, Schop RF, et al. High-resolution genomic analysis in Waldenstrom's macroglobulinemia identifies disease-specific and common abnormalities with marginal zone lymphomas. Clin Lymphoma Myeloma [Internet]. 2009;9(1):39–42. Available from: http://www.ncbi.nlm.nih.gov/pubmed/19362969%5Cn; http://ac.els-cdn.com/S1557919011701603/1-s2.0-S1557919011701603-main.pdf?_tid=73d096bc-fa07-11e2-b15c-00000aacb35f&acdnat=1375292249_11028b6cf6af66b08b75953daafa6969
120. Nguyen-Khac F, Lambert J, Chapiro E, Grelier A, Mould S, Barin C, Daudignon A, Gachard N, Struski S, Henry C, Penther D, Mossafa H, Andrieux J, Eclache V, Bilhou-Nabera C, Luquet I, Terre C, Baranger L, Mugneret F, Chiesa J, Mozziconacci MJ, Callet-Bauchu LV. Chromosomal aberrations and their prognostic value in a series of 174 untreated patients with Waldenström's macroglobulinemia. Haematologica. 2013;98(4):649–54.
121. Treon SP, Xu L, Yang G, Zhou Y, Liu X, Cao Y, et al. MYD88 L265P somatic mutation in Waldenström's macroglobulinemia. N Engl J Med [Internet]. 2012;367(9):826–33. Available from: http://www.nejm.org/doi/abs/10.1056/NEJMoa1200710
122. Wu X, Ivanova G, Merup M, Jansson M, Stellan B, Grandér D, et al. Molecular analysis of the human chromosome 5q13.3 region in patients with hairy cell leukemia and identification of tumor suppressor gene candidates. Genomics [Internet]. 1999;60(2):161–71. Available from: http://www.scopus.com/inward/record.url?eid=2-s2.0-0033199405&partnerID=tZOtx3y1
123. Andersen CL, Gruszka-Westwood A, Østergaard M, Koch J, Jacobsen E, Kjeldsen E, et al. A narrow deletion of 7q is common to HCL, and SMZL, but not CLL. Eur J Haematol. 2004;72(6):390–402.
124. Cawley JC. The pathophysiology of the hairy cell. Hematol Oncol Clin North Am. 2006;20:1011–21.
125. Mason EF, Brown RD, Szeto DP, Gibson CJ, Jia Y, Garcia EP, Jacobson CA, Dal Cin P, Kuo FC, Pinkus GS, Lindeman NI, Sholl LM, Aster JC, Morgan EA. Detection of activating MAP2K1 mutations in atypical hairy cell leukemia and hairy cell leukemia variant. Leuk Lymphoma. 2017;58(1):233–6.
126. Weinberg OK, Ai WZ, Mariappan MR, Shum C, Levy R, Arber DA. "Minor" BCL2 breakpoints in follicular lymphoma: frequency and correlation with grade and disease presentation in 236 cases. J Mol Diagn [Internet]. 2007;9(4):530–7. Available from: http://www.ncbi.nlm.nih.gov/entrez/query.fcgi?cmd=Retrieve&db=PubMed&dopt=Citation&list_uids=17652637
127. Vega F, Medeiros J, Luthra R. Taqman PCR in the detection and quantification of chromosomal translocations in follicular lymphoma, mantle cell lymphoma and chronic myeloid leukemia: taqman real-time PCR assay. Internet J Pathol. 2002;2(1). Available from: http://www.ispub.com/IJPA/2/1/5239.

128. Guo Y, Karube K, Kawano R, Suzumiya J, Takeshita M, Kikuchi M, et al. Bcl2-negative follicular lymphomas frequently have Bcl6 translocation and/or Bcl6 or p53 expression. Pathol Int [Internet]. 2007;57(3):148–52. Available from: http://www.ncbi.nlm.nih.gov/entrez/query.fcgi?cmd=Retrieve&db=PubMed&dopt=Citation&list_uids=17295647
129. Guo Y, Karube K, Kawano R, Yamaguchi T, Suzumiya J, Huang GS, et al. Low-grade follicular lymphoma with t(14;18) presents a homogeneous disease entity otherwise the rest comprises minor groups of heterogeneous disease entities with Bcl2 amplification, Bcl6 translocation or other gene aberrances. Leukemia [Internet]. 2005;19(6):1058–63. Available from: http://www.ncbi.nlm.nih.gov/entrez/query.fcgi?cmd=Retrieve&db=PubMed&dopt=Citation&list_uids=15815725
130. Katzenberger T, Ott G, Klein T, Kalla J, Müller-Hermelink HK, Ott MM. Cytogenetic alterations affecting BCL6 are predominantly found in follicular lymphomas grade 3B with a diffuse large B-cell component. Am J Pathol [Internet]. 2004;165(2):481–90. Available from: http://www.sciencedirect.com/science/article/pii/S0002944010633135
131. Karube K, Guo Y, Suzumiya J, Sugita Y, Nomura Y, Yamamoto K, et al. CD10-MUM1+ follicular lymphoma lacks BCL2 gene translocation and shows characteristic biologic and clinical features. Blood [Internet]. 2007;109(7):3076–9. Available from: http://www.ncbi.nlm.nih.gov/entrez/query.fcgi?cmd=Retrieve&db=PubMed&dopt=Citation&list_uids=17138820
132. Bouska A, Zhang W, Gong Q, Iqbal J, Scuto A, Vose J, et al. Combined copy number and mutation analysis identifies oncogenic pathways associated with transformation of follicular lymphoma. Leukemia. 2016;8(June 2015):1–9.
133. d'Amore F, Chan E, Iqbal J, Geng H, Young K, Xiao L, et al. Clonal evolution in t(14;18)-positive follicular lymphoma, evidence for multiple common pathways, and frequent parallel clonal evolution. Clin Cancer Res [Internet]. 2008;14(22):7180–7. Available from: http://www.ncbi.nlm.nih.gov/entrez/query.fcgi?cmd=Retrieve&db=PubMed&dopt=Citation&list_uids=19010834
134. Schwaenen C, Viardot A, Berger H, Barth TF, Bentink S, Dohner H, et al. Microarray-based genomic profiling reveals novel genomic aberrations in follicular lymphoma which associate with patient survival and gene expression status. Genes Chromosom Cancer [Internet]. 2009;48(1):39–54. Available from: http://www.ncbi.nlm.nih.gov/entrez/query.fcgi?cmd=Retrieve&db=PubMed&dopt=Citation&list_uids=18828156
135. Leich E, Ott G, Rosenwald A. Pathology, pathogenesis and molecular genetics of follicular NHL. Best Pr Res Clin Haematol [Internet]. 2011;24(2):95–109. Available from: http://www.ncbi.nlm.nih.gov/entrez/query.fcgi?cmd=Retrieve&db=PubMed&dopt=Citation&list_uids=21658611
136. Cheung KJ, Johnson NA, Affleck JG, Severson T, Steidl C, Ben-Neriah S, et al. Acquired TNFRSF14 mutations in follicular lymphoma are associated with worse prognosis. Cancer Res [Internet]. 2010;70(22):9166–74. Available from: http://www.ncbi.nlm.nih.gov/entrez/query.fcgi?cmd=Retrieve&db=PubMed&dopt=Citation&list_uids=20884631
137. Casulo C, Burack W, Friedberg J. Transformed follicular non Hodgkin lymphoma. Blood [Internet]. 2014;125(1):40–8. Available from: http://europepmc.org/abstract/med/25499449
138. Ozawa MG, Bhaduri A, Chisholm KM, Baker SA, Ma L, Zehnder JL, Luna-Fineman S, Link MP, Merker JD, Arber DA, Ohgami RS. A study of the mutational landscape of pediatric-type follicular lymphoma and pediatric nodal marginal zone lymphoma. Mod Pathol. 2016;39(10):1212–20.
139. Bouska A, McKeithan TW, Deffenbacher KE, Lachel C, Wright GW, Iqbal J, et al. Genome-wide copy-number analyses reveal genomic abnormalities involved in transformation of follicular lymphoma. Blood. 2014;123(11):1681–90.
140. Kramer MH, Hermans J, Wijburg E, Philippo K, Geelen E, van Krieken JH, et al. Clinical relevance of BCL2, BCL6, and MYC rearrangements in diffuse large B-cell lymphoma. Blood [Internet]. 1998;92(9):3152–62. Available from: http://www.ncbi.nlm.nih.gov/entrez/query.fcgi?cmd=Retrieve&db=PubMed&dopt=Citation&list_uids=9787151
141. Tibiletti MG, Martin V, Bernasconi B, Del Curto B, Pecciarini L, Uccella S, et al. BCL2, BCL6, MYC, MALT 1, and BCL10 rearrangements in nodal diffuse large B-cell lymphomas:

a multicenter evaluation of a new set of fluorescent in situ hybridization probes and correlation with clinical outcome. Hum Pathol [Internet]. 2009;40(5):645–52. Available from: http://www.ncbi.nlm.nih.gov/entrez/query.fcgi?cmd=Retrieve&db=PubMed&dopt=Citation&list_uids=19144384
142. Bosga-Bouwer AG, Haralambieva E, Booman M, Boonstra R, van den Berg A, Schuuring E, et al. BCL6 alternative translocation breakpoint cluster region associated with follicular lymphoma grade 3B. Genes Chromosom Cancer [Internet]. 2005;44(3):301–4. Available from: http://www.ncbi.nlm.nih.gov/entrez/query.fcgi?cmd=Retrieve&db=PubMed&dopt=Citation&list_uids=16075463
143. Pasqualucci L, Dalla-Favera R. The genetic landscape of diffuse large B-cell lymphoma. Semin Hematol. 2015;52:67–76.
144. Li S, Lin P, Fayad LE, Lennon PA, Miranda RN, Yin CC, et al. B-cell lymphomas with MYC/8q24 rearrangements and IGH@BCL2/t(14;18)(q32;q21): an aggressive disease with heterogeneous histology, germinal center B-cell immunophenotype and poor outcome. Mod Pathol [Internet]. 2012;25(1):145–56. Available from: http://www.ncbi.nlm.nih.gov/entrez/query.fcgi?cmd=Retrieve&db=PubMed&dopt=Citation&list_uids=22002575
145. Pasqualucci L, Trifonov V, Fabbri G, Ma J, Rossi D, Chiarenza A, et al. Analysis of the coding genome of diffuse large B-cell lymphoma. Nat Genet [Internet]. 2011;43(9):830–7. Available from: http://www.pubmedcentral.nih.gov/articlerender.fcgi?artid=3297422&tool=pmcentrez&rendertype=abstract
146. Muppidi JR, Schmitz R, Green JA, Xiao W, Larsen AB, et al. Loss of signalling via Gα13 in germinal centre B-cell-derived lymphoma. Nature [Internet]. 2014;516(7530):254–8. Available from: http://www.ncbi.nlm.nih.gov/pubmed/25274307
147. Barriga F, Kiwanuka J, Alvarez-Mon M, Shiramizu B, Huber B, Levine P, et al. Significance of chromosome 8 breakpoint location in Burkitt's lymphoma: correlation with geographical origin and association with Epstein-Barr virus. Curr Top Microbiol Immunol [Internet]. 1988;141:128–37. Available from: http://www.ncbi.nlm.nih.gov/entrez/query.fcgi?cmd=Retrieve&db=PubMed&dopt=Citation&list_uids=2850892
148. Pelicci PG, Knowles DM 2nd, Magrath I, Dalla-Favera R. Chromosomal breakpoints and structural alterations of the c-myc locus differ in endemic and sporadic forms of Burkitt lymphoma. Proc Natl Acad Sci U S A [Internet]. 1986;83(9):2984–8. Available from: http://www.ncbi.nlm.nih.gov/entrez/query.fcgi?cmd=Retrieve&db=PubMed&dopt=Citation&list_uids=3458257
149. Shiramizu B, Barriga F, Neequaye J, Jafri A, Dalla-Favera R, Neri A, et al. Patterns of chromosomal breakpoint locations in Burkitt's lymphoma: relevance to geography and Epstein-Barr virus association. Blood [Internet]. 1991;77(7):1516–26. Available from: http://www.ncbi.nlm.nih.gov/entrez/query.fcgi?cmd=Retrieve&db=PubMed&dopt=Citation&list_uids=1849033
150. Gutierrez MI, Bhatia K, Barriga F, Diez B, Muriel FS, de Andreas ML, et al. Molecular epidemiology of Burkitt's lymphoma from South America: differences in breakpoint location and Epstein-Barr virus association from tumors in other world regions. Blood [Internet]. 1992;79(12):3261–6. Available from: http://www.ncbi.nlm.nih.gov/entrez/query.fcgi?cmd=Retrieve&db=PubMed&dopt=Citation&list_uids=1317726
151. Schmitz R, Young RM, Ceribelli M, Jhavar S, Xiao W, Zhang M, et al. Burkitt lymphoma pathogenesis and therapeutic targets from structural and functional genomics. Nature [Internet]. 2012;490(7418):116–20. Available from: http://www.pubmedcentral.nih.gov/articlerender.fcgi?artid=3609867&tool=pmcentrez&rendertype=abstract
152. Love C, Sun Z, Jima D, Li G, Zhang J, Miles R, et al. The genetic landscape of mutations in Burkitt lymphoma. Nat Genet [Internet]. 2012;44(12):1321–5. Available from: http://www.pubmedcentral.nih.gov/articlerender.fcgi?artid=3674561&tool=pmcentrez&rendertype=abstract
153. Richter J, Schlesner M, Hoffmann S, Kreuz M, Leich E, Burkhardt B, et al. Recurrent mutation of the ID3 gene in Burkitt lymphoma identified by integrated genome, exome and tran-

scriptome sequencing. Nat Genet [Internet]. 2012;44(12):1316–20. Available from: http://www.ncbi.nlm.nih.gov/pubmed/23143595
154. Yoo HY, Kim P, Kim WS, Lee SH, Kim S, Kang SY, et al. Frequent CTLA4-CD28 gene fusion in diverse types of T-cell lymphoma. Haematologica. 2016;101(6):757–63.
155. Attygalle AD, Feldman AL, Dogan A. ITK/SYK translocation in Angioimmunoblastic T-cell lymphoma. Am J Surg Pathol. 2013;37(9):1456–7.
156. Pechloff K, Holch J, Ferch U, Schweneker M, Brunner K, Kremer M, et al. The fusion kinase ITK-SYK mimics a T cell receptor signal and drives oncogenesis in conditional mouse models of peripheral T cell lymphoma. J Exp Med [Internet]. 2010 [cited 2018 Nov 13];207(5):1031–44. Available from: http://www.ncbi.nlm.nih.gov/pubmed/20439541
157. Dobay MP, Lemonnier F, Missiaglia E, Bastard C, Vallois D, Jais J-P, et al. Integrative clinicopathological and molecular analyses of angioimmunoblastic T-cell lymphoma and other nodal lymphomas of follicular helper T-cell origin. Haematologica [Internet]. 2017 [cited 2018 Nov 13];102(4):e148–51. Available from: http://www.ncbi.nlm.nih.gov/pubmed/28082343
158. Nelson M, Horsman DE, Weisenburger DD, Gascoyne RD, Dave BJ, Loberiza FR, et al. Cytogenetic abnormalities and clinical correlations in peripheral T-cell lymphoma. Br J Haematol [Internet]. 2008;141(4):461–9. Available from: http://www.ncbi.nlm.nih.gov/entrez/query.fcgi?cmd=Retrieve&db=PubMed&dopt=Citation&list_uids=18341637
159. Fujiwara SI, Yamashita Y, Nakamura N, Choi YL, Ueno T, Watanabe H, et al. High-resolution analysis of chromosome copy number alterations in angioimmunoblastic T-cell lymphoma and peripheral T-cell lymphoma, unspecified, with single nucleotide polymorphism-typing microarrays. Leukemia [Internet]. 2008;22(10):1891–8. Available from: http://www.ncbi.nlm.nih.gov/entrez/query.fcgi?cmd=Retrieve&db=PubMed&dopt=Citation&list_uids=18633432
160. Thorns C, Bastian B, Pinkel D, Roydasgupta R, Fridlyand J, Merz H, et al. Chromosomal aberrations in angioimmunoblastic T-cell lymphoma and peripheral T-cell lymphoma unspecified: a matrix-based CGH approach. Genes Chromosom Cancer [Internet]. 2007;46(1):37–44. Available from: http://www.ncbi.nlm.nih.gov/entrez/query.fcgi?cmd=Retrieve&db=PubMed&dopt=Citation&list_uids=17044049
161. Sakata-Yanagimoto M, Enami T, Yoshida K, Shiraishi Y, Ishii R, Miyake Y, et al. Somatic RHOA mutation in angioimmunoblastic T cell lymphoma. Nat Genet [Internet]. 2014;46(2):171–5. Available from: http://www.ncbi.nlm.nih.gov/pubmed/24413737%5Cn; http://www.nature.com/ng/journal/v46/n2/pdf/ng.2872.pdf
162. Yoo HY, Sung MK, Lee SH, Kim S, Lee H, Park S, et al. A recurrent inactivating mutation in RHOA GTPase in angioimmunoblastic T cell lymphoma. Nat Genet [Internet]. 2014;46(4):371–5. Available from: http://www.ncbi.nlm.nih.gov/pubmed/24584070%5Cn; http://www.nature.com/ng/journal/v46/n4/pdf/ng.2916.pdf
163. Rohr J, Guo S, Huo J, Bouska A, Lachel C, Li Y, et al. Recurrent activating mutations of CD28 in peripheral T-cell lymphomas. Leukemia [Internet]. 2016;30(5):1062–70. Available from: http://www.ncbi.nlm.nih.gov/pubmed/26719098
164. Lee SHL, Kim JS, Kim J, Kim SJ, Kim WS, Lee S, et al. A highly recurrent novel missense mutation in CD28 among angioimmunoblastic T-cell lymphoma patients. Haematologica. 2015;100:e505–7.
165. Odejide O, Weigert O, Lane AA, Toscano D, Lunning MA, Kopp N, et al. A targeted mutational landscape of angioimmunoblastic T-cell lymphoma. Blood [Internet]. 2014 [cited 2018 Nov 13];123(9):1293–6. Available from: http://www.ncbi.nlm.nih.gov/pubmed/24345752
166. Couronne L, Bastard C, Bernard OA. TET2 and DNMT3A mutations in human T-cell lymphoma. N Engl J Med [Internet]. 2012;366(1):95–6. Available from: http://www.ncbi.nlm.nih.gov/entrez/query.fcgi?cmd=Retrieve&db=PubMed&dopt=Citation&list_uids=22216861
167. Dang L, White DW, Gross S, Bennett BD, Bittinger MA, Driggers EM, et al. Cancer-associated IDH1 mutations produce 2-hydroxyglutarate. Nature [Internet]. 2010;465(7300):966. Available from: http://www.ncbi.nlm.nih.gov/entrez/query.fcgi?cmd=Retrieve&db=PubMed&dopt=Citation&list_uids=20559394

168. Cairns RA, Iqbal J, Lemonnier F, Kucuk C, de Leval L, Jais JP, et al. IDH2 mutations are frequent in angioimmunoblastic T-cell lymphoma. Blood [Internet]. 2012;119(8):1901–3. Available from: http://www.ncbi.nlm.nih.gov/entrez/query.fcgi?cmd=Retrieve&db=PubMed&dopt=Citation&list_uids=22215888
169. Feldman AL, Dogan A, Smith DI, Law ME, Ansell SM, Johnson SH, et al. Discovery of recurrent t(6;7)(p25.3;q32.3) translocations in ALK-negative anaplastic large cell lymphomas by massively parallel genomic sequencing. Blood [Internet]. 2011;117(3):915–9. Available from: http://www.ncbi.nlm.nih.gov/entrez/query.fcgi?cmd=Retrieve&db=PubMed&dopt=Citation&list_uids=21030553
170. Parrilla Castellar ER, Jaffe ES, Said JW, Swerdlow SH, Ketterling RP, Knudson RA, et al. ALK-negative anaplastic large cell lymphoma is a genetically heterogeneous disease with widely disparate clinical outcomes. Blood. 2014;124(9):1473–80.
171. Boddicker R, Razidlo G, Dasari S, Zeng Y, Hu G, Knudson RA, Greipp PT, Davila JI, Johnson SH, Porcher JC, Smadbeck JB, Eckloff BW, Billadeau DD, Kurtin PJ, McNiven MA, Link BK, Ansell SM, Cerhan JR, Asmann YW, Vasmatzis GFAL. Integrated mate-pair and RNA sequencing identifies novel, targetable gene fusions in peripheral T-cell lymphoma. Blood. 2016;128(9):1234–45.
172. Crescenzo R, Abate F, Lasorsa E, Tabbo' F, Gaudiano M, Chiesa N, et al. Convergent mutations and kinase fusions lead to oncogenic STAT3 activation in anaplastic large cell lymphoma. Cancer Cell. 2015;27(4):516–32.
173. Vasmatzis G, Johnson SH, Knudson RA, Ketterling RP, Braggio E, Fonseca R, et al. Genome-wide analysis reveals recurrent structural abnormalities of TP63 and other p53-related genes in peripheral T-cell lymphomas. Blood [Internet]. 2012 [cited 2018 Nov 13];120(11):2280–9. Available from: http://www.ncbi.nlm.nih.gov/pubmed/22855598
174. Iida S, Rao PH, Butler M, Corradini P, Boccadoro M, Klein B, et al. Deregulation of MUM1/IRF4 by chromosomal translocation in multiple myeloma. Nat Genet [Internet]. 1997 [cited 2018 Nov 13];17(2):226–30. Available from: http://www.nature.com/articles/ng1097-226
175. Feldman AL, Law M, Remstein ED, Macon WR, Erickson LA, Grogg KL, et al. Recurrent translocations involving the IRF4 oncogene locus in peripheral T-cell lymphomas. Leukemia [Internet]. 2009;23(3):574–80. Available from: http://www.ncbi.nlm.nih.gov/entrez/query.fcgi?cmd=Retrieve&db=PubMed&dopt=Citation&list_uids=18987657
176. Ohgami RS, Ma L, Merker JD, Martinez B, Zehnder JL, Arber DA. STAT3 mutations are frequent in CD30+ T-cell lymphomas and T-cell large granular lymphocytic leukemia. Leukemia. 2013;27(11):2244–7.
177. Blombery P, Thompson ER, Jones K, Arnau GM, Lade S, Markham JF, Li J, Deva A, Johnstone RW, Khot A, Prince HM, Westerman D. Whole exome sequencing reveals activating JAK1 and STAT3 mutations in breast implant-associated anaplastic large cell lymphoma anaplastic large cell lymphoma. Haematologica. 2016;101(9):e387–90.
178. Di Napoli A, Jain P, Duranti E, Margolskee E, Arancio W, Facchetti F, Alobeid B, Santanelli di Pompeo F, Mansukhani MB. Targeted next generation sequencing of breast implant-associated anaplastic large cell lymphoma reveals mutations in JAK/STAT signalling pathway genes, TP53 and DNMT3A. Br J Haematol. 2018;180(5):741–4. https://doi.org/10.1111/bjh.14431.
179. Savage KJ, Harris NL, Vose JM, Ullrich F, Jaffe ES, Connors JM, et al. ALK- anaplastic large-cell lymphoma is clinically and immunophenotypically different from both ALK+ ALCL and peripheral T-cell lymphoma, not otherwise specified: report from the International Peripheral T-Cell Lymphoma Project. Blood [Internet]. 2008;111(12):5496–504. Available from: http://www.ncbi.nlm.nih.gov/entrez/query.fcgi?cmd=Retrieve&db=PubMed&dopt=Citation&list_uids=18385450
180. Oishi N, Brody GS, Ketterling RP, Viswanatha DS, He R, Dasari S, et al. Genetic subtyping of breast implant–associated anaplastic large cell lymphoma. Blood [Internet]. 2018 [cited 2018 Nov 13];132(5):544–7. Available from: http://www.ncbi.nlm.nih.gov/pubmed/29921615

181. Boi M, Rinaldi A, Kwee I, Bonetti P, Todaro M, Tabbò F, et al. PRDM1/BLIMP1 is commonly inactivated in anaplastic large T-cell lymphoma. Blood [Internet]. 2013;122(15):2683–93. Available from: http://www.ncbi.nlm.nih.gov/pubmed/24004669
182. Streubel B, Vinatzer U, Willheim M, Raderer M, Chott A. Novel t(5;9)(q33;q22) fuses ITK to SYK in unspecified peripheral T-cell lymphoma. Leukemia [Internet]. 2006;20(2):313–8. Available from: http://www.ncbi.nlm.nih.gov/pubmed/16341044
183. Nakagawa M, Nakagawa-Oshiro A, Karnan S, Tagawa H, Utsunomiya A, Nakamura S, et al. Array comparative genomic hybridization analysis of PTCL-U reveals a distinct subgroup with genetic alterations similar to lymphoma-type adult T-cell leukemia/lymphoma. Clin Cancer Res [Internet]. 2009 [cited 2018 Nov 13];15(1):30–8. Available from: http://www.ncbi.nlm.nih.gov/pubmed/19118030
184. Hartmann S, Gesk S, Scholtysik R, Kreuz M, Bug S, Vater I, et al. High resolution SNP array genomic profiling of peripheral T cell lymphomas, not otherwise specified, identifies a subgroup with chromosomal aberrations affecting the *REL* locus. Br J Haematol [Internet]. 2010 [cited 2018 Nov 13];148(3):402–12. Available from: http://www.ncbi.nlm.nih.gov/pubmed/19863542
185. Wang C, McKeithan TW, Gong Q, Zhang W, Bouska A, Rosenwald A, et al. IDH2R172 mutations define a unique subgroup of patients with angioimmunoblastic T-cell lymphoma. Blood [Internet]. 2015 [cited 2018 Nov 13];126(15):1741–52. Available from: http://www.ncbi.nlm.nih.gov/pubmed/26268241
186. Palomero T, Couronne L, Khiabanian H, Kim MY, Ambesi-Impiombato A, Perez-Garcia A, et al. Recurrent mutations in epigenetic regulators, RHOA and FYN kinase in peripheral T cell lymphomas. Nat Genet [Internet]. 2014;46(2):166–70. Available from: http://www.ncbi.nlm.nih.gov/pubmed/24413734%5Cn; http://www.nature.com/ng/journal/v46/n2/pdf/ng.2873.pdf
187. Abate F, da Silva-Almeida AC, Zairis S, Robles-Valero J, Couronne L, Khiabanian H, Quinn SA, Kim MY, Laginestra MA, Kim C, Fiore D, Bhagat G, Piris MA, Campo E, Lossos IS, Bernard OA, Inghirami G, Pileri S, Bustelo XR, Rabadan R, Ferrando AA, Palomero T. Activating mutations and translocations in the guanine exchange factor VAV1 in peripheral T-cell lymphomas. Proc Natl Acad Sci U S A. 2017;pii:20160.
188. Kristensen T, Larsen M, Rewes A, Frederiksen H, Thomassen M, Møller MB. Clinical relevance of sensitive and quantitative STAT3 mutation analysis using next-generation sequencing in T-cell large granular lymphocytic leukemia. J Mol Diagnostics. 2014;16(4):382–92.
189. Jerez A, Clemente MJ, Makishima H, Koskela H, LeBlanc F, Ng KP, et al. STAT3 mutations unify the pathogenesis of chronic lymphoproliferative disorders of NK cells and T-cell large granular lymphocyte leukemia. Blood. 2012;120(15):3048–57.
190. Koskela HL, Eldfors S, Ellonen P, van Adrichem AJ, Kuusanmäki H, Andersson EI, et al. Somatic STAT3 mutations in large granular lymphocytic leukemia. N Engl J Med [Internet]. 2012;366(20):1905–13. Available from: http://www.pubmedcentral.nih.gov/articlerender.fcgi?artid=3693860&tool=pmcentrez&rendertype=abstract
191. Rajala HL, Eldfors S, Kuusanmäki H, van Adrichem AJ, Olson T, Lagström S, et al. Discovery of somatic STAT5b mutations in large granular lymphocytic leukemia. Blood. 2013;121(22):4541–50.
192. Rajala HL, Olson T, Clemente MJ, Lagström S, Ellonen P, Lundan T, et al. The analysis of clonal diversity and therapy responses using STAT3 mutations as a molecular marker in large granular lymphocytic leukemia. Haematologica. 2015;100(1):91–9.
193. Andersson EI, Rajala HLM, Eldfors S, Ellonen P, Olson T, Jerez A, et al. Novel somatic mutations in large granular lymphocytic leukemia affecting the STAT-pathway and T-cell activation. Blood Cancer J [Internet]. 2013;3(12):e168. Available from: http://www.pubmedcentral.nih.gov/articlerender.fcgi?artid=3877422&tool=pmcentrez&rendertype=abstract
194. Stengel A, Kern W, Zenger M, Perglerová K, Schnittger S, Haferlach T, et al. Genetic characterization of T-PLL reveals two major biologic subgroups and JAK3 mutations as prognostic marker. Genes Chromosomes and Cancer. 2016;55:82–94.

195. Madani A, Choukroun V, Soulier J, Cacheux V, Claisse J, Valensi F, et al. Expression of p13MTCP1 is restricted to mature T-cell proliferations with t(X;14) translocations. Blood [Internet]. 1996 [cited 2018 Nov 13];87(5). Available from: http://www.bloodjournal.org/content/87/5/1923?sso-checked=true
196. Virgilio L, Isobe M, Narducci MG, Carotenuto P, Camerini B, Kurosawa N, et al. Chromosome walking on the TCL1 locus involved in T-cell neoplasia. Proc Natl Acad Sci U S A [Internet]. 1993;90(20):9275–9. Available from: http://www.ncbi.nlm.nih.gov/entrez/query.fcgi?cmd=Retrieve&db=PubMed&dopt=Citation&list_uids=8415691
197. Suzuki R, Matsushita H, Kawai H, Matsuzawa H, Tsuboi K, Watanabe S, et al. Identification of a novel SEPT9-ABL1 fusion gene in a patient with T-cell prolymphocytic leukemia. Leuk Res Reports. 2014;3(2):54–7.
198. Durig J, Bug S, Klein-Hitpass L, Boes T, Jons T, Martin-Subero JI, et al. Combined single nucleotide polymorphism-based genomic mapping and global gene expression profiling identifies novel chromosomal imbalances, mechanisms and candidate genes important in the pathogenesis of T-cell prolymphocytic leukemia with inv(14)(q11q32). Leukemia [Internet]. 2007;21(10):2153–63. Available from: http://www.ncbi.nlm.nih.gov/entrez/query.fcgi?cmd=Retrieve&db=PubMed&dopt=Citation&list_uids=17713554
199. Kiel MJ, Velusamy T, Rolland D, Sahasrabuddhe AA, Chung F, Bailey NG, et al. Integrated genomic sequencing reveals mutational landscape of T-cell prolymphocytic leukemia. Blood. 2014;124(9):1460–72.
200. Bug S, Durig J, Oyen F, Klein-Hitpass L, Martin-Subero JI, Harder L, et al. Recurrent loss, but lack of mutations, of the SMARCB1 tumor suppressor gene in T-cell prolymphocytic leukemia with TCL1A-TCRAD juxtaposition. Cancer Genet Cytogenet [Internet]. 2009;192(1):44–7. Available from: http://www.ncbi.nlm.nih.gov/entrez/query.fcgi?cmd=Retrieve&db=PubMed&dopt=Citation&list_uids=19480937
201. Moffitt AB, Ondrejka SL, McKinney M, Rempel RE, Goodlad JR, Teh CH, et al. Enteropathy-associated T cell lymphoma subtypes are characterized by loss of function of SETD2. J Exp Med [Internet]. 2017 [cited 2018 Nov 14];214(5):1371–86. Available from: http://www.ncbi.nlm.nih.gov/pubmed/28424246
202. Tomita S, Kikuti YY, Carreras J, Kojima M, Ando K, Takasaki H, et al. Genomic and immunohistochemical profiles of enteropathy-associated T-cell lymphoma in Japan. Mod Pathol [Internet]. 2015;28(10):1286–96. Available from: http://www.nature.com/doifinder/10.1038/modpathol.2015.85%5Cn; http://www.ncbi.nlm.nih.gov/pubmed/26226842
203. Wilson AL, Swerdlow SH, Przybylski GK, Surti U, Choi JK, Campo E, et al. Intestinal γδ T-cell lymphomas are most frequently of type II enteropathy-associated T-cell type. Hum Pathol. 2013;44(6):1131–45.
204. deLeeuw RJ, Zettl A, Klinker E, Haralambieva E, Trottier M, Chari R, et al. Whole-genome analysis and HLA genotyping of enteropathy-type T-cell lymphoma reveals 2 distinct lymphoma subtypes. Gastroenterology. 2007;132(5):1902–11.
205. Roberti A, Dobay MP, Bisig B, Vallois D, Boéchat C, Lanitis E, et al. Type II enteropathy-associated T-cell lymphoma features a unique genomic profile with highly recurrent SETD2 alterations. Nat Commun [Internet]. 2016;7:12602. Available from: http://www.nature.com/doifinder/10.1038/ncomms12602
206. Kataoka K, Nagata Y, Kitanaka A, Shiraishi Y, Shimamura T, Yasunaga J, et al. Integrated molecular analysis of adult T cell leukemia/lymphoma. Nat Genet [Internet]. 2015 [cited 2018 Nov 17];47(11):1304–15. Available from: http://www.nature.com/articles/ng.3415
207. Kataoka K, Iwanaga M, Yasunaga J, Nagata Y, Kitanaka A, Kameda T, et al. Prognostic relevance of integrated genetic profiling in adult T-cell leukemia/lymphoma. Blood [Internet]. 2018 [cited 2018 Nov 17];131(2):215–25. Available from: http://www.bloodjournal.org/lookup/doi/10.1182/blood-2017-01-761874
208. Pancewicz J, Taylor JM, Datta A, Baydoun HH, Waldmann TA, Hermine O, et al. Notch signaling contributes to proliferation and tumor formation of human T-cell leukemia virus type 1-associated adult T-cell leukemia. Proc Natl Acad Sci [Internet]. 2010 [cited

2018 Nov 17];107(38):16619–24. Available from: http://www.pnas.org/cgi/doi/10.1073/pnas.1010722107

209. Yeh C-H, Bellon M, Pancewicz-Wojtkiewicz J, Nicot C. Oncogenic mutations in the FBXW7 gene of adult T-cell leukemia patients. Proc Natl Acad Sci [Internet]. 2016 [cited 2018 Nov 17];113(24):6731–6. Available from: http://www.ncbi.nlm.nih.gov/pubmed/27247421
210. Nagata Y, Kontani K, Enami T, Kataoka K, Ishii R, Totoki Y, et al. Variegated RHOA mutations in adult T-cell leukemia/lymphoma. Blood [Internet]. 2016 [cited 2018 Nov 17];127(5):596–604. Available from: http://www.bloodjournal.org/cgi/doi/10.1182/blood-2015-06-644948
211. Koo GC, Tan SY, Tang T, Poon SL, Allen GE, Tan L, et al. Janus kinase 3–activating mutations identified in natural killer/T-cell lymphoma. Cancer Discov [Internet]. 2012 [cited 2018 Nov 14];2(7):591–7. Available from: http://www.ncbi.nlm.nih.gov/pubmed/22705984
212. Lee S, Park HY, Kang SY, Kim SJ, Hwang J, Lee S, et al. Genetic alterations of JAK/STAT cascade and histone modification in extranodal NK/T-cell lymphoma nasal type. Oncotarget [Internet]. 2015 [cited 2018 Nov 14];6(19):17764–76. Available from: http://www.ncbi.nlm.nih.gov/pubmed/25980440
213. Küçük C, Jiang B, Hu X, Zhang W, Chan JKC, Xiao W, et al. Activating mutations of STAT5B and STAT3 in lymphomas derived from γδ-T or NK cells. Nat Commun [Internet]. 2015;6:6025. Available from: http://www.ncbi.nlm.nih.gov/pubmed/25586472
214. Jiang L, Gu Z-H, Yan Z-X, Zhao X, Xie Y-Y, Zhang Z-G, et al. Exome sequencing identifies somatic mutations of DDX3X in natural killer/T-cell lymphoma. Nat Genet [Internet]. 2015 [cited 2018 Nov 14];47(9):1061–6. Available from: http://www.ncbi.nlm.nih.gov/pubmed/26192917
215. Dobashi A, Tsuyama N, Asaka R, Togashi Y, Ueda K, Sakata S, et al. Frequent *BCOR* aberrations in extranodal NK/T-Cell lymphoma, nasal type. Genes Chromosomes Cancer [Internet]. 2016 [cited 2018 Nov 14];55(5):460–71. Available from: http://www.ncbi.nlm.nih.gov/pubmed/26773734

Index

L. J. Tafe, M. E. Arcila (eds.), *Genomic Medicine*,
https://doi.org/10.1007/978-3-030-22922-1

Q

R

S

T

U

MIX
Papier aus verantwortungsvollen Quellen
Paper from responsible sources
FSC® C105338

If you have any concerns about our products,
you can contact us on
ProductSafety@springernature.com

In case Publisher is established outside the EU,
the EU authorized representative is:
Springer Nature Customer Service Center GmbH
Europaplatz 3, 69115 Heidelberg, Germany

Printed by Libri Plureos GmbH
in Hamburg, Germany